Family Nurse Practitioner
Certification Review

Family Nurse Practitioner Certification Review

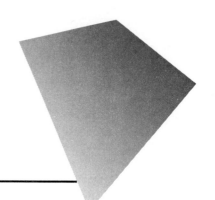

Second Edition

JoAnn Zerwekh, EdD, RN, FNP, APRN, BC
Faculty
University of Phoenix Online
Phoenix, Arizona

Executive Director
Nursing Education Consultants
Midlothian, Texas

Jo Carol Claborn, MS, RN, CS
Executive Director
Nursing Education Consultants
Midlothian, Texas

SAUNDERS
An Imprint of Elsevier

An Imprint of Elsevier

11830 Westline Industrial Drive
St. Louis, Missouri 63146

NOTICE

Nursing is an ever-changing field. Standard safety precautions must be followed, but as new research and clinical experience broaden our knowledge, changes in treatment and drug therapy may become necessary or appropriate. Readers are advised to check the most current product information provided by the manufacturer of each drug to be administered to verify the recommended dose, the method and duration of administration, and contraindications. It is the responsibility of the licensed health care provider, relying on experience and knowledge of the patient, to determine dosages and the best treatment for each individual patient. Neither the publisher nor the editor assumes any liability for any injury and/or damage to persons or property arising from this publication.

Previous editions copyrighted 1999

ISBN-13: 978-0-7216-8249-5
ISBN-10: 0-7216-8249-9

Executive Publisher: Barbara Nelson Cullen
Senior Developmental Editor: Victoria Bruno
Publishing Services Manager: John Rogers
Project Manager: Helen Hudlin
Design Manager: Amy Buxton

Printed in the United States of America

Last digit is the print number: 9   8   7   6   5

Dedication

We dedicate this book to our parents

CHARLES GRAHAM AND HAZEL COOPER, who have provided us a lifetime of unconditional love and support

Reviewers

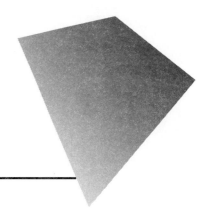

RHONDA LARIMORE, RN, FNP-CERTIFIED, MSN
Western Carolina University
Asheville, North Carolina

BRENDA S. RAPP, MSN, CS, FNP-C
Health Texas Provider Network (Baylor System)
Waxahachie, Texas

CATHERINE ELIZABETH COHILL TURNER, RN, MSN, FNP-C, CDR, USN
Halyburton Naval Hospital
Cherry Point, North Carolina

Contributors

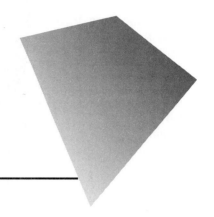

MARY ATTARDO
Easton, Massachusetts

KATHRYN A. BLAIR, PhD, RN, FNP
Professor
Graduate Coordinator FNP Program
University of Northern Colorado
Greeley, Colorado

MARY BOYLE, MSN, RN, FNP, BCADM, CDE, CS
Mayo Clinic
Scottsdale, Arizona

SUSAN CHANEY, EdD, APRN, FNP-C, BC
Professor/FNP Coordinator
College of Nursing
Texas Women's University
Dallas, Texas
Family Nurse Practitioner
Homeless Outreach Medical Services
Parkland Health & Hospital System
Dallas, Texas

SHARON G. CHILDS, MS, APRN-BC, CS, ONC
Adult Nurse Practitioner
Orthopedic Trauma/Critical Care–Clinical Nurse
Specialist
Baltimore, Maryland

CYNDY CHURGIN, RN-C, FNP, CNM
Casa Blanca Medical Group
Mesa, Arizona

SHARON DECKER, MSN, RN, CS, CCRN
Professor & Director of Clinical Simulations
School of Nursing
Texas Tech University Health Science Center
Lubbock, Texas

GAIL KOELKER, MSN, RN-C, FNP
Certified Family Nurse Practitioner
Good Shepherd Health System
Longview, Texas
Faculty
University of Phoenix Online
BSN Program
Phoenix, Arizona

ELA-JOY LEHRMAN, PhD, MS, MAED, RN, CNM
Professor & Chair, Nursing & Health Sciences
Southern Arizona Campus
University of Phoenix
Phoenix, Arizona

MARGARET A. LYNCH, MSN, BA
Family Nurse Practitioner
The Cambridge Hospital
Cambridge, Massachusetts

MARY D. MACKENBURG, MS, RN, CPNP
Assistant Professor, Department of Nursing
College of St. Catherine
St. Paul, Minnesota
Nurse Practitioner
Emergency Department
Children's Hospital and Clinics
St. Paul, Minnesota

JOYCE A. MEADOR, MSN, RN, ARNP-BC, GNP
Faculty
University of Phoenix Online
BSN Program
Phoenix, Arizona

DIANE TODD PACE, PhD, APRN, BC
Nurse Practitioner/Researcher
Health Science Department
University of Tennessee
Assistant Clinical Professor, College of Nursing
Assistant Professor, Department of Preventative
Medicine
Memphis, Tennessee
Assistant Professor
Union University
Jackson, Tennessee
Faculty
University of Phoenix Online
Phoenix, Arizona

PATRICIA SHANNON, MS, MA, RN, CS, PNP
Faculty
University of Phoenix
Phoenix, Arizona
Adjuct Faculty
Grand Canyon University
Phoenix, Arizona

SCOTT W. SHIFFER, MSN, FNP
Head, Family Practice Department
Naval Hospital
Rota, Spain

TAMARA R. TRIPP, MSN, ANP/GNP-C
Medical Plaza Family Physicians
Charlotte, North Carolina

CYNTHIA M. WILBORNE, MSN, FNP
Family Nurse Practitioner Board Certified
Danville Urologic Clinic
Danville, Virginia
Faculty
University of Phoenix Online
Phoenix, Arizona

Preface

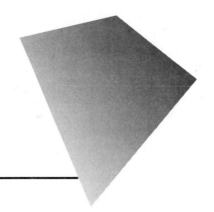

With the dawn of the role of the nurse practitioner, there is an increasing need for additional reference information and study materials for the certification examinations. Nurse practitioners are playing a vital role in the changing health care delivery system in the United States. The numbers of candidates for the certification examinations is rapidly increasing as more nursing programs implement the nurse practitioner curriculum in their graduate programs. *Family Nurse Practitioner Certification Review*, second edition, has been developed to assist the advanced practice nurse to prepare for the FNP certification examination. Extensive efforts have been made to include current information that is representative of the content, based on the blueprints for the certification exams. This book of questions is not intended to be an exhaustive review of the content but an adjunct to the review process.

Test-taking strategies are included in Chapter 1. As a candidate prepares for the examination, it is vitally important to be familiar with and to practice good testing strategies. Testing strategies can prevent the candidate from making mistakes and selecting the wrong answer. As the review process begins, a review of the testing strategies chapter and the practice of good testing strategies is critical. With many years experience in the field of testing, we have consistently identified the importance practice testing plays in the review process. Practice questions give the candidate an opportunity to review questions written from different perspectives. To enhance the review process, answers with

complete rationales are provided at the end of each chapter. Not only does the candidate increase his/her knowledge of the subject area, but also, with more practice, testing skills become fine-tuned. Good testing skills make the candidate more comfortable and help to decrease the stress associated with certification exams.

This book also includes chapters reviewing important concepts related to Growth & Development and Health Promotion & Maintenance. These chapters provide questions that test information related to growth and development, general health supervision, and health maintenance. The clinical chapters are developed using a systems approach (i.e., cardiovascular, respiratory, endocrine, etc.). In each of these chapters, the test questions are divided into three areas: Physical Examination & Diagnostic Tests, Disorders, and Pharmacology. This format assists the candidate to easily locate specific questions. The last three chapters in the text are on Research & Theory, Issues & Trends, and Legal & Ethical Issues. The test questions in these chapters focus on professional competencies inherent in the role and function of the FNP.

Our thanks to the many nurse practitioners across the country who provided questions and insight into the role of the nurse practitioner. We wish to thank Victoria Bruno, our editor at Elsevier, for her support and suggestions in our preparation of the manuscript. Thank you also goes to the nurse practitioners who took time from their busy schedules to review the questions for content and clarity.

Acknowledgments

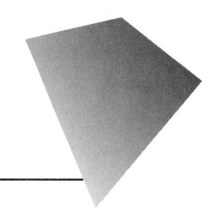

We are continually grateful for the contributions and efforts of our test item contributors who provided their expertise and knowledge for this nurse practitioner certification review series.

We thank the staff at Elsevier: Barbara Nelson Cullen, Executive Publisher, and Victoria Bruno, Senior Developmental Editor, for their calmness and patience; Helen Hudlin, who managed the book's production; and Roger McWillians for copy-editing the manuscript. What a job to keep track of thousands of questions!

Last, but certainly not least, we want to thank our children, Tyler and Ashley Zerwekh, Jaelyn Conway, Michael Brown, and Kim Aultman, for teasing their mothers about writing so many books!! We thank Tom Gaglione and Robert Claborn for their encouragement, support, and love. We love you all.

Contents

xvi   Contents

Test-Taking Strategies

Testing Strategies

Knowing how to take an examination is a skill that is developed through practice and experience. Being able to take an examination effectively is almost as important as the basic knowledge required to answer the question. Everyone has taken an examination only to find in the review of the exam that questions were missed due to inadequate testing skills.

Nurse practitioner programs provide the graduate student with a comprehensive base of knowledge; how you utilize this knowledge will determine your success on a certification examination. The certification examination is an objective test that covers knowledge, understanding, and application of professional nursing theory and practice. When you register for the examination, you will receive a "Candidate Handbook" or information materials from the Certification Board administering the examination. This handbook will have helpful information to assist you in preparing, such as important registration information, test content outline, sample test questions, and in some cases a bibliography. This important information can assist you in your review process.

Read the information in this chapter carefully and make sure you understand the strategies discussed. This chapter is designed to help you identify problem areas in testing skills and learn how to use strategy and judgment in selecting correct answers.

It is important for you to practice testing skills if you are going to be able to utilize these skills on the certification examination.

Question Characteristics

A. Multiple-choice questions
1. Scene or scenario—establishes the setting of the question. Not all questions will have a scenario; if a scenario is included, consider the appropriateness of the answer to the information provided.
2. Stem—states the question that is being asked.
3. Options—there are four options from which to choose an answer.
   a. Distracters—designed to distract you from the correct answer.
   b. Correct answer—correctly answers the question asked in the stem.
   c. There are only four options in any item; there are no combinations of options to consider.
   d. There is only one correct response; no partial credit is given for another answer.
B. Questions are derived from common clinical situations in practice setting

Strategies for Multiple-Choice Questions

1. Cover the options with your hand or a piece of scratch paper. This strategy makes you focus on the content of the question and prevents your eyes from "darting" to look at the distracters. If you peruse the distracters before you completely understand the question, key words in the distracters will influence your interpretation of the question. If you practice this during your preparation for the examination, when you are testing on the computer you will be less likely to go to the answers before you understand the question.

2. Do not read extra meaning into the question. The question is asking for specific information; if it appears to be simple "common sense," then assume it is simple. Do not look for a hidden meaning in what appears to be an easy question.

E X A M P L E

The nurse practitioner understands that the most common form of facial paralysis in the adult client is:

1. Facial nerve fasciitis.
2. Trigeminal neuralgia.
3. Bell's palsy.
4. Herpes zoster.

The correct answer is Option #3. Be careful not to "read into" the question and add pain to the facial paralysis symptom. The most common form of facial paralysis is Bell's palsy, which is a disorder affecting the facial nerve and characterized by muscle flaccidity of the affected side of the face. Trigeminal neuralgia is a disorder of cranial nerve V characterized by an abrupt onset of pain in the lower and upper jaw, cheek, and lips. Herpes zoster affects the dermatomes and does not cause a paralysis, but pain is possible with postherpetic neuralgia.

E X A M P L E

When administering skin tests to an immunocompromised client, the nurse practitioner must consider:

1. The importance of not applying more than one skin test at a time.
2. The skin test possibly reacting more aggressively than expected.
3. The use of a known allergen for the client as a control.
4. The immunocompromised client should not be skin tested.

The correct answer is Option #3. Do not read into the question and make it more difficult by trying to make the client sicker (e.g., full-blown AIDS). It is important to remember to apply controls when skin testing the immunocompromised client. Ask clients what diseases they believe they have immunity to, such as measles. Apply the "known" allergen and the skin test to be performed. If the client is unable to mount an immune response, the known allergen will not react. By not applying the controls, the nurse practitioner may assume a skin test is negative, when in fact the client's immune system is unable to respond.

3. Read the stem correctly. Make sure you understand exactly what information the question is asking. It is important to understand the question before reviewing the options for the correct answer.

E X A M P L E

The nurse practitioner would refer to a pediatric cardiologist for workup and evaluation in 1–2 weeks for a child with:

1. Signs of exercise intolerance, dyspnea, and elevated pulse.
2. Poor feeding, increased cyanosis with crying, and dizziness.
3. Nonfunctional heart murmur, respiratory crackles, and retarded growth and development.
4. Systolic ejection murmur, grade II, which disappears on sitting.

The question asks you to determine which child's symptoms would require a referral to a pediatric cardiologist in the next 1–2 weeks. Options #1, #2, and #3 are considered unstable and acute and should be immediately referred to a pediatric cardiologist. In Option 4, children with a murmur need to be further evaluated, but it is not considered an emergency as long as they are asymptomatic, have normal activity and exercise, and are growing normally.

4. Before considering the options, think about the characteristics of this condition and the critical concepts to consider. Begin by assessing each option with regard to the concepts of the condition.

E X A M P L E

A mother who is 3 days postpartum has been complaining of soreness and fullness in her breasts and that she wants to stop breast-feeding her infant until her breasts feel better. The nurse practitioner:

1. Shows the client how to apply a breast binder to decrease the discomfort and the production of milk.
2. Tells the client that breast fullness may be a sign of infection and to stop breast-feeding.
3. Suggests to the client that she decrease her fluid intake for the next 24 hours to suppress lactation temporarily.
4. Explains to the client that the breast discomfort is normal and that the infant's sucking will promote the flow of milk.

Formulate in your mind critical information for the care of this client. Think to yourself, "Is it normal to have fullness and soreness in the breasts during the first 3 days of lactation?" If you are unsure, go back and reassess the question. In this instance, Option #4 is correct. Initially, breast soreness may occur for about 2–3 minutes during each feeding until the let-down reflex is established.

5. Identify what type of response the question is asking. A positive stem requires identification of three false items and one correct answer.

EXAMPLE

Clients who believe they have been exposed to human immunodeficiency virus (HIV) should have an HIV antibody test how soon after the exposure?

1. The next day and 2 months later.
2. 6 months after exposure and again at 12 months.
3. 6 to 12 weeks after exposure and again at 6 months.
4. 4 weeks and 12 weeks.

The correct answer is Option #3. This question requires you to identify three incorrect responses and one correct response. The HIV antibody develops between 6 and 12 weeks after exposure. Because of the variability of antibody development, it is recommended that the test be repeated in 6 months to confirm the findings.

6. Identify questions that require identification of something the practitioner should not or would not do (i.e., unsafe action, contraindication, inappropriate action).

EXAMPLE

The nurse practitioner is prescribing astemizole (Hismanal) for a geriatric client's allergy problems. When considering the client's current medications, which medication would be a contraindication to the administration of astemizole (Hismanal)?

1. Erythromycin ethylsuccinate (E.E.S.).
2. Verapamil (Calan).
3. Propranolol (Inderal).
4. Captopril (Capoten).

The correct answer is Option #1. Macrolides and Hismanal should not be administered concurrently. The nurse practitioner is required to identify a medication that should not be ordered.

7. Questions may also be analytical. These questions may ask the nurse practitioner to identify findings, identify statements that are consistent/inconsistent with the client's presenting problem, and/or differentiate between them.

EXAMPLE

A child is being evaluated for attention deficit hyperactivity disorder (ADHD). Which test is helpful in evaluating the difference between ADHD and a learning disability?

1. Standardized IQ achievement test.
2. Denver Developmental Screening Test.
3. Audiologic and visual testing.
4. Complete neurologic examination.

Before you examine the options in this question, it is important to think about the differences between ADHD and learning disabilities. The correct answer is Option #1. Children with learning disabilities and ADHD are often impulsive, inattentive, and overactive. Usually, children with ADHD do not have lower IQ achievement scores; however, children with a learning disability usually demonstrate a level of educational achievement substantially below that of the IQ.

8. Identify key words that affect your understanding of the question. Make sure you understand exactly what information the question is asking. Be aware of questions in which the stem includes words such as *except, contraindicated, avoid, least, not applicable,* and *does not occur.* These words change the direction of the question. It may help to rephrase the question in your own words to better understand what information is being requested.

EXAMPLE

Clients with arteriosclerotic heart disease (ASHD) go through several stages before becoming severely compromised. Which does not occur in the early stages of ASHD?

1. Decreased urine output.
2. Dyspnea on exercise.
3. Anginal pain relieved by rest.
4. Increased serum triglyceride levels.

Rephrase the question: "In early stages of ASHD, which of the following does not occur?" It is important that you identify the key point "early stages of ASHD" and the key words "does not occur." If you miss these essential points, you do not understand the question, and chances are you will not choose the correct answer. The correct answer is Option #1: a decrease in urine output occurs when cardiac disease is advanced enough to cause a severe decrease in cardiac output and renal perfusion.

9. As you read the options, eliminate those you know are not correct. Now that you understand the question, begin eliminating the incorrect answers. This will help narrow the field of choice. When you select an answer or eliminate a distracter, you should have a specific reason for doing so. Don't try to predict a correct answer; it is distressing if the answer you want is not a selection.

EXAMPLE

A 45-year-old female complains of knee pain when kneeling and a "clicking" noise when walking up steps. On examination, there is a slight knee effusion and tenderness when palpating the patella against the condyles. The diagnosis for this client is:

1. Anterior cruciate tear. (*No, the client generally cannot bear weight on the extremity without it buckling or giving way.*)
2. Dislocated patella. (*No, there would be considerable effusion and locking of the knee in flexion.*)
3. Chondromalacia patella. (*Yes, there is clicking and anterior knee pain around or under the kneecap aggravated by knee extensor stress.*)
4. Tendinitis. (*No, there would be no clicking sound with movement.*)

After systematically evaluating the options, Option #3 is the correct answer.

10. Identify similarities in the distracters. Frequently, three distracters will contain similar information, and one will be different. The different one may be the correct answer.

EXAMPLE

An elderly client is to be encouraged to increase her intake of protein. The addition of which of these

foods to 100 ml of milk will provide the greatest amount of protein?

1. 50 ml light cream and 2 tbsp corn syrup.
2. 30 gm powdered skim milk and one egg.
3. 1 small scoop (90 gm) ice cream and 1 tbsp chocolate syrup.
4. 2 egg yolks and 1 tbsp sugar.

Options #1, #3, and #4 all contain a simple sugar. The correct answer, Option #2, has more protein. Notice that three of the options are similar; the one that is different may be the correct answer. This strategy is not a substitute for basic knowledge but may help you figure out the answer.

11. Select the most comprehensive answer. All the options may be correct, but **one** will include the other three options or will need to be considered first.

EXAMPLE

A new mother tells the nurse practitioner that her infant was born HIV positive. She asks the nurse practitioner how long her baby has to live. The nurse practitioner's response would be based on the knowledge that:

1. The antibodies present in the baby's blood may reflect the antibodies received from the mother at birth.
2. If antibodies are present at birth, the baby has acquired immunodeficiency syndrome (AIDS) in an active form.
3. Since the baby is HIV positive, the child will develop full-blown AIDS within 3 years.
4. The antibodies detected at birth indicate presence of the HIV; the test does not indicate when or if the child will develop AIDS.

The correct answer is Option #4. It is important to give the mother as much hope as possible but still be realistic about the condition. There is no way to tell when or if the child will convert to active AIDS. Many infants seroconvert to HIV-negative status.

12. Select the best answer that is most specific to what the question asks. All the options may be correct, but **one** is more specific or essential.

EXAMPLE

When a child comes in for a health maintenance clinic visit, what is essential for the nurse practitioner to do?

1. Order routine laboratory tests.
2. Perform vision and auditory screening.

3. Plot height and weight on charts.

4. Review immunization record.

It is absolutely essential that the immunization record be reviewed. The other options are important but are not essential for a health maintenance visit. Recognize key words that identify the question that is asking for a priority of care—first, initial, best, most. The correct answer is Option #4; the other alternatives may be correct but should be prioritized.

13. Watch questions in which the options contain several items to consider. After you are sure you understand what information the question is requesting, evaluate each part of the distracter. Is it appropriate to what the question is asking? If an option contains one incorrect item, the entire option is incorrect. **All** the items listed in the selection must be correct if it is to be the answer to the question.

EXAMPLE

Diagnostic studies used in the differential diagnosis of systemic lupus erythematosus (SLE) include:

1. Complete blood count (CBC), electrolyte panel, and erythrocyte sedimentation rate (ESR).
2. Chest x-ray and coagulation profile.
3. Antinuclear antibodies (ANA), ESR, and C-reactive protein.
4. CBC, urinalysis (UA), and chest x-ray.

The correct answer is Option #3. In a methodical evaluation of the items in the options, you can eliminate items in options #1, #2, and #4. Although all the tests included in the answer may be included in a complete physical examination, the laboratory test specific to the diagnosis of SLE includes the ANA, ESR, and C-reactive protein. During flares, ESR and C-reactive protein are elevated. The ANA titer in a client with SLE is positive at a 1:80 ratio.

14. Be alert to relevant information contained in previous questions. Sometimes as you are answering questions, you will find information similar to the question being tested. Previous questions may assist you in identifying relevant information in the current question.

EXAMPLE

The American College of Physicians (ACP) recommends that healthy adults receive a tetanus-diphtheria (Td) booster vaccination:

1. Every 5 years.
2. At age 75.

3. At age 65.

4. Every 10 years.

The ACP recommends that adults receive a Td booster every 10 years or a single booster at age 50 for clients who have completed full pediatric series, including teenage and young adult boosters. The correct answer is Option #4. In another question involving immunizations, you read the following question:

EXAMPLE

In taking the history of an alert older adult, the nurse practitioner determines the client is an avid gardener and spends much of his time outside. He had a pneumococcal vaccination last year and states he cannot remember when he had a tetanus vaccination. A health maintenance recommendation for this client would be to obtain:

1. Pneumococcal vaccine.
2. Tetanus vaccine.
3. Hepatitis B vaccine.
4. No recommendation.

The correct answer is Option #2. A clue to the answer to this question may be found in the previous question. Older adults who enjoy gardening and outdoor activities should have a Td booster once every 10 years, as recommended by ACP. Some professionals advocate that high-risk populations (e.g., gardeners, construction workers, others who work outdoors) should have a Td booster every 5 years. When you are taking the test on computer, it is more difficult to remember previous questions because you cannot go back and change answers.

15. Multiple-choice mathematical computations may be included in the exam. Mathematical computations may include calculations of IM, PO, and IV dosages; calculations of pediatric dosage; determining creatinine clearance; and conversion of units of measurement.

EXAMPLE

The nurse practitioner is ordering amoxicillin (Amoxil) for a child with otitis media. The child weighs 22 lb. How would the order be written?

1. Amoxicillin 250 mg/5 ml Sig: 5 ml PO tid × 10 days.
2. Amoxicillin 500 mg Sig: 1 tab PO tid × 3 days.
3. Amoxicillin 350 mg/5 ml Sig: 5 ml PO bid × 14 days.
4. Amoxicillin 125 mg/5 ml Sig: 5 ml PO tid × 10 days.

First, you must convert the lb to kg, which is 2.2 lb/kg. This child weighs 10 kg. The dose for amoxicillin is 30–50 mg/kg/day for a child. 10 kg ¥ 40 mg/kg/day = 400 mg/day. Amoxicillin is supplied in 125 mg/5 ml and 250 mg/5 ml. The correct dose for this child would be the 125 mg/5 ml. The answer closest to that dosage is Option #4.

16. Evaluate priority questions carefully. Frequently, all the answers are appropriate to the situation. You need to decide which of the actions you should do first.

EXAMPLE

While attending a rural public school, a 7-year-old child was bitten on the hand by a raccoon. At the rural clinic the nurse practitioner cleansed the wound. The next action is:

1. Administer tetanus antitoxin.
2. Contact local animal control authorities.
3. Administer rabies immune globulin (RIG) and human diploid cell vaccine (HDCV).
4. Teach the family how to do hourly soaks to the hand using normal saline and peroxide.

The correct answer is Option #3. Any type of animal bite that might be associated with an animal that may harbor rabies (skunks, bats, raccoons, foxes, coyotes, rats) should be treated with both active and passive rabies immunization. The priority action is to prevent rabies. Tetanus antitoxin would be indicated if the child was not current on the immunization. Animal authorities would be called after the initial treatment to locate the animal and sacrifice it so that the brain can be examined for rabies.

Techniques to Increase Critical Thinking Skills

Memory aids and mindmapping™ are tools that assist in drawing associations from other ideas with the use of visual images. **Mnemonics** are words, phrases, or other techniques that help you remember information. **Imagery** is a tool that helps you identify a problem and visualize a mental picture. Learning content that uses these techniques will assist you to recall information more effectively.

Mindmapping™ is a method of organizing important information that is in sharp contrast to the traditional outline format. A thought or concept is written in the center of the page, and images and color are added to information as ideas begin to flow from the center focus (Figure 1–1).

FIGURE 1–1   EXAMPLE OF MINDMAPPING™: PERITONITIS "HOT BELLY"
From Zerwekh J, Claborn J, Miller CJ: *Memory Notebook of Nursing*, Vol I, 2nd ed. Dallas: Nursing Education Consultants Publishing, 2000, p 85.

FIGURE 1–2   ACRONYM MEMORY AID: THE "6-PS" OF DYSPNEA
From Zerwekh J, Claborn J, Miller CJ: *Memory Notebook of Nursing*, Vol II, 2nd ed. Dallas: Nursing Education Consultants Publishing, 2003, p 22.

Acronyms help you to recall information through word associations or letter arrangements to recall specific information. Examples of these are the "6-Ps" of dyspnea (Figure 1–2), the "5-Ps" of circulatory assessment (Figure 1–3), and the "ABCD" of malignant melanoma (Figure 1–4).

Acrostics are catchy phrases in which the first letter of each word stands for something to recall. For example, in remembering the use of canes and walkers, think of "Wandering Wilma's Always Late" (**W**alker **W**ith **A**ffected **L**eg) (Figure 1–5). Everyone remembers the cranial nerve mnemonic (Figure 1–6).

Memory aids/images are pictures or caricatures that help you to recall information more effectively (Figure 1–7).

Rhymes are phrases or words spoken in a rhythmic or musical manner that increase recall, such as the rhyme for hypoglycemia versus hyperglycemia (Figure 1–8). Another rhyme, "fingers, nose, penis, toes," identifies the areas where lidocaine with epinephrine is contraindicated as a local anesthetic. "Two is too much" may help you remember toxic levels of lithium, digoxin, and theophylline, which have a narrow margin of safety (Figure 1–9). Books are available on these helpful aids (see References at the end of this chapter).

Testing Skills for Paper and Pencil Tests

Because your certification tests are available on computer, the following skills are applicable for paper-and-pencil tests that you may encounter while a student in your program.

1. Go through the exam and mark all the answers that you know are correct. This ensures you have adequate time to answer the questions you know. Go back and evaluate those questions for which you did not readily recognize the answer.

2. Do not indiscriminately change answers. If you go back and change an answer, you should have a specific reason for doing so. You may remember information and realize you answered the question incorrectly. Frequently, test-takers "talk themselves out of" the correct answer and change it to an incorrect one.

3. After you have completed the exam, go back and check your booklet and make sure all the questions are answered. Answer all the questions, even if you must guess.

FIGURE 1–3 CIRCULATION ASSESSMENT: THE "5-PS"
From Zerwekh J, Claborn J, Miller CJ: *Memory Notebook of Nursing*, Vol II, 2nd ed. Dallas: Nursing Education Consultants Publishing, 2003, p 27.

Successful Test Taking

1. Listen carefully to the instructions given at the beginning of the examination. Make sure you understand all the information given and exactly how to mark your answers and/or how to use the keyboard.

2. Watch your timing. Do not spend too much time on one question. It is very important that you practice your timing on the sample exams. You will not be able to review your questions and answers on completion of the computer testing. Do it right the first time and there is no need to review the entire test again. Watch your timing on computer tests; make use of a computer clock if available.

3. Be aware of your "first hunch." It is frequently the correct answer. Sometimes information is processed by the brain without your aware-ness. If something about an answer "feels right" or if you have a "gut feeling," pay attention to it.

4. Eliminate distracters that assume the client "would not understand" or "is ignorant of" the situation or those that "protect them from worry." For example, "The client should not be told she has cancer because it would upset her too much."

5. Be aware of distracters that contain the words always and never.

6. There is no pattern of correct answers. Both computer and paper-and-pencil examinations are compiled by computer, and the position of the correct answers is selected at random.

7. Watch the length of the options to consider. The number of words required to adequately state the correct answer is sometimes longer then the other options.

HINTS TO MALIGNANT MELANOMA

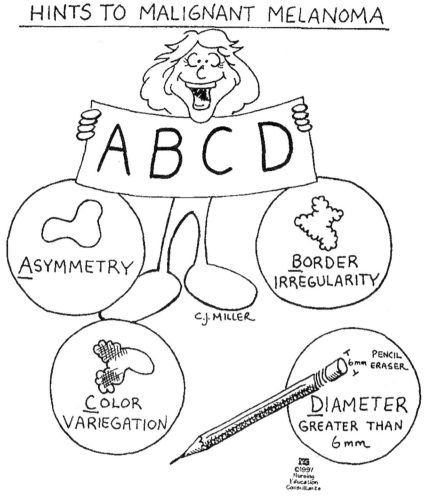

FIGURE 1–4 INDICATIONS OF POSSIBLE MALIGNANT MELANOMA: "ABCD"

From Zerwekh J, Claborn J, Miller CJ: *Memory Notebook of Nursing*, Vol II, 2nd ed. Dallas: Nursing Education Consultants Publishing, 2003, p 137.

Decrease Anxiety

Your activities on the day of the examination strongly influence your level of anxiety. By carefully planning ahead, you will be able to eliminate some anxiety-provoking situations. If you are a diabetic or have special needs, contact the certification agency ahead of time to make arrangements to have food or other accommodations that you might require.

1. Visit the examination site prior to the day of the exam. Evaluate travel time, parking, and time to reach the designated area. Get an early start to allow extra time.

2. If you have to travel some distance to the examination site, try to spend the night in the immediate vicinity.

3. Do something pleasant the evening before the examination. This is not the time to "crash study."

4. Anxiety is contagious. If those around you are extremely anxious, avoid contact with them before the examination.

5. Make your meal before the test a light, healthy one.

6. Avoid eating highly spiced or different foods. This is not the time for a gastrointestinal upset.

7. Wear comfortable clothes. This is not a good time to wear tight clothing or new shoes.

8. Wear clothing of moderate weight. It is difficult to control the temperature to keep everyone comfortable. Take a sweater or wear layered clothes that can be removed if you get too warm.

9. Wear soft-soled shoes; this decreases the noise in the testing area.

10. Make sure you have the papers that are required to gain admission to the exam site. Do not forget your reading glasses, if you wear them.

FIGURE 1–5   MNEMONICS FOR CANES ("COAL") AND WALKERS ("WWAL")
From Zerwekh J, Claborn J, Miller CJ: *Memory Notebook of Nursing*, Vol II, 2nd ed. Dallas: Nursing Education Consultants Publishing, 2003, p 8.

11. Do not take study material to the exam site. You cannot take it into the exam area, and it is too late to study.

12. Do not panic when you encounter content with which you are unfamiliar in a question. Use good test-taking strategies, select an answer, and continue. Remember, you are not going to know all of the right answers.

13. Reaffirm to yourself that you know the material. It is not time for any self-defeating behavior or negative self-talk. **You will pass!** Build your confidence by visualizing yourself in 6 months working in the area you desire. Create that mental picture of where you want to be and who you want to be— certified nurse practitioner. Use your past successes to bring positive energy and "vibes" to your certification. **We know you can do it!**

Study Habits

Enhancing Study Skills

- Decide on a realistic study schedule; write it down and stick with it.
- Divide the review material into segments—pediatrics, well woman, geriatric, and so forth.
- Prioritize the segments; review first the areas in which you seem deficient or weak.
- Identify areas that will require additional review.
- Establish a realistic schedule; study in short segments or "bursts." Avoid marathon sessions.
- Plan on achieving your study goal several days prior to the examination.

CRANIAL NERVE MNEMONIC

S = Sensory	M = Motor	B = Both

O Olfactory	O On	S Some
O Optic	O Old	S Say
O Oculomotor	O Olympus'	M Marry
T Trochlear	T Tiny	M Money
T Trigeminal	T Tops	B But
A Abducens	A A	M My
F Facial	F Finn	B Brother
A Acoustic	A And	S Says
G Glossopharyngeal	G German	B Bad
V Vagus nerve	V Viewed	B Business
S Spinal	S Some	M Marry
H Hypoglossal	H Hops	M Money

© 1994 Nursing Education Consultants

FIGURE 1–6 CRANIAL NERVE MNEMONIC

From Zerwekh J, Claborn J, Miller CJ: *Memory Notebook of Nursing*, Vol I, 2nd ed. Dallas: Nursing Education Consultants Publishing, 2000, p 91.

FIGURE 1–7 IMAGE AS MEMORY AID FOR THE SIGNS/SYMPTOMS OF HYPERTHYROIDISM

From Zerwekh J, Claborn J, Miller CJ: *Memory Notebook of Nursing*, Vol I, 2nd ed. Dallas: Nursing Education Consultants Publishing, 2000, p 46.

BLOOD SUGAR MNEMONIC

Hot & Dry = Sugar High

Cold & Clammy = Need Some Candy

FIGURE 1–8   BLOOD SUGAR RHYME
From Zerwekh J, Claborn J, Miller CJ: *Memory Notebook of Nursing*, Vol I, 2nd ed. Dallas: Nursing Education Consultants Publishing, 2000, p 50.

FIGURE 1–9   "TWO IS TOO MUCH": TOXIC LEVELS OF LITHIUM, DIGOXIN, AND THEOPHYLLINE
From Zerwekh J, Claborn J, Miller CJ: *Memory Notebook of Nursing*, Vol II, 2nd ed. Dallas: Nursing Education Consultants Publishing, 2003, p 43.

- Do not study when you are tired or when there are frequent distractions or interruptions.
- Review general concepts of practice from a variety of resources.

Group Study

- Keep the group limited to four or five people.
- Group members should be mature and serious about studying.
- The group should agree on the planned study schedule.
- If the group makes you anxious, or if you do not think the group meets your study needs, do not continue to participate.

Testing Practice

- Include testing practice in your schedule.
- Select about 50 questions for a practice testing session of 1 hour. This will allow you to evaluate the pace of the exam (i.e., approximately a question per minute).

- Try to answer the questions as if you were taking the real examination. Do not look up the right answer immediately after answering the question. Complete all the questions you have selected, then go back and grade the questions.
- Utilize the testing strategies described in this chapter.
- Evaluate the practice exams for problem areas: testing skills and knowledge base.
- Evaluate the questions you answer incorrectly. Review the rationale for the right answer and understand why you missed it.
- Utilize the questions at a later point to review the information again.

References

Beitz J: Unleashing the power of memory: the mighty mnemonic. *Nurse Educator*, 22(2):25–28, 1997.

Bloomingfield R: *Mnemonics, Rhetorics, and Poetics for Medics*. Salem, NC: Harbinger Medical Press, 1982.

Rayfield S, Manning L: *Nursing Made Insanely Easy*. Shreveport, La: ICAN Publishing, 2002.

Zerwekh J, Claborn J: Test-taking strategies. In *NCLEX-RN®: A Comprehensive Study Guide*, 5th ed. Dallas: Nursing Education Consultants Publishing, 2002.

Zerwekh J, Claborn J, Miller CJ: *Memory Notebook of Nursing*, Vol I, 2nd ed. Dallas: Nursing Education Consultants Publishing, 2000.

Zerwekh J, Claborn J, Miller CJ: *Memory Notebook of Nursing*, Vol II, 2nd ed. Dallas: Nursing Education Consultants Publishing, 2003.

Growth & Development

Physical Assessment

1. The following sequence is recommended for well-child examinations up to the age of 5 years:

   1. 2 weeks, 2 months, 4 months, 6 months, 1 year, 15 months, 18 months, and every year from ages 2–5.

   2. 2 months, 4 months, 6 months, 9 months, and annually from years 1–5.

   3. 2 weeks, 2 months, 4 months, 6 months, 9 months, 12 months, 15 months, 18 months, and annually years 2–5.

   4. The same intervals recommended for immunizations.

2. An appropriate treatment for overweight children under 8 years of age would include:

   1. Administer an appetite suppressant.

   2. Eliminate all carbohydrates in the diet.

   3. Plan a program of activity and exercise.

   4. Use vitamin therapy and herbal teas.

3. The nurse practitioner is seeing a 2-week-old newborn on the first clinic visit. She notes dysmorphic facial features. The nurse practitioner's evaluation includes:

   1. Ordering a chromosome analysis.

   2. Complete postnatal history.

   3. Detailed physical examination and perinatal history. ✓

   4. Avoiding discussion with parents until diagnostic studies are completed.

4. An 18-month-old's feet turn inward. The mother is concerned, although the child is unaware of the problem. The differential diagnosis includes all except:

   1. Femoral anteversion.

   2. Metatarsus adductus.

   3. Legg-Calvé-Perthes disease.

   4. Adducted great toe.

5. The characteristics of an innocent heart murmur in children include:

    1. Asymptomatic, loud diastolic rumble, grade I–V.

    2. Midsystolic, no thrill, and asymptomatic.

    3. Asymptomatic with an S$_4$ heard at left lower sternal border.

    4. May disappear on sitting and following any type of physical activity.

6. The nurse practitioner is examining a 6-month-old infant. What would be the anticipated findings on examining the infant's fontanels?

    1. Both anterior and posterior should be open.

    2. The anterior should be open, the posterior closed.

    3. Both anterior and posterior should be closed.

    4. The anterior should be closed, the posterior open.

7. Genu varum up to 20 degrees is normal until age:

    1. 18 years.

    2. 5 years.

    3. 18 months.

    4. 6 months.

8. When approaching a toddler to complete a cardiac assessment, the nurse practitioner would:

    1. Allow the toddler to handle the stethoscope while the history is being taken.

    2. Explain in detail what you are going to do and get the toddler involved.

    3. Keep the child warm and covered to minimize discomfort.

    4. Approach the child by cheerfully calling his name out.

9. In performing a physical examination, the nurse practitioner first allows the child to touch the medical equipment and then begins by examining the extremities. This sequence would be most appropriate for a client in what age group?

    1. Infant.

    2. Toddler.

    3. School-age child.

    4. Adolescent.

10. An appropriate test to check for color perception in a preschooler would be:

    1. Ishihara's test. *color*

    2. Bruchner's test. *RR*

    3. Hirschberg's test. *light reflex*

    4. Jaeger's test. *near vision*

11. When assessing the cranial nerves in a young child, the nurse practitioner should:

    1. Obtain help from the parents to enlist the child's cooperation.

    2. Defer assessing the cranial nerve until the child is older.

    3. Modify the technique of examination based on the child's developmental level.

    4. Expect minimal variations among age groups.

12. The nurse practitioner understands the following about the Denver Developmental Screening Test Revised (DDST-R or Denver II):

    1. It is a measurement of intelligence (IQ).

    2. It screens personal/social history, fine and gross motor skills, and language.

    3. It is conducted when the examiner pronounces words and the child repeats.

    4. It is used for ages 0–36 months.

13. Genu valgum is considered normal from:

    1. 1–2 years old.

    2. 2–6 years old. *Knock Kneed*

    3. 8–10 years old.

    4. 12–16 years old.

14. An African American mother and her newborn are seen by the nurse practitioner for a well-baby visit. The mother is responsive to the baby's cries, and the baby comforts easily and makes frequent eye contact with the mother. On examination the nurse practitioner notes the following: height and weight are at the 75th percentile on growth charts, there is a strong sucking reflex, and there is a large blue-black macular lesion over the lumbosacral area. The nurse practitioner should:

    1. Contact a social worker and report the mother to Child Protective Services immediately.

2. Refer the mother and infant to a dermatologist.

3. Recognize that the blue-black spot is a mongolian spot, and counsel the mother that no treatment is necessary.

4. Prescribe clotrimazole cream 1% (Mycelex) bid for 4 weeks.

15. The plantar fat pad, which makes a young child appear to have pes planus, is normal until:

1. 1–2 years old.

2. 2–3 years old.

3. 2–6 years old.

4. 6–8 years old.

16. Growth hormone secretion tests along with a history and physical examination have indicated a positive diagnosis for delayed puberty. The next step for the nurse practitioner is:

1. Treat with hormone replacement.

2. Refer to pediatric endocrinologist.

3. Treat with hormone stimulation therapy.

4. Refer for possible pituitary tumor.

17. During the physical examination of a 13-year-old female, it is developmentally important that the nurse practitioner:

1. Maintain a comfortable silence.

2. Verbally affirm normalcy.

3. Discuss only the major areas of abnormality.

4. Verbally address problems of sexually transmitted diseases.

18. At a school clinic, a 14-year-old girl comes in complaining of dizziness midmorning and a second episode in class that morning. The practitioner should question the adolescent regarding diet/nutrition, drug use, and:

1. Asthma.

2. Pregnancy.

3. Heart disease.

4. Stress.

19. The nurse practitioner understands that sulfa medications are not recommended for children less than which age?

1. 18 months.

2. 12 months.

3. 6 months.

4. 2 months.

Growth & Development

20. The major influence on the timing of puberty is:

1. Exposure to light.

2. Genetics.

3. General health.

4. Nutrition.

21. A 14-year-old girl is seen in the clinic by the nurse practitioner because she has not achieved menarche. Examination reveals axillary and pubic hair and breast buds with increased size of areola. Based on these findings the most appropriate intervention would be:

1. Bone age studies.

2. Labs for luteinizing hormone (LH) and follicle-stimulating hormone (FSH) levels.

3. Chromosome analysis to rule out Turner's syndrome.

4. Reassurance that she is developing normally.

22. A 13-year-old male is seen by the nurse practitioner for a sports physical. The genital exam reveals straight dark pubic hair at the base of the penis and testicular enlargement. Using the Tanner scale, the nurse practitioner would record these findings as:

1. Tanner stage I.

2. Tanner stage II.

3. Tanner stage III.

4. Tanner stage IV.

23. An 11-year-old girl who has just begun to show signs of breast development asks the nurse practitioner when she will start having

periods like her friends. The nurse practitioner's response is based on the knowledge that:

1. The average age of menarche is 12.8 years.

2. Most girls will have a growth spurt following the onset of menarche.

3. Menarche usually occurs about 3–6 months after the onset of breast development.

4. Menarche usually occurs about 18–24 months after the onset of breast development.

24. A teenage girl with curly pubic hair on the mons pubis and breast enlargement without secondary contour would be classified on the Tanner scale as:

1. Tanner stage I.

2. Tanner stage II.

3. Tanner stage III.

4. Tanner stage IV.

25. A mother of a 2-year-old brings her child to see the nurse practitioner because he has been irritable and has a small "knot" under his left ear. The child has no history of fever, upper respiratory infection, or pulling at his ears. The most likely reason for these symptoms is:

1. Otitis media.

2. Teething.

3. Tonsillitis.

4. Otitis externa.

26. A routine well-child visit for a healthy full-term infant should include a hemoglobin and hematocrit at:

1. 1 month of age.

2. 4 months of age.

3. 6–9 months of age.

4. 1 year of age.

27. The mother of a 3-month-old infant is concerned because her baby seems to sleep most of the time. The nurse practitioner's response is based on the knowledge that a 3-month-old infant usually spends:

1. 10 hours in 24 sleeping.

2. 15–16 hours in 24 sleeping.

3. 18–19 hours in 24 sleeping.

4. Most of the 24 hours sleeping, waking only to eat.

28. What advice should the nurse practitioner give a mother who reports during a routine well-child exam that her 5-month-old (weight, 15 lb) who was sleeping all night at 3 months of age is now waking up in the middle of the night hungry. A diet history reveals that the infant is taking six 6-oz bottles of formula in a 24-hour period and has 2 tbsp of rice cereal in the morning.

1. Increase the amount of formula at each feeding to 8 oz.

2. Take the child off formula and switch to homogenized milk.

3. Decrease the amount of formula to 32 oz in 24 hours and add fruits, cereals, and juices.

4. Continue the same amount of formula and introduce a variety of baby foods.

29. The father of a 12-year-old male tells the nurse practitioner that he is afraid that his son is "getting fat." The child is at the 50th percentile for height and the 75th percentile for weight on the growth chart. The most appropriate response would be:

1. Reassure the father that the son is not "fat."

2. Assess family for presence of obesity.

3. Suggest a low-calorie, low-fat diet.

4. Explain that this is typical of the growth pattern of boys at this age.

30. A mother asks the nurse practitioner if an infant walker will help her 6-month-old to learn to walk faster. The nurse practitioner's response is based on the knowledge that:

1. Infant walkers help to strengthen the infant's extremities and prepare them to walk.

2. Infants who are placed in walkers usually walk about 1 month earlier than other infants.

3. Infant walkers are dangerous and should not be recommended for use.

4. There have been very few injuries related to the use of infant mobile walkers.

31. The mother of a 6-month-old infant tells the nurse practitioner that the baby was spitting up his formula so she put him on goat milk. The nurse practitioner is concerned because goat milk places the infant at risk of developing:

    1. Rickets.

    2. Scurvy.

    3. Megaloblastic anemia secondary to folic acid deficiency.

    4. Botulism.

32. A 1-year-old reaches for the nurse practitioner's stethoscope with his left hand and the father says, "It looks like he's going to be a lefty, just like his old man!" The nurse's response is based on the knowledge that:

    1. Male infants usually have the same hand preference as their fathers.

    2. Hand preference is well established by 9 months of age.

    3. Children will not demonstrate a hand preference until about age 6.

    4. Children usually develop handedness by 18–24 months.

33. A mother is concerned that her 7-month-old breast-fed infant is not getting enough to eat. The infant weighed 7 lb 8 oz at birth and was 19 inches long. At 6 months of age, he weighed 15 lb and was 25 inches long. He now weighs 15 lb and is 25 1/2 inches long. The nurse practitioner's response is based on the knowledge that:

    1. Infants should gain 2–4 oz/wk and 1/2 inch in height a month during the first 6 months of life.

    2. Infants should triple their birth weight by 6 months of age.

    3. Infants should gain 3–4 oz/wk and 1/2 inch in height a month from 6–12 months of age.

    4. Infants should gain 1–2 oz/wk and 1 inch in height a month from 6–12 months of age.

34. A child will be able to do which of the following fine motor skills first?

    1. Imitate a circle.

    2. Imitate a square.

    3. Copy a triangle.

    4. Copy a diamond.

35. The nurse practitioner would expect a child to follow a one-step command given without a gesture and using only four to six individual words at what age?

    1. 7 months.

    2. 9 months.

    3. 14 months.

    4. 20 months.

36. The nurse practitioner knows that language is the best single measure of normal cognitive development in early childhood. At what age do children begin to combine two words together?

    1. 8–10 months.

    2. 10–12 months.

    3. 12–15 months.

    4. 14–23 months.

37. A mother of 2-year-old twins is concerned that the twins do not talk very much and seem to have their own "private" language. The nurse practitioner should:

    1. Tell the mother to spend some individual time with the twins so that they learn language skills.

    2. Perform a pure-tone audiometry.

    3. Tell the mother that this is normal for twins or siblings that are close in age.

    4. Refer to a speech pathologist for further testing.

38. The nurse practitioner notices that a 9-month-old infant who was born 2 months prematurely only reaches for an object with his left hand. The nurse would:

    1. Record these findings as normal for a premature infant.

    2. Refer the infant for further evaluation.

    3. Order a muscle biopsy to rule out muscular dystrophy.

    4. Make a note on the chart that the child will probably be left-handed.

39. The mother of a 6-month-old infant tells the nurse practitioner that her infant is now taking homogenized milk instead of an iron-fortified infant formula. The nurse practitioner's response would be based on the knowledge that:

    1. Homogenized milk has the same solute load as formula and is a safe alternative to iron-fortified formula if vitamin supplements are given.

    2. There is an increased incidence of occult gastrointestinal bleeding and the development of iron deficiency anemia in infants fed homogenized milk before 1 year of age.

    3. Once the infant is taking solid foods regularly, there is no need to continue offering iron-fortified formula.

    4. Homogenized milk has too high of a fat content and needs to be diluted 2:1 with water.

40. The development of the male sexual characteristics in utero is dependent on:

    1. Estrogen.

    2. Progesterone.

    3. Prolactin.

    4. Testosterone.

41. The production of sperm usually begins during the:

    1. Eighth week of gestation.

    2. Beginning of puberty.

    3. End of puberty.

    4. Eighth month of gestation.

42. What is true about the developmental process of sperm or spermatozoa?

    1. Each mature sperm contains 23 chromosomes.

    2. Sperm become motile immediately at maturation.

    3. Spermatogenesis takes place in the prostate.

    4. Higher than body temperature contributes to sperm production.

43. What is produced by the testes?

    1. Alkaline phosphate.

    2. Gonadotropin.

    3. Testosterone.

    4. Acid phosphate.

44. Which statement is correct concerning healthy sexual developmental tasks?

    1. At 9 years of age, children are less self-conscious and readily expose themselves to younger children or parents of the opposite sex.

    2. At 16 years of age, adolescents are significantly influenced by the media in terms of sexual content and conduct.

    3. At 4 years of age, children distinguish organs associated with each sex and demonstrate increased sexual curiosity.

    4. At 5 years of age, children begin to have concerns about body image and begin to investigate their own sexual organs.

45. The nurse practitioner understands the following about birth defects and growth and developmental problems in mothers with prenatal alcohol exposure:

    1. If alcohol is ingested late in the pregnancy, there is a higher incidence of postmaturity syndrome.

    2. The practice of drinking alcohol while eating a meal significantly reduces the risk of fully expressed fetal alcohol syndrome.

    3. If alcohol is ingested in large amounts early in the pregnancy, there is an increased incidence of fully expressed clinical features of fetal alcohol syndrome.

    4. Growth retardation is associated with early trimester alcohol consumption and postmaturity syndrome.

46. In response to a young adult male's question concerning the production of sperm, the nurse practitioner knows that sperm is produced in the:

    1. Epididymis.

    2. Vas deferens.

    3. Prostate.

    4. Seminiferous tubules.

47. An adolescent female with breast budding and sparse, straight, lightly pigmented pubic hair

along medial border of labia is at which Tanner stage of sexual maturity?

1. Stage I.
2. Stage II.
3. Stage III.
4. Stage IV.

48. Precocious puberty is defined as:

1. Onset of puberty before age 8 in females and 9 in males.
2. Onset of puberty before age 5 in females and 7 in males.
3. Onset of puberty before age 10 in females and 12 in males.
4. Onset of puberty for either gender before older siblings enter puberty.

49. The mother of a 5-month-old infant brings her child to the clinic because the infant awakens frequently at night and cries. The nurse practitioner understands that the most common cause of night awakening in healthy infants is:

1. Night terrors and nightmares.
2. Separation anxiety.
3. Trained night crying.
4. Hunger pain and wet diaper.

50. A 10-day-old breast-fed infant is brought to the clinic because the mother is concerned about the infant's "yellow-orange" color. History and findings are as follows: Mother's blood type AB-positive, infant's blood type B-negative, total bilirubin 15 mg/dl. The nurse practitioner understands that this is most likely caused by:

1. Hemolytic jaundice.
2. Breast-fed jaundice.
3. Obstructive jaundice.
4. Physiologic jaundice.

51. A new mother presents to the clinic inquiring about when she should start feeding her 2-month-old infant solid foods. The nurse practitioner should recommend that the mother:

1. Start the infant on meat and eggs now.

2. Wait until the infant is 1 year old before introducing solid foods.
3. Start the infant on cereals now.
4. Introduce one new food at a time when the infant is 4–6 months old.

Aging

52. As an individual ages, which physiologic change would affect responses to pharmacologic agents?

1. Increased gastric emptying.
2. Increased glomerular filtration rate.
3. Decreased percentage of body fat.
4. Decreased albumin concentration.

53. The number one cause of accidental death in clients older than 65 years of age is:

1. Motor vehicle accidents.
2. Poisoning.
3. Falls.
4. Drowning.

54. The nurse practitioner selects which assessment tool to evaluate balance and gait problems in elderly clients?

1. Lawton & Brody Balance and Coordination Scale.
2. Tinetti Balance and Gait Evaluation.
3. Instrumental Activities of Daily Living Scale.
4. Index of Independence of Activities of Daily Living.

55. In assessing the nutritional status of an elderly client, the nurse practitioner identifies the common physiologic change in the gastrointestinal system to be:

1. Increased peristalsis.
2. Decreased absorption of iron.
3. Maintenance of normal fat metabolism.
4. Increased drug metabolism.

56. What are the normal physiologic changes in the thyroid gland that occur with aging?

    1. Hypertrophy with a decrease in triiodothyronine (T3) and thyroxine (T4).

    2. Normal size with increase in thyroid-stimulating hormone (TSH) and decrease in T4.

    3. Atrophy of the gland with a decrease in TSH, T3, and T4.

    4. Increase in nodularity with normal TSH and T4. ✓

57. The aging process causes what normal physiologic changes in the heart?

    1. Heart size stays the same, and the valves thicken and become rigid secondary to fibrosis and sclerosis.

    2. Cardiomegaly occurs along with prolapse of the mitral valve and regurgitation.

    3. Dilatation of the right ventricle with sclerosis of pulmonic and tricuspid valves.

    4. Hypertrophy of the right ventricle with decreasing capacity and compromised efficiency of the coronary arteries.

58. Which pulmonary physiologic change is commonly associated with the aging process?

    1. Increased cough response.

    2. Decrease in vital capacity.

    3. Decreased anteroposterior (AP) diameter of thorax.

    4. Increase in residual carbon dioxide partial pressure (pCO_2).

59. Which of these clinical findings would indicate a deviation from the normal age-related changes in the neurologic system that may have some diagnostic significance for the older client?

    1. Decreased sense of touch.

    2. Increased tolerance to pain.

    3. Decreased short-term memory.

    4. Decreased ability to maintain balance.

60. During a teaching session the nurse practitioner instructs the client regarding normal skin lesions in the older population. These would include:

    1. Seborrheic dermatitis.

    2. Senile keratosis.

    3. Senile lentigines.

    4. Squamous cell.

61. Which assessment is a normal physiologic change of the respiratory system that occurs with aging?

    1. Decreased residual lung volume (RV). ✓

    2. Hyperresonance.

    3. Increased forced vital capacity (FVC).

    4. Increased tactile fremitus.

62. The nurse practitioner indicates an understanding of the normal aging process with which documentation of the gastrointestinal (GI) system in the physical examination?

    1. Increase in the size of the liver (16 cm).

    2. Absent bowel sounds.

    3. Femoral bruit.

    4. Increased adipose tissue. ✓

63. During the physical examination of an older client, the nurse practitioner indicates an understanding of deviations in the neurologic system from the normal aging processs with which clinical finding?

    1. Decrease in short-term memory.

    2. Decrease in deep tendon and superficial reflexes.

    3. Decreased sense of touch.

    4. Positive Romberg's sign.

64. Which functional assessment tool should the nurse practitioner use to evaluate the safety for a cerebrovascular accident (CVA) client planning to return to his home environment?

    1. OARS ADL Scale.

    2. Bennet Social Isolation Scale.

    3. Mini Mental State Examination.

    4. Norton Scale.

65. The nurse practitioner understands which factor is most influential in the driving ability of an older adult?

    1. Ability to coordinate the transmissions.

    2. Acuity of vision.

    3. Comprehension of the details of the road rules.

    4. Reaction times. ✓

66. As an individual ages, which physiologic change would affect sleep?

    1. Decreased rapid-eye-movement (REM) sleep.

    2. Increased delta or stage IV sleep.

    3. Decreased nocturnal awakenings.

    4. Decreased sleep latency.

67. When treating an infection in the older adult, the nurse practitioner must consider:

    1. Thymus-derived immunity is increased.

    2. Immune function declines with age. ✓

    3. Immune function increases with age.

    4. Antibody production increases.

68. The diminished immunity of the older adult can be attributed to a decline in:

    1. B-cell function.

    2. T-cell production. ✓

    3. B-cell production.

    4. T-cell function.

69. Which physiologic factor of aging contributes to incontinence in elderly persons?

    1. Decreased vascularity of the bladder mucosa.

    2. Increased urethral closing pressure.

    3. Increased ability to concentrate urine.

    4. Decreased bladder capacity.

70. The nurse practitioner understands that as the client ages changes occur in the cells of the immune system. Which statement reflects these changes?

    1. The cells are able to proliferate as they would in the younger client.

    2. The total number of T cells is decreased.

    3. There is an increased ability to respond to infections with previously produced "remembered" antibodies.

    4. The immune system is able to respond to antigenic stimulation as in the younger client.

Answers & Rationales

Physical Assessment

1. **(3)** These are the recommended health evaluation intervals for children to obtain regular assessment information regarding growth and development and to administer recommended immunizations.

2. **(3)** An approach with a well-balanced diet, activity, and exercise is necessary for weight reduction. This allows for a slow approach to weight loss that incorporates healthy behavior habits.

3. **(3)** The first and most important part of all data gathering starts with a detailed history and physical examination. A detailed, objective description of the dysmorphic features is essential for comparison to textbook descriptions and other data. Although chromosome analysis will probably be ordered, it is not done initially. Parents should be included in the discussion of findings and be kept informed of the progress throughout the evaluation process.

4. **(3)** In-toeing is a common problem and can result from femoral anteversion, adduction of the great toe, medial tibial torsion, and metatarsus adductus. Legg-Calvé-Perthes disease is commonly seen in older children (ages 4–8 years) with loss of hip medial rotation.

5. **(2)** Characteristics of innocent murmurs include: midsystolic, asymptomatic, less than a grade III, loudest in pulmonic area (2–3 left intercostal space at the left sternal border), no radiation to other areas, may disappear on sitting, may intensify with fever, activity, anemia, and stress. Any S_4 sound is considered pathologic in children, as well as adults.

6. **(2)** The posterior fontanel is usually closed by 2 months of age; the anterior fontanel closes about 24 months of age.

7. **(3)** Genu varum (bowleg) of 20 degrees is normal up to the age of 18 months.

8. **(1)** Toddlers like to make the first move (i.e., let them move closer and initiate eye contact first; do not call out their name because this may frighten them). Allowing them to handle the stethoscope will decrease their fear. Option #2 is more appropriate when assessing a school-age child.

9. **(2)** Allow a toddler to explore the instruments and start with the extremities. Save the most invasive examination (of the head) for last. In infants, auscultate the heart and lungs while the infant is quiet, then proceed to do a head-to-toe assessment. In the school-age and adolescent a head-to-toe sequence is preferred.

10. **(1)** Ishihara's: tests for color perception; Bruchner's: tests for the red reflex; Hirschberg's: tests corneal light reflex; Jaeger's: tests near vision.

11. **(3)** Because assessing cranial nerves can be a challenging task, the nurse practitioner should employ techniques that consider the child's developmental level.

12. **(2)** The DDST-R is used for infants through age 5 1/2 years. It is interpreted as normal, suspect, or untestable and measures personal/social area, fine and gross motor skills, and language. Option #3 is the Denver Articulation Screening Exam (DASE), and

Option #4 refers to the age group used for the Early Language Milestone Scale (ELM).

13. **(2)** Genu valgum (knock knee) is considered normal from age 2 to age 6 years.

14. **(3)** Mongolian spots are often found in African American, Hispanic, Native American, and Oriental infants. These spots are benign and tend to fade and disappear by age 3, requiring no intervention or treatment. Abuse is not suspected because signs of a healthy mother-infant relationship are noted (e.g., mother and infant respond positively to each other, baby is thriving).

15. **(2)** The plantar fat pad is normal up to 2–3 years old.

16. **(2)** Once the tentative diagnosis is made, the nurse practitioner should refer to a pediatric endocrinologist for further workup. It is beyond the scope of the practitioner's practice to treat at this point.

17. **(2)** Early adolescence is a time when the child undergoing great physical changes continually wonders if these are normal. Verbal affirmation of areas of normalcy during the exam can decrease anxiety.

18. **(2)** Although all areas would be assessed, pregnancy is a common reason for midmorning syncope in adolescents, associated with altered nutrition.

19. **(4)** Newborns and infants up to age 2 months may develop kernicterus as sulfas displace bilirubin from the plasma proteins.

Growth & Development

20. **(2)** Genetics is the primary determinant of the timing of puberty. Factors such as geographic location, exposure to light, nutritional status, and health status play a role, but genetics is the major influence.

21. **(4)** Menarche usually occurs about 18–24 months after the onset of breast development. Bone age and laboratory studies are not necessary because development is within normal limits. Findings do not indicate a

chromosomal abnormality, so chromosome analysis is unnecessary.

22. **(2)**

Stage	Pubic Hair
I	None
II	Countable; straight; increased pigmentation and length
III	Darker; begins to curl; increased quantity
IV	Increased quantity; coarser texture; covers most of pubic area
V	Adult distribution; spread to medial thighs and lower abdomen
	Genital Development
I	Prepubertal
II	Testicular enlargement; slight rugation of scrotum
III	Further testicular enlargement; penile lengthening begins
IV	Testicular enlargement continues; increased rugation of scrotum; increased penile length
V	Adult

23. **(4)** Menarche usually occurs about 18–24 months after the onset of breast development. Although the average age of menarche is 12.8 years, this should not be the basis for the nurse practitioner's response. Most girls have a growth spurt at Tanner stage IV.

24. **(3)**

Stage	Pubic Hair
I	None
II	Countable; straight; increased pigmentation and length
III	Darker; begins to curl; increased quantity on mons pubis
IV	Increased quantity; coarser texture; labia and mons well covered
V	Adult distribution; with feminine triangle and spread to medial thighs
	Breast Development
I	None
II	Breast bud present; increased areolar size
III	Further enlargement of breast; no secondary contour
IV	Areolar area forms secondary mound on breast contour
V	Mature; areolar area of part of breast contour; nipples project

25. **(2)** At approximately 20 months of age the lower second molars erupt, and at 24 months the upper second molars erupt. With a history

of irritability and lymph node enlargement without fever or other symptoms, teething is the most likely cause of discomfort.

26. **(3)** It is important in a healthy infant to check the hemoglobin and hematocrit between 6 and 9 months of age, when the maternal hemoglobin stores have been depleted. Before 4 months of age the infant has not depleted hemoglobin stores. One would not want to wait until 1 year of age to check hemoglobin.

27. **(2)** Normally, 3-month-old infants sleep 15–16 hours in a 24-hour period.

28. **(3)** Consumption of 32 oz of formula per day is usually an indicator of the need for solids. Formula is recommended for the first year of life. Nutritional requirements are 110–120 cal/kg/day. Introduction of solids usually occurs between 4 and 6 months of age.

29. **(4)** It is normal for boys at this age to appear heavier before they get their "growth spurt." Reassuring the father, although appropriate, is not the best response. Since the findings are within normal limits, it would not be necessary to assess the family for the presence of obesity. Low-calorie, low-fat diets are contraindicated for the growing child.

30. **(3)** The American Academy of Pediatrics (AAP) Committee on Injury and Poison Control issued a policy statement on the use of infant walkers (*Pediatrics* 108:790-792). Because data indicate a considerable risk of major and minor injury and even death from the use of infant walkers, and because there is no clear benefit from their use, AAP recommends a ban on the manufacture and sale of mobile infant walkers. If a parent insists on using a mobile infant walker, it is vital that they choose a walker that meets the performance standards of ASTM F977-96 to prevent falls down stairs. Stationary activity centers should be promoted as a safer alternative to mobile infant walkers.

31. **(3)** Goat milk can cause folic acid deficiency, which can lead to megaloblastic anemia. Rickets is caused by the lack of vitamin D. Scurvy is caused by a lack of ascorbic acid in the diet. Botulism is food poisoning caused by an endotoxin produced by the bacillus *Clostridium botulinum*. Most botulism occurs after eating improperly canned or cooked foods. Infants have been known to develop botulism

from raw honey that is placed on their pacifiers.

32. **(4)** Children usually develop handedness by 18–24 months. The hand preference is usually fixed after 5 years of age.

33. **(3)** Infants should gain 3–4 oz/wk and 1/2 inch in height a month from 6–12 months of age. This child also doubled his birth weight by 6 months of age, as expected.

Age	Weight	Length/Height
0–6 months	6–8 oz/wk (doubles birth weight by 5–7 months)	1 in/mo
6–12 months	3–4 oz/wk (triples birth weight by 1 year)	1/2 in/mo

34. **(1)** A child should be able to imitate a circle at 30 months, copy a square at 4 years, copy a triangle at 5 years, and copy a diamond at 6 years.

35. **(3)** A child should be expected to follow a one-step command (using no gestures and using only four to six individual words) between 10.5 and 16.5 months of age.

36. **(4)** Two-word combinations are expected at 14–23 months of age.

37. **(3)** It is normal for twins or siblings close in age to develop a "private" language understood only by them. Although it is important for the mother to spend individual time with each child, this is not what the question is asking. Pure-tone audiometry is done after age 3. There is no need for a referral to a speech pathologist at this time.

38. **(2)** The infant should be referred for further evaluation. Handedness before 1 year of age may be an early sign of cerebral palsy. The history of prematurity could be an indication of anoxia at birth and would warrant further investigation. The earlier a child is diagnosed, the earlier intervention can be started.

39. **(2)** Homogenized milk does not have the same solute load as formula and is not a safe alternative to iron-fortified formula, even if vitamin supplements are given. The solute load of whole milk is too much for the infant's immature kidneys. The infant needs to

continue taking iron-fortified formula for the first year of life, if possible. There is an increased incidence of occult gastrointestinal bleeding and iron deficiency anemia in infants fed homogenized milk before 1 year of age.

40. **(4)** The most important sex hormone during embryonic development is the primary male sex hormone, testosterone. Testosterone is produced by the gonads of the genetic male embryo, causing the male gonads to develop into two testes, which produce sperm. The other hormones are female hormones. Estrogen, the major female hormone, is produced by the ovaries (ovarian follicle and corpus luteum) and cortices of the adrenal glands and placenta during pregnancy. Progesterone, the second major female hormone, is produced by the corpus luteum. Prolactin is an anterior pituitary hormone and one of the somatotropic hormones that are secreted by lactotropic cells and that target the breast to cause milk production.

41. **(3)** Between the ages of 9 and 12 years the gonads produce more of the sex hormones, which triggers sexual maturation or puberty. Puberty in males begins at approximately age 11 and lasts for 2–3 years, ending with the first ejaculation that contains mature sperm.

42. **(1)** Each mature sperm develops from mitotic division of diploid (46-chromosome) germ cells (spermatogonium) found on the basement membrane of each seminiferous tubule and become primary spermatocytes with 23 chromosomes each. Each of these two cells further divides into two more cells (spermatids), each of which has 23 chromosomes. Motility depends on the biochemicals in semen and in the female reproductive tract. Sperm production needs a temperature that is less than body temperature by at least 1°–2°F.

43. **(2)** The testes have two functions: production of gonadotropin (androgens and testosterone) and production of gametes (sperm). The sperm are produced in the seminiferous tubules of the testes. The androgens and testosterone are produced mainly by Leydig cells of the testes (androgens and testosterone are also produced by the adrenal glands).

44. **(2)** Adolescents are greatly influenced by the media and tend to identify with their parents as sexually functioning people. At age 9,

children are more interested in their own body and are quite self-conscious. Option #3 is true for 6-year-olds, not 4-year-olds. Option #4 is true for 10-year-olds.

45. **(3)** Large amounts of alcohol early in the pregnancy have the most devastating effects on the maturing fetus. There is no safe, established dose for alcohol in pregnancy. Food consumption along with alcohol intake does not reduce the risk of defects. Ingesting alcohol in the later months of pregnancy is associated with an increased incidence of premature and small-for-gestational-age neonates.

46. **(4)** Sperm is produced in the seminiferous tubules of the testes.

47. **(2)** Tanner has five stages of sexual maturity for both males and females. Stage I for both is preadolescent, and stage V for both is mature or adult development. Stages II, III, and IV chronicle development of breasts, pubic hair distribution, penis, and testes. This young female is demonstrating characteristics of Tanner stage II. (See table in rationale for Question 24.)

48. **(1)** Precocious puberty is defined as beginning at age 8 for females and age 9 for males.

49. **(3)** Trained night crying can become a problem in infants who are not allowed to learn to "self-quiet." Activities such as rocking to sleep, exciting play activities before bedtime, and picking the infant up as soon as he cries can lead to trained night crying. Separation anxiety occurs in infants after 6 months of age. The majority of infants after 4 months of age are able to sleep through the night. Nightmares and night terrors occur at a later age.

50. **(2)** This is a type of exaggerated physiologic jaundice that occurs frequently in breast-fed babies due to the infant's inadequate caloric intake before the mother's milk comes in. It typically occurs between 7 and 15 days of life, whereas physiologic jaundice occurs most often after the third day of life. Hemolytic jaundice occurs in an Rh-negative mother who has an Rh-positive infant who becomes isoimmunized.

51. **(4)** Solid foods are not recommended until the infant is 4–6 months old. Cereals should be introduced first, followed by fruits, vegetables,

meats, and eggs. All foods should be introduced based on the readiness of the child.

Aging

52. **(4)** Medications are often protein bound (not fat bound); albumin decreases with age. A low albumin level decreases the number of protein-binding sites, causing an increase in the amount of free drug in the plasma. Drug overdose may occur in elderly clients. Gastric emptying and glomerular filtration rate *decrease* with the aging process.

53. **(3)** Falls are the major cause of morbidity and mortality in the elderly. A fall is often the precipitating event for a cascade of problems leading to death. Complications from falls include fractures, pneumonia, pressure ulcers, pain, and immobility.

54. **(2)** The Tinetti Balance and Gait Evaluation is an activity-based test that asks the client to perform tasks, such as sitting and rising from a chair, turning, and bending. It requires no more than 15–20 minutes to perform. Another appropriate test for assessment of falls is the timed "Up and Go" test, which assesses balance and gait speed. The Instrumental Activities of Daily Learning assesses complex tasks such as shopping, laundry, and food preparation. The Index of Independence of Activities of Daily Living helps to identify daily activities with which the client needs assistance.

55. **(2)** Decreased hydrochloric acid, which occurs with aging, leads to decreased absorption of iron and vitamin B_{12}. Fat absorption would decrease, as would peristalsis and drug metabolism.

56. **(4)** There is usually adequate secretion of TSH and a normal serum concentration of T_4. Aging may produce fibrosis and increased nodularity, but overall the thyroid function remains within normal limits.

57. **(1)** The heart does not increase in size with normal aging. An enlarged heart is a result of cardiac dysfunction. Dilatation of the left ventricle occurs with myocardial infarction and altered cardiac functioning secondary to cardiac disease, not from normal aging. The

aging process does cause fibrosis and sclerosis of the cardiac valves; all valves are equally affected.

58. **(2)** A decrease in the vital capacity, along with a 50% increase in residual volume, occurs during the aging process. Other aging changes include a less effective cough, impaired ciliary action, and weaker respiratory muscles. Increased AP diameter is associated with aging and in chronic obstructive pulmonary disease (COPD) clients. Po_2 usually decreases, but pco_2 usually remains unchanged.

59. **(4)** This may indicate a cerebellar complication. The first three findings are normal age-related changes.

60. **(3)** The senile lentigo is a gray-brown, irregular, macular lesion on sun-exposed areas of the face, arms, and hands that are normal skin lesions. The other lesions are common abnormal skin lesions in the older adult.

61. **(2)** A normal age-related change is an increase in the anteroposterior diameter that results in hyperresonance. Age-related changes result in an increase in the RV and decrease in the FVC. An increased tactile fremitus is a deviation that is of diagnostic significance.

62. **(4)** Common age-related changes in the GI system include increased adipose tissue, decreased liver size, reduced motility and peristalsis, decreased acid secretions and motor activity of stomach, and decreased glomerular filtration rate. Absence of bowel sounds after 5 full minutes and bruits are deviations of clinical significance.

63. **(4)** Romberg's sign indicates the inability to maintain balance, which indicates a need for further evaluation. Options #1, #2, and #3 are normal age-related changes. If it affects the client's functional ability, a decrease in short-term memory would be considered a deviation.

64. **(1)** OARS ADL Scale is the more appropriate screening tool for identifying at-risk populations. The Bennet Social Isolation Scale would be appropriate to evaluate social interactions and resources. The Mini Mental State Examination is used to evaluate memory, orientation, and attention. The Norton Scale is used to evaluate pressure ulcer risk.

65. **(2)** The most age-dependent factor is sensory change. The elderly client being assessed for driving capacity should use any prescribed corrective devices for optimal performance. Poor hearing by itself is generally not a limiting factor for motor vehicle operation, and vision assessment has received the greatest emphasis in assessing older drivers. Documenting the best-corrected binocular visual acuity, color perception, and dark vision is basic in assessing driving visual acuity. Laboratory performance studies have not clearly demonstrated that the other factors are highly applicable to the on-the-road skills of the elderly driver.

66. **(1)** REM sleep begins approximately 120 minutes from sleep onset and recurs in three or four regularly spaced, 10- to 15-minute cycles. REM sleep, associated with skeletal muscle atonia and dreaming, decreases with aging. Delta sleep, or stage IV, is deep sleep and also decreases with age. Nocturnal wakening and sleep latency increase. Sleep is generally less efficient in older clients, who spend more time in bed and less time sleeping.

67. **(2)** Immune function declines with age, making the older adult more susceptible to infection. The older adult has less thymus-derived immunity due to the shrinking of the thymus gland, thus making it more difficult for the older adult to produce antibodies.

68. **(4)** The older adult has diminished cell-mediated immunity because of a decline in T-cell function. The T cells have a decreased ability to produce cytokines, which are needed to facilitate B-cell growth and maturation, and have a decreased ability to proliferate in response to an antigen.

69. **(4)** Decreased bladder capacity, decreased ability to concentrate urine, and decreased urethral closing pressure after menopause lead to incontinence. Other factors are depression, decreased mobility, decreased vision, and lack of attention to bladder cues of fullness.

70. **(3)** Elderly clients are able to respond to infections with previously produced "remembered" antibodies, but they are less able to respond to antigenic stimulation (new antigens) than younger clients. In the elderly client the cells of the immune system also are less likely to proliferate. The total number of T cells remains the same with age, but cell function decreases and cells have decreased cytotoxicity.

Health Promotion & Maintenance

1. What are the current American Cancer Society dietary recommendations for cancer prevention?

    1. Maintaining a desirable body weight and eating a variety of foods, including fruits and vegetables and foods that are high in fiber.

    2. Increasing the amount of protein in the diet.

    3. Alcohol use in small to moderate amounts.

    4. Increase in fresh fruits, fish, and diary products.

2. In the presence of dyslipidemia and diabetes, the National Cholesterol Education Program guidelines set the goal for lipid levels as:

    1. LDL <130 mg/dl and triglyceride levels <200 mg/dl.

    2. LDL <160 mg/dl and triglyceride levels <240 mg/dl.

    3. LDL <100 mg/dl and triglyceride levels <180 mg/dl.

    4. LDL <150 mg/dl and triglyceride levels <220 mg/dl.

3. The American Diabetes Association recommends screening adults starting at age 45 with a fasting plasma glucose (FPG) test every:

    1. 1 year.

    2. 3 years.

    3. 5 years.

    4. 10 years.

4. What are tertiary prevention activities for an elderly woman who has had a cerebrovascular accident (CVA)?

    1. Annual influenza vaccination. 1° prevention

    2. Physical therapy program.

    3. Annual mammogram. 2°

    4. Annual ophthalmologic examination to evaluate for glaucoma.

5. A client is continuing his recovery at home after an extensive surgery. The practitioner would instruct the client to increase his intake of what foods to promote healing?

    1. Tomatoes, rice, whole-bran cereal.

    2. Milk, poultry, yellow vegetables.

    3. Red meat, oranges, green beans.

    4. Liver, corn, eggs.   *protein*

6. When an elderly client has an alteration in the sensory-perceptual function of hearing, which plan would be most appropriate for the nurse practitioner to implement during a health promotion session?

    1. Increase the pitch of the voice.

    2. Stand behind the client when speaking.

    3. Speak in a tone that does not include shouting.

    4. Use typical complex sentences to prevent insulting the client.

7. Which of the following management plans demonstrates an understanding of primary prevention of falls among elderly persons?

    1. Evaluate need for assistive devices for ambulation after the client has been injured in a fall.

    2. Provide resources to correct hazards contributing to falling in the home environment.

    3. Reinforce the need to use prescribed eyeglasses to prevent further injury from falls.

    4. Provide information about medications, side effects, and interactions.

8. Which of these health promotion screenings should be completed annually for the elderly client over 65?

    1. Chest x-ray.

    2. Pneumococcal vaccination.

    3. Colonoscopy.

    4. Stool guaiac test.

9. While teaching a class to a group of senior citizens, which would be most important for the nurse practitioner to consider during the presentation?

    1. Provide increased overhead lighting to enhance visualization.

    2. Provide handouts on blue paper with black print.

    3. Review a video narrated by a woman.

    4. Recognize that past life experiences are beneficial in learning new information.

10. What is the most common occupationally related health problem?

    1. Repetitive motion injury.

    2. Hearing loss.

    3. Lung disease.

    4. Cancer.

11. Which of the following best describes the benefit of sports screening physicals?

    1. Screening for undiagnosed cardiomyopathy.

    2. Assessment of drug and alcohol use.

    3. Estimation of aerobic capacity.

    4. Identification of unresolved injuries.

12. A 48-year-old male presents to the clinic after having his cholesterol checked at a health fair. He states that they told him it was over 300 and that he needed to see his primary care provider for further testing. Appropriate interventions for the nurse practitioner include:

    1. Prescribing a cholesterol-lowering agent.

    2. Ordering an electrocardiogram (ECG) and an exercise stress test.

    3. Starting the client on an exercise program.

    4. Performing a thorough history and physical and drawing a lipid profile.

13. In preparing a client for colorectal screening, the nurse practitioner should instruct the client to:

    1. Eat at least two servings of meat daily prior to collecting samples.

    2. Avoid antibiotics, aspirin, iron, and anti-inflammatory medications.

    3. Avoid taking extra vitamin and mineral supplements prior to the test.

    4. Eat extra servings of high-fiber foods and water to ensure good samples.

14. Teaching testicular self-examination should be targeted to which age group?

    1. 10–14 years.

    2. 15–25 years.

    3. 30–40 years.

    4. 45–65 years.

15. According to the American Dietetics Association, how many servings of the bread/cereal/pasta/rice group should be included each day?

    1. 6–11 servings.

    2. 2–4 servings.

    3. 3–5 servings.

    4. 2–3 servings.

16. At what age should routine screening mammography begin for women who have no increased risk of breast cancer?

    1. 30 years old.

    2. 35 years old.

    3. Begin at age 40.

    4. Before age 50.

17. Which of the following components should be included when taking a history from a client who is new to the clinic?

    1. Past medical and surgical history, family medical and surgical histories, psychosocial history, diet and exercise habits, chemical use, sexual practices, review of systems.

    2. Interval history, past medical history, family medical history, dietary habits, substance use, sexual practices.

    3. Past medical and surgical histories, family medical history, psychosocial history, physical activity, tobacco and other substance use, sexual practices.

    4. The history listed on the form provided to clients for completion before the physical examination is sufficient, and no interview needs to be done.

18. A 50-year-old female presents to the clinic for a first-visit checkup. She states she is in good health and takes no medications. She was adopted and does not know her family history. She is 62 inches tall and weighs 175 lb. She is a secretary and admits to a sedentary lifestyle. She does not smoke and drinks 4-5 alcoholic beverages per week. Which of the following interventions would be most appropriate for the nurse practitioner to recommend in this client's plan of care?

    1. Recommend that she start an exercise program that includes jogging and weight training.

    2. Prescribe vitamin supplements to her diet while eliminating alcoholic beverages.

    3. Discuss possible job changes that that will increase her daily amount of exercise.

    4. Suggest that she keep a daily record of her food intake and bring it to her next visit.

19. Which group is at greatest risk for alterations in immune functions related to nutritional status?

    1. Young adults.

    2. Adults.

    3. Premature infants.

    4. Older adults.

20. The most common cause of infant deaths worldwide is:

    1. Pneumonia.

    2. Dehydration.

    3. Acquired immunodeficiency syndrome (AIDS).

    4. Beta-streptococcal infections.

21. The nurse practitioner is discussing making lifestyle changes that will decrease the geriatric client's risks for cardiovascular disease. Which of the following is most important to include in this discussion?

    1. Decrease smoking; increase vitamin supplements; increase protein intake.

    2. Control hypertension; stop smoking; maintain normal weight; exercise regularly.

    3. Maintain normal levels of serum blood sugar; decrease cholesterol intake.

    4. Have a yearly physical examination; increase fiber in diet; exercise regularly.

22. The nurse practitioner is discussing anticipatory guidance with the parents of a 26-week-gestation premature infant who is now 2 months old and being discharged from the NICU. Which of the following would be most important to include in the discussion?

    1. Fluoride supplement due to lack of breast-feeding.
    2. Lights to be on 24 hours a day.
    3. Decreased handling and stimulation.
    4. Bright colors and continuous music for stimulation.

23. Which of the following is an example of a community health promotion activity?

    1. High school–based family planning clinic.
    2. Work-site urgent care clinic.
    3. Asthma follow-up clinic in an elementary school.
    4. Employer-sponsored multiphasic health screening.

24. Which of the following is most important for the nurse practitioner to do each time a child comes in for a health maintenance clinic visit?

    1. Order routine laboratory tests.
    2. Perform vision and auditory screening.
    3. Plot height and weight on charts.
    4. Review immunization record.

25. Which of the following guidelines should the nurse practitioner follow when developing educational materials?

    1. Present the most important material first using all capital letters for emphasis.
    2. Provide the information in English along with three other languages.
    3. Keep sentences short and to the point using graphic images for clarification.
    4. Keep a readability level of at least 8 (eighth-grade level.)

26. In explaining the purpose of primary prevention programs to a group of nursing students, the nurse practitioner states that primary prevention programs:

    1. Work to lower the incidence of birth defects.
    2. Emphasize early diagnosis and treatment of pediatric anomalies.
    3. Minimize the handicapping effect of mental retardation.
    4. Focus on the prevention of complications and rehabilitation.

27. A healthy 4-month-old infant weighing 13 lb 3 oz has started waking up at night after previously sleeping for periods of 9–11 hours. The infant takes 32 oz of formula in a 24-hour period. The nurse practitioner recommends:

    1. Increase the formula to 38 oz in a 24-hour period.
    2. Start introducing one food item at a time, beginning with vegetables.
    3. Maintain current formula intake and start small amounts of rice cereal.
    4. Change over to whole milk instead of formula.

28. The nurse practitioner understands that the infant mortality rate is:

    1. The number of infant deaths per 1000 live births.
    2. The total number of infant deaths per 1000 persons in the population.
    3. The number of infant deaths attributed to specific illnesses.
    4. The monthly infant death rate per 100 live births.

29. A father (height 74 inches, onset of puberty age 16) is concerned that his 15-year-old son is going to be short. On physical examination the nurse practitioner finds Tanner stage II, height 62 inches, and physical exam essentially normal for a well-nourished adolescent. After reviewing his growth records, which indicate a growth pattern of height at the fifth percentile, the most likely diagnosis is:

    1. Constitutional growth delay.
    2. Familial short stature.
    3. Hypopituitarism.
    4. Idiopathic gonadotropin deficiency.

30. Which of the following is most important to include in the anticipatory guidance of a family with a 9-month-old child?

   1. Keep buttons, beads, and coins out of the child's reach.

   2. Turn the handles of pots on the stove inward.

   3. Encourage self-feeding with silverware.

   4. Encourage weaning to a cup and eliminating pacifier use.

31. Anticipatory guidance for the family with a 4-year-old includes:

   1. Avoid fluoride supplements to prevent staining of teeth and dental caries.

   2. Continue to use a car seat until the child weighs 60 lb or head is higher than the backseat.

   3. Instruct parents to use bottled drinking water when traveling to different parts of the country.

   4. Serve only three regular meals with no snacks to prevent development of poor nutrition habits.

32. In teaching a new mother about fevers, the nurse practitioner knows that:

   1. Fevers over 40°C (104°F) can cause brain damage.

   2. Most fevers over 40°C (104°F) are usually of bacterial origin.

   3. Children under 6 months of age are especially susceptible to brain damage from a fever.

   4. Fevers may precipitate convulsions in children between 6 months and 6 years of age.

33. A new mother asks about the differences between human milk and cow's milk. The nurse practitioner explains that:

   1. Human milk has more lipase and linoleic acid.

   2. Human milk has more calcium, phosphorus, sodium, and potassium.

   3. Cow's milk has low protein and casein content.

   4. Cow's milk has high linoleic acid and low saturated fatty acids.

34. The nurse recognizes the following as correct for the frequency and quantity of formula feedings:

   1. 1 month: 9–10 feedings/24 hr of 2–3 oz.

   2. 6 months: 8–10 feeding/24 hr of 4–5 oz.

   3. 10 months: 3–4 feedings/24 hr of 7–8 oz.

   4. 12 months: 6–8 feedings/24 hr of 8–9 oz.

35. According to the American Academy of Pediatrics (AAP), infants may be fed whole cow's milk once they reach:

   1. 6 months of age.

   2. 8 months of age.

   3. 12 months of age.

   4. 18 months of age.

36. A mother states that the iron-fortified formula her 3-month-old infant is on has been causing constipation. The nurse practitioner recommends:

   1. Discontinuing the iron-fortified formula.

   2. Starting the infant on rice cereal.

   3. Adding 1–2 tsp of dark corn syrup to formula.

   4. Adding apple or white grape juice to daily intake.

37. Which of the following best describes lactose intolerance?

   1. Symptoms typically include intestinal dilatation, bloating, increased flatulence, and pain followed eventually by diarrhea in children 4–6 years of age.

   2. An abrupt onset of nausea, vomiting, and diarrhea within 30 minutes after consuming milk products in children 12–18 months of age.

   3. Its presentation is the same as cow's milk intolerance.

   4. Its prevalence is highest among the Caucasian population.

38. A 1-year-old child who had a normal physical examination has a lead level of 15 µg/dl. Which of the following actions should the nurse practitioner take?

   1. Repeat the test because it may be a false result.

   2. Hospitalize for immediate chelation therapy.

3. Investigate possible sources of lead and repeat in 6 months.

4. Repeat the test in 1 year.

39. The recommended time for introduction of solid foods into an infant's diet is:

1. Age 2 months.

2. Age 3 months.

3. Age 4–6 months.

4. Age 6–8 months

40. The nurse practitioner is aware that fluoride levels in drinking water should be:

1. 0.6 ppm in temperate and cold climates.

2. 1.0 ppm in temperate and 0.6 ppm in cold climates.

3. 1.0 ppm in temperate and cold climates.

4. 0.6 ppm in temperate and 1.0 ppm in cold climates.

41. A 20-day-old infant is brought to the clinic by her parents. She has not been eating well and has a temperature of 38.2°C (100.8°F). Examination reveals no focal bacterial infection; laboratory tests indicate white blood cell (WBC) count of 12,000/mm³ with 1480 bands/mm³; urinalysis is normal; and no diarrhea is noted. Which of the following is the most appropriate management plan for this infant?

1. Treat at home with antipyretics and fluids.

2. Hospitalize for a septic workup.

3. Treat at home with antipyretics and ampicillin.

4. Do a urine culture and have the infant return in 24 hours.

42. Which of the following is most important to remember when teaching fifth-through eighth-grade children about health promotion behaviors?

1. Girls are more extrinsically motivated.

2. Both boys and girls are highly influenced by family.

3. Boys are more extrinsically motivated.

4. High maternal education levels affect both.

43. In the preparation of reading and education materials for clients and parents, the nurse practitioner is aware that the reading level of most adults is at the:

1. Twelfth-grade level.

2. Tenth-grade level.

3. Sixth-grade level.

4. Fourth-grade level.

44. A child presenting with vague symptoms and a serum lead level of 28 μg/dl would be managed by:

1. Removal of the child from the lead source.

2. Removal of the environmental lead hazard.

3. Chelation therapy treatment.

4. Rescreening and referral to physician.

45. Which of the following should be included when discussing primary injury prevention with the parents of a 2-month-old child?

1. Set water heater thermostat at <120°F.

2. Make sure crib rails are no more than 3¼ inches apart.

3. Use a rear-facing car seat until the child is >40 lb.

4. Apply sunscreen for when outside and temperature is 75°F.

46. A Hispanic child presents with symptoms of weakness, irritability, weight loss, constipation, and mild ataxia and a history of elevated lead level. Which of the following homeopathic substances would the nurse practitioner suspect had been used?

1. White willow bark.

2. Arnica root.

3. Mexican yam root.

4. Azarcon and greta.

47. Which lifestyle modifications are most effective in controlling hypertension in the older client?

1. Maintain normal weight; decrease sodium in diet; exercise regularly.

2. Increase dietary protein; decrease weight; use stress reduction techniques.

3. Consume high-complex carbohydrate, low-sodium diet; decrease stress.

4. Reduce weight; increase vitamin supplements; exercise regularly.

Immunizations

48. A child is in first grade. How many doses of inactivated poliovirus vaccine (IPV) will he have received?

   1. 2 doses.

   2. 3 doses.

   3. 4 doses.

   4. 5 doses.

49. Before giving a child the measles-mumps-rubella (MMR) trivalent vaccine, it is recommended to wait how long after cancer chemotherapy has stopped?

   1. 30 days.

   2. 2 months.

   3. 3 months.

   4. 6 months.

50. The National Childhood Vaccine Injury Act requires standardized consent forms for the administration of vaccines to children. The content on the form for the medical record includes the vaccine lot number, nurse signature, injection/inoculation site, and:

   1. Signature of parent or legal guardian.

   2. Education provided.

   3. Absence of contraindications.

   4. Vaccine expiration date.

51. The mother of a 15-year-old who has not had chickenpox is concerned and wants her daughter to be vaccinated. The recommendations are:

   1. Not recommended for children over age 12.

   2. One-time dose.

   3. Two doses 4–8 weeks apart.

   4. Three doses 2 months apart.

52. Consultation with the mother of an 18-month-old who has received no immunizations reveals that the child was exposed to measles 48 hours prior to the visit. At this time the practitioner would:

   1. Discharge the client with care instructions.

   2. Administer live attenuated measles vaccine.

   3. Administer 0.5 ml/kg immunoglobulin G (IgG).

   4. Administer half the regular measles vaccine dose.

53. Which statement about the polyvalent pneumococcal vaccine is true?

   1. It is recommended children with chronic diseases, including diabetes.

   2. It is recommended to prevent otitis media (OM) and other pneumococcal infections in children less than 2 years of age.

   3. It may not be given concurrently with other vaccines.

   4. Severe systemic reactions are common after immunization.

54. The influenza vaccination is recommended annually for high-risk groups. The nurse practitioner knows that the greatest need for this vaccination would be for:

   1. Adults with chronic disease.

   2. Residents of long-term care facilities.

   3. Dialysis clients.

   4. Health care employees.

55. The nurse practitioner understands that the only contraindication to hepatitis B vaccination is:

   1. Pregnancy and lactation.

   2. History of poliomyelitis.

   3. Prior anaphylaxis or severe hypersensitivity.

   4. Mild viral illness.

56. Immunizations and chemoprophylaxis offered routinely to clients 65 years of age or older are:

   1. Diphtheria, tetanus toxoid, and pertussis absorbed (DPT); influenza; and Pneumovax.

   2. Tetanus toxoid and diphtheria (Td), influenza, and pneumococcal vaccine.

   3. Td and influenza; for those with chronic diseases, offer the pneumococcal vaccine.

   4. Influenza and pneumococcal pneumonia and Td to those who have not had vaccine in last 10 years.

57. The nurse practitioner understands that the following is considered an attenuated live-virus vaccination:

   1. Rubella and measles.

   2. Mumps and hepatitis B.

   3. Poliomyelitis and hepatitis B.

   4. Rubella and rabies.

58. The nurse practitioner understands that children who are at high risk to the measles vaccine are children who have severe allergic reactions to:

   1. Fungi.

   2. Pollen.

   3. Pets.

   4. Food.

59. What type of immunity does a child develop after contracting chickenpox?

   1. Active natural immunity.

   2. Active artificial immunity.

   3. Passive natural immunity.

   4. Passive artificial immunity.

60. The nurse practitioner is assessing an 8-month-old infant in an immunization clinic. By this time, the infant should have received which immunizations?

   1. All three hepatitis B shots, all the DPT series, two doses of the polio series.

   2. Hepatitis B first and second dose, all the DPT and polio series, MMR.

   3. DPT first and second dose, MMR first dose, all the hepatitis B series.

   4. Varicella, DPT first dose, hepatitis B first dose.

61. Which of the following client situations requires the use of inactivated (not live) vaccines?

   1. History of nonspecific allergies.

   2. Immunocompromised adult.

   3. Concurrent antimicrobial therapy.

   4. Mild acute illness.

62. In taking the history of a healthy 50-year-old man, the nurse practitioner determines the client is an avid gardener and spends much of his time enjoying outdoor activities. A health maintenance recommendation for this client is to obtain a:

   1. Pneumococcal vaccine.

   2. Tetanus vaccine.

   3. Hepatitis B vaccine.

   4. Varicella vaccine.

63. The Advisory Committee on Immunization Practices (ACIP) recommends that healthy adults receive a diphtheria and tetanus toxoid (Td) booster vaccination:

   1. Every 5 years.

   2. Every 8 years.

   3. At age 60.

   4. Every 10 years.

64. Which statement most correctly describes tetanus toxoid?

   1. Tetanus toxoid (Td) induces more persistent antitoxin antibody titers.

   2. DPT and diphtheria and tetanus toxoid absorbed (DT) are safe to give to adults.

   3. The recommended dose for the adult is 0.75 ml IM.

   4. Tetanus toxoid fluid provides the same antitoxin antibody titers as tetanus toxoid.

65. Immunizations recommended for healthy young adults include:

    1. Measles, rubella, varicella, and hepatitis B.

    2. Pneumovax, influenza, and rubella.

    3. Tetanus, influenza, varicella, Pneumovax, and hepatitis B.

    4. Influenza, hepatitis B, rubella, measles, and tetanus.

66. A 2-month-old infant received his immunizations, and 12 hours later the mother calls and says the infant has a fever of 101°F. What is the most likely cause of the fever?

    1. Vaccination for the measles, mumps, and rubella.

    2. Combination of the diphtheria and the polio vaccinations.

    3. Presence of an infection when immunizations were given.

    4. Pertussis immunization.

Answers & Rationales

1. **(1)** The American Cancer Society (ACS) recommends maintenance of a desirable body weight; research has shown an association between increased mortality from various cancers and varying degrees of being overweight. Another recommendation is to eat a wide variety of foods, consistent with the Food Guide Pyramid of the U.S. Department of Agriculture and U.S. Department of Health and Human Services. A variety of fruits and vegetables should be included in the daily diet (5–9 servings/day) because research has shown an association between lower cancer rates and high fruit and vegetable consumption. High-fiber foods are also recommended; a lower risk of colon cancer is seen in those who consume a high-fiber diet. There are no recommendations to increase the amount of protein in the diet at this time. Due to the high consumption of red meat in the American diet, many people are already receiving large quantities in their current diets. ACS recommends limiting the daily consumption of alcohol to two drinks for males, one drink for females, and no drinks for pregnant females. They also state that ideally, no alcohol should be consumed; regular alcohol consumption has been shown to increase the risk of various cancers.

2. **(1)** The recommendation is low-density lipoprotein (LDL) <130 mg/dl and triglyceride levels <200 mg/dl. All other choices have inaccuracies of goals.

3. **(2)** The American Diabetes Association recommends screening adults starting at age 45 every 3 years.

4. **(2)** The physical therapy program will assist her in restoring her optimum level of functioning after a CVA. Option #1 is a primary prevention activity nonspecific to a CVA. Options #3 and #4 are examples of secondary prevention activities nonspecific to a CVA.

5. **(3)** The client needs an increased intake of protein and vitamin C to promote healing. Red meat, citrus fruits, and green vegetables will give the highest amounts of these elements from the selections offered.

6. **(3)** Shouting increases the pitch of the voice. In presbycusis, or hearing loss in elderly persons, high-pitched consonant sounds are the first to be affected, and the change may occur gradually. The nurse practitioner should face the client when speaking. If the nurse needs to stand behind the client, touch is used to get the client's attention. Simple sentences should be used to facilitate understanding.

7. **(4)** This information will prevent complications that may result in a fall. Options #1 and #2 are appropriate for tertiary prevention. Option #3 is appropriate for secondary prevention, which is to prevent the client from experiencing another fall.

8. **(4)** This evaluation will assist in identifying any problems with bleeding. Option #1 is not necessary. Option #2 is not a screening and would not be administered annually. A colonoscopy is recommended every 3–5 years for clients over 50.

9. **(4)** Using past life experiences applies the concept of adult educational principles. Overhead lighting may produce an increase in the glare, which can decrease visualization. There is an alteration of color perception (e.g., blue appears green-blue) as an individual ages. As individuals age, the ability to hear women's and children's voices decreases because these are high-pitched voices. This video would not enhance the program if the clients frequently have presbycusis as a result of the normal aging process.

10. **(3)** All these disorders can be associated with workplace exposure, but currently, lung disease is still the most common occupationally related disease. Musculoskeletal injuries are on the rise.

11. **(4)** The only proven benefit of a sports screening examination is to determine the athletes at risk for orthopedic injuries secondary to previously unresolved injuries. A thorough history with the screening exam will increase the likelihood of identifying underlying health problems but has not been shown to be very effective.

12. **(4)** The client's history and physical will reveal the presence of any coronary heart disease (CHD) risk factors (age, family history of CHD, diabetes, current cigarette smoking, blood pressure, height/weight, cardiovascular exam). A lipid profile is also recommended to assess the level of risk and consists of total cholesterol, high-density lipoprotein (HDL), low-density liproprotein (LDL), and triglyceride levels. It would be prudent to have a precise cholesterol level done, since the previous result was from a screening health fair and has no written record. These parameters should be assessed first before a cholesterol-lowering agent, ECG, or stress test is ordered. An exercise program is also important but should only be done after a history and physical and lipid profile results are known; if the lipid profile or the exam results are abnormal, stress testing may be appropriate before undertaking a new exercise program.

13. **(2)** Screening for colorectal cancer includes annual fecal occult blood screening for individuals over age 50. Avoiding medications that can cause gastrointestinal irritation and bleeding can help avoid false-positive results. Rare meat and vegetables that are high in peroxidase will cause false-positive results, whereas vitamin C can cause false-negative results.

14. **(2)** The 15- to 25-year-old group is most often affected by testicular cancer.

15. **(1)** The recommended servings for each of the food groups are as follows:

Food Group	Servings
Bread/cereal/rice/pasta	6–11 servings
Fruit	2–4 servings
Vegetable	3–5 servings
Meat/poultry/fish, dry beans, eggs, nuts	2–3 servings
Fats/oils/sweets	Sparing use

16. **(3)** In summer 1997 the National Institutes of Health (NIH) and American Cancer Society changed the recommendation to begin yearly mammography at age 40.

17. **(1)** All these areas are important to probe in the initial interview of a new client. The history will help determine the necessary components of the physical examination and laboratory or radiologic studies that are ordered and the counseling that is done during the appointment.

18. **(4)** An account of the client's usual intake is necessary so that problem areas can be identified. Before beginning any exercise program, a physical examination should be done to assess the client's physical condition and to aid in the proper selection of a specific exercise plan. A dietary assessment needs to be completed before recommending vitamin and protein supplements; the client may already be receiving adequate amounts in her diet. A more active job would be ideal; however, most people do not have options regarding their choice of job, so increasing her activity outside of work would be most appropriate.

19. **(4)** The older adult is at greatest risk for altered immune function related to nutrition. The older adult often does not receive enough nutrition for a variety of reasons, including altered taste, eating alone, ability to prepare meals, and malabsorption. Adequate nutrition in the older adult has been shown to improve immune status and antibody response to influenza vaccine.

20. **(2)** Dehydration results in the deaths of more infants worldwide than any other syndrome.

21. **(2)** Hypertension, smoking, and hyperlipidemia are the major risk factors in the development of cardiovascular disease. Controlling hyperglycemia, high dietary fiber intake, and vitamin supplements assist in maintaining a healthy lifestyle but are not as important in preventing cardiovascular disease.

22. **(2)** Premature infants who have spent an extended period in the neonatal intensive care unit (NICU) take 6–10 months to be deinstitutionalized to the noise and light. These must be decreased slowly over time.

23. **(4)** Multiphasic health screening is a form of periodic health surveillance in which participants undergo a battery of laboratory or diagnostic tests to determine risk factors and disease detection. The other three settings described are not examples of community health promotion activities; they are secondary care settings. The locations of the two clinics are in community settings.

24. **(4)** It is essential that the immunization record be reviewed. The other options are important but not essential for a health maintenance visit.

25. **(3)** Printed materials must be written to a level of readability so that they can be understood. Do not use all capital letters because such words are difficult to read. In addition, it is helpful to write in the active versus the passive voice, to use one- and two-syllable words, to avoid complex grammatical structures, and to express only one idea in each sentence. Well-chosen and easily understood graphics can significantly enhance the literature.

26. **(1)** Primary prevention programs exist to prevent disease, malfunctioning, or maladaptation from occurring. Examples of these types of programs include the promotion of a healthy diet, practice of safe sex, and avoidance of alcohol and tobacco. Secondary prevention is early diagnosis and treatment (e.g., screening for tuberculosis or sickle cell disease, breast and testicular self-examination). Tertiary prevention is the prevention of complications and rehabilitation after the disease or condition has occurred (e.g., cardiac rehabilitation, complete blood count done before chemotherapy).

27. **(3)** If the infant has been satisfied up to this point (by sleeping for long intervals), he probably needs additional calories in the form of rice cereal. Adding increased amounts of formula can lead to iron deficiency anemia.

28. **(1)** This frequently used ratio is calculated as follows:

$$\frac{\text{No. of deaths} <1 \text{ year of age in a year}}{\text{No. of live births in the same year}} \times 1000 = \text{Infant mortality rate}$$

29. **(1)** Familial short stature is not indicated here because the father is of normal height. Hypopituitarism would be associated with other findings (micropenis, small testes, immature facies, olfactory defects). Gonadotropin deficiency might be a possibility, but considering all the findings in the situation and based on the father having a pubertal onset at age 16 and achieving an average height, the more likely diagnosis is constitutional growth delay.

30. **(4)** Children should be using a cup and ideally not using a pacifier at 12 months of age. At 9 months the child does not have the mobility to reach the pot handles on the stove. Self-feeding should be encouraged at this age, but silverware is not used until the second year of life. Keeping buttons, beads, and coins out of the child's reach should have been done since this child was about 4 months of age.

31. **(2)** Car safety and use of a car seat continues to be a priority for the 4-year-old. Bottled drinking water is not necessary when traveling, unless it is outside the United States. A fluoridated dentifrice should be used in a small amount (pea size), and children under 6 should be supervised so that they do not swallow too much toothpaste, which would put them at risk for fluoridosis. Three regular meals and two snacks are recommended for the busy 4-year-old. Snacks should be rich in complex carbohydrates and low in fat. Avoid candy, chips, and soft drinks.

32. **(4)** Febrile seizures are benign and do not lead to brain damage. Most febrile illnesses in children result from a virus rather than bacteria and are associated with a high fever.

33. **(1)** Human milk has more lipase and linoleic acid. Cow's milk is not as good of a nutritional source as human milk because cow's milk has more mineral content (calcium, phosphorus, sodium, potassium), which causes a larger renal solute load. In addition, cow's milk is high in protein, casein, and saturated fat and lower in carbohydrates.

34. **(3)** Usual frequency and quantity of formula feedings are as follows:

0–1 month	6–8 feedings/24 hr of 2–4 oz
2 months	4–5 feedings/24 hr of 5 oz
3 months	4–5 feedings/24 hr of 5–6 oz
4 months	4–5 feedings/24 hr of 6–7 oz
7–10 months	3–4 feedings/24 hr of 8 oz
11–12 months	3 feedings/24 hr of 8 oz

35. **(3)** At 1 year of age, infants may be fed whole cow's milk. The purpose for waiting is that it has been shown that cow's milk is low in iron, linoleic acid, and vitamin E, as well as being high in protein, sodium, and potassium.

36. **(3)** The American Academy of Pediatrics does not recommend low-iron formulas but does recommend, if stools are hard, to treat for constipation. Typical treatment includes giving 1–2 tsp of dark corn syrup including fruit juices (prune, pineapple, apricot), nonstarchy vegetables, and water and avoiding rice cereal.

37. **(1)** These are characteristics of lactose intolerance. Symptoms occur from 2 hours up to 12 hours after milk or milk product ingestion. The prevalence is highest in African Americans, Native Americans, and Asians. Cow's milk intolerance occurs in infancy with symptoms of blood in the stools often accompanied by allergies (e.g., eczema, hives, asthma).

38. **(3)** Although 15 µg/dl is an elevated count (normal is <10 µg/dl), chelation therapy in children with a normal exam is not usually conducted until the level is >25 µg/dl. It is important at this level to identify the source of the elevation and to monitor the child frequently.

39. **(3)** Solid food does not need to be introduced before 4–6 months of age. The first foods introduced are cereals. New foods are introduced one at a time at weekly intervals. In this way the infant's digestive system can adapt to the food, and any reaction can be easily detected.

40. **(4)** The recommended levels of 0.6 ppm in temperate climates and 1.0 ppm in cold climates are based on the rationale that people in temperate climates drink more fluids. Intake is determined at 1 L/day. Below this level, children need supplements, which cannot be prescribed without knowing the exact fluoride/water concentration.

41. **(2)** Practice guidelines recommend that even if they meet low-risk criteria, febrile infants less than 28 days of age should have a sepsis evaluation.

42. **(1)** Fifth-grade through eighth-grade girls are more motivated by peers and family. Boys are more intrinsically motivated, with family and peers having less influence. Peers are also more influential for girls in the high school years. High maternal education level is not an influential factor for boys.

43. **(3)** The reading level of most American adults is at the sixth-grade level.

44. **(4)** Recommendations of the Centers for Disease Control and Prevention (CDC) for a serum lead level greater than 10 µg/dl are for rescreening and referral to a physician. Rescreening is done before removal of the child/family from the hazard, although a thorough environmental assessment is essential at rescreening.

45. **(1)** The water heater should not be set over 120°F to prevent scald burns. Crib rails should be no more than 2 3/8 inches apart. The rear-facing infant seat is applicable to 20 lb of weight or 1 year of age. Sunscreen should be applied whenever there is sun exposure.

46. **(4)** Azarcon and greta are traditional Hispanic remedies that contain lead, which can result in increased lead levels and eventual poisoning. The other substances will not cause the symptoms described. The Mexican yam root is used for menopausal symptoms and is a source of natural progesterone.

47. **(1)** These three modifications are the most effective in maintaining normal blood pressure.

Immunizations

48. **(3)** It is recommended that the child receive the IPV at 2 months, 4 months, the third dose between 6 and 18 months, and the fourth dose between 4 and 6 years of age.

49. **(3)** The MMR is a live-virus vaccine. Children severely immunosuppressed due to cancer therapy should not receive live-virus vaccines

for 3 months after chemotherapy has been stopped (American Academy of Pediatrics, 2000, p. 60).

50. **(1)** The law calls for the parental signature to be maintained in the clinical record.

51. **(3)** Children over the age of 13 years who have not had chickenpox and have not been previously immunized are recommended to have two doses 4–8 weeks apart for effective immunity.

52. **(2)** If given within 72 hours of exposure, the live attenuated measles vaccine will provide protection in most cases. The dose of IgG would be 0.25 ml/kg, given within 6 days of exposure.

53. **(1)** Polyvalent pneumococcal vaccine is recommended for children with chronic diseases. It is not recommended for use to prevent OM and other pneumococcal diseases; it can be given concurrently with other vaccines; and it does not cause severe systemic reactions. It will occasionally cause mild local reactions (American Academy of Pediatrics, 2000, pp. 458-459).

54. **(2)** Influenza outbreaks may affect 60% of those in long-term care, and mortality rates are high. All the other groups listed are appropriate for the influenza vaccine but are not as high a priority.

55. **(3)** Prior anaphylaxis and severe hypersensitivity would be considered a contraindication; a mild viral illness would not. The client who is pregnant or lactating may be immunized.

56. **(4)** Pneumococcal and annual influenza immunizations are recommended for those age 65 and older. Adult Td is offered to those who have not had a booster in the last 10 years.

57. **(1)** Attenuated live-virus vaccines are available for the following communicable diseases: measles, mumps, rubella, poliomyelitis, yellow fever, and smallpox. Rabies vaccine is a killed virus, and hepatitis B is a purified viral antigen obtained from the blood of an infected client and then inactivated when manufactured into a vaccination.

58. **(4)** Atopic (allergic) children who have severe food allergy are at increased risk for the development of an allergic reaction to the measles vaccine. Children with food allergy should be observed for at least 90 minutes in a setting equipped for emergency medical treatment.

59. **(1)** A child who contracts chickenpox for the first time develops antibodies during the period of infection. These antibodies create a naturally acquired, lifelong type of active immunity. Artificially acquired active immunity occurs with immunizations. Natural passive immunity occurs with placental transfer. Artificial passively acquired immunity occurs with an injection of human or animal serum (antitoxin).

60. **(1)** Hepatitis B #1 should be given at birth. HPV #2 should be given at least 4 weeks after that with HPV #3 given 16 weeks after the first dose. By 8 months of age, all 3 doses of the hepatitis B series should have been given (American Academy of Pediatrics, 2000).

61. **(2)** Live vaccine can produce serious disseminated disease in clients with immunocompromised status (e.g., leukemia, lymphoma, HIV/AIDS) and in those undergoing cancer chemotherapy. Mild acute illness, concurrent antimicrobial therapy, and a history of nonspecific allergies are not contraindications for use of a live vaccine.

62. **(2)** Adults who enjoy gardening and outdoor activities should have a tetanus vaccine at least every 10 years due to the high-risk activities. A pneumoccocal vaccine is recommended for adults age 65 or older and for those with a chronic illness or in an immunosuppressed state. Most older adults had chickenpox as a child and do not require the vaccine.

63. **(4)** The ACIP recommends that adults receive a Td booster every 10 years or a single booster at age 50 for clients who have completed the full pediatric series, including teenage and young adult boosters.

64. **(1)** Tetanus toxoid induces more persistent antitoxin antibody titers than tetanus toxoid fluid. DPT and DT are for use in children under age 7 years and should *not* be used in adults. The recommended dose of DT alone for an adult is 0.5 ml IM.

65. **(4)** From 5% to 20% of young adults are susceptible to measles and/or rubella. Influenza and hepatitis B are recommended for students who have exposure to a large number of people. Tetanus is recommended every 10 years, especially in high-risk situations (young adults who participate in outdoor sports). Pneumovax is indicated in a young adult who has a chronic disease (e.g., diabetes, chronic pulmonary disease, chronic cardiovascular disease) and is also indicated for young adults who are immunocompromised.

66. **(4)** The most common cause of fever at the 2-month immunization series is the pertussis. This vaccine causes reactions in about 75% of the infants. MMR is not given until 12–15 months of age.

Reference

American Academy of Pediatrics, Committee on Infectious Diseases: *Red Book*, 25th ed. Elk Grove, Ill: The Academy, 2000.

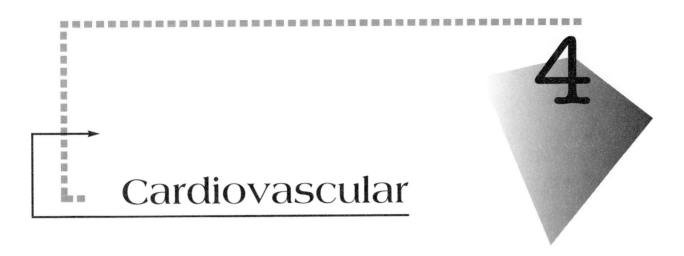

Cardiovascular

Physical Examination & Diagnostic Tests

1. The practitioner is performing a physical examination on a healthy adult male. On auscultation, the stethoscope would be placed in what areas to best hear the characteristic heart sounds S_1 and S_2?

   1. S_1 is best heard at the apex and S_2 at the base of the heart.

   2. Both are heard equally well at the right midclavicular line.

   3. On the left side, S_1 is at the area of pulmonic valve and S_2 at the aortic valve.

   4. Both sounds are best heard at Erb's point.

2. On the general assessment of an adult client, the practitioner determines the presence of the apical impulse at the point of maximal impulse (PMI) on the client's chest wall. Where on the chest wall is the PMI normally found?

   1. Second intercostal space at the midclavicular line on the left side.

   2. Right lower sternal border, fifth intercostal space.

   3. Left side at fifth intercostal space on the midclavicular line.

   4. Left fifth intercostal space, lateral to the midclavicular line.

3. The nurse practitioner is auscultating the carotids. What is the correct procedure?

   1. Use the diaphragm of the stethoscope.

   2. Use the bell of the stethoscope.

   3. Place the stethoscope 1 inch off the area above the sternocleidomastoid muscle.

   4. Position the client at a 30-degree angle, and press firmly with bell of the stethoscope.

4. When inspecting the precordium, the nurse practitioner is checking for:

   1. Scars and anatomic landmarks.

   2. Pulsations and retractions.

   3. Heaves and cardiac dullness.

   4. Pericardial friction rub and lifts.

5. While examining a client in a left lateral decubitus position, the nurse practitioner auscultates a third heart sound (S_3). The nurse practitioner knows:

   1. This sound is considered normal in children and young adults.

   2. This rarely is associated with myocardial failure in the older adult.

   3. This client should be immediately referred to a cardiologist for evaluation.

   4. This is considered a normal splitting of the S_2 during inspiration.

6. The nurse practitioner knows that the correct ausculatory site for the aortic area is the:

   1. Midclavicular line, fifth interspace, left side.

   2. Left fourth interspace close to the sternum.

   3. Right second interspace close to the sternum.

   4. Midclavicular line, second interspace, left side.

7. The nurse practitioner should include which statement in client teaching when ordering a lipid profile on a client?
Eat a typical diet over the next week and:

   1. Eat a normal breakfast the morning of the exam.

   2. Fast for 12 hours prior to the exam.

   3. There are no restrictions on alcohol for this test.

   4. Take any current medications with a few sips of water before the test.

8. When auscultating the heart sounds of a 72-year-old client with a history of hypertension, the nurse practitioner notes an S_4. This finding could indicate:

   1. Normal variant in people 65 years and older.

   2. Beginning of ventricular failure.

   3. Decreased resistance to ventricular filling.

   4. Severely failing heart.

9. A 55-year-old client has a blood pressure (BP) of 168/100. This is classified as:

   1. Moderate hypertension.

   2. Mild hypertension.

   3. High-normal BP.

   4. Severe hypertension.

10. The nurse practitioner is examining a client with a history of rheumatic fever who is being followed for the development of carditis. During the cardiac auscultation, where on the chest wall is the stethoscope placed to determine the most common murmurs associated with this condition?

   1. At the left sternal border, fourth left intercostal space.

   2. Fifth intercostal space, left side, at the midclavicular line.

   3. Second or third intercostal space at the left of the sternal border.

   4. Second intercostal space on the right of the sternal border.

11. A client presents with unusual coolness in the left hand compared with the right hand. What is the next step in the examination?

   1. Palpate the radial pulse on both hands for a full minute.

   2. Perform Allen's test on both hands.

   3. Feel the forearms with the backs of the fingers.

   4. Hold the hand in a dependent position then reexamine.

12. S_1 and S_2 are identified when the nurse practitioner auscultates for cardiac sounds. The physiology responsible for the production of these heart sounds is:

   1. Closure of atrioventricular (AV) valves produces S_1; closure of semilunar valves forms S_2.

   2. Closure of aortic valve produces S_2; opening of mitral valve produces S_1.

   3. Opening of AV valves produces S_1; closure of semilunar valves produces S_2.

   4. Opening of tricuspid valve produces S_1; closure of pulmonic valve forms S_2.

13. The nurse practitioner is assessing a cardiac client who is experiencing an atrial dysrhythmia. The pulse rate is irregular at 110 beats/min, and there is concern regarding a

pulse deficit. How is a pulse deficit determined in this client?

1. A 12-lead electrocardiogram (ECG) is necessary to determine the presence and length of the PR intervals.

2. The apical pulse is counted, then the radial pulse is counted; the pulse deficit is determined by the difference in the two rates.

3. The apical pulse is counted, and an increase or decrease is correlated with the phases of the respiratory cycle.

4. The apical pulse and radial pulse are determined simultaneously; a pulse deficit is established if the apical rate is higher than the radial rate.

14. The nurse practitioner notes a grade V systolic murmur while examining a client's precordium. Which characteristics describe this type of murmur?

1. Barely audible, faint with bell of the stethoscope.

2. Heard only with diaphragm of the stethoscope.

3. Heard with the stethoscope partly off the chest.

4. Heard without the aid of the stethoscope.

15. Normal physiology changes in the geriatric population that affect conductivity and contractility of the myocardium include:

1. Increased automaticity and excitability.

2. Increased contractility and conductivity.

3. Decreased excitability and conductivity.

4. Decreased automaticity and contractility.

16. When assessing the temperature of an extremity as part of a client's peripheral vascular assessment, which part of the hand is the most sensitive?

1. Palm.

2. Fingertips.

3. Back of the wrist.

4. Back of the fingers.

17. A 45-year-old male's lipid profile results are sent to the nurse practitioner, with levels as follows: total cholesterol = 287 mmol/L; high-density lipoprotein (HDL) = 30 mg/dl; low-density lipoprotein (LDL) = 165 mg/dl; triglyceride = 238 mg/dl. The nurse practitioner interprets these results as:

1. Abnormal; the elevated triglyceride level is of the most concern.

2. Borderline; this is considered to be a borderline risk lipid profile.

3. Abnormal; total cholesterol and LDL levels are elevated, and HDL level is too low.

4. Normal; these results are of no concern; follow up with client in 1 year.

18. On examination of a child, the nurse practitioner notes weak femoral pulses. This finding is associated with what condition?

1. Patent ductus arteriosus.

2. Coarctation of the aorta.

3. Tetralogy of Fallot.

4. Pulmonary stenosis.

19. A client returns to the chest pain clinic 3 weeks post–myocardial infarction (MI) complaining of pericardial pain and elevated temperature. Physical examination reveals a pericardial friction rub. What diagnostic studies are indicated?

1. 24-hour Holter monitoring.

2. Echocardiogram.

3. Complete blood count (CBC) with differential.

4. Cardiac enzymes with myoglobin.

20. In doing a cardiac assessment of a 4-month-old infant, the nurse practitioner notes a machinery-like murmur. This finding is consistent with a diagnosis of:

1. Coarctation of the aorta.

2. Patent ductus arteriosus.

3. Ventricular septal defect.

4. Aortic stenosis.

21. On assessment of a geriatric client, the nurse practitioner notes bilateral pulsations and distention of the jugular veins when the client's head is elevated 45 degrees. What further assessment needs to be done at this time?

    1. Estimate the level of venous pressure by measuring from the sternal angle to the highest level of venous pulsations.

    2. Place the client in a supine position and determine effect of position change on distention and pulsations of jugular vein.

    3. Measure carotid pulses, because of the increased left ventricular pressure.

    4. Have the client hold his/her breath to facilitate evaluation for the presence of carotid bruits.

22. The nurse practitioner is examining a woman with a known history of mitral valve disease. What type of murmur heard on auscultation supports a history of mitral stenosis?

    1. Diastolic murmur, heard loudest at the apex with the client on her left side.

    2. Midsystolic ejection murmur heard loudest over the left lower sternal border. *aortic stenosis*

    3. Holosystolic murmur, heard loudest over the apex and left axillary area. *mitral regurg*

    4. Diastolic murmur, heard loudest with client in sitting position leaning forward. *aortic regurg*

23. The nurse practitioner is doing an assessment of a client who is 2 weeks post-MI affecting the left ventricle. The nurse practitioner would pay particular attention to what area of the physical assessment?

    1. Lower extremities and the jugular vein.

    2. Area on the chest where the PMI is heard.

    3. Presence of dyspnea and auscultation of crackles in the lungs.

    4. Level of dependent edema and fluid intake over the past 24 hours.

24. Which symptoms would indicate to the nurse practitioner that the client is experiencing intermittent claudication?

    1. Petechiae and itching of the lower part of the leg.

    2. Extensive discoloration and edema of the upper leg.

    3. Profuse rash and discoloration from the trunk down to the feet.

    4. Complaints of pain on walking, relieved by sitting down.

25. Stress testing, or the exercise tolerance test, is the most widely used diagnostic test in ischemic heart disease. It is most accurate, up to 98%, in what client population?

    1. Males under age 40 with atypical agina pectoris.

    2. Asymptomatic premenopausal females without risk factors.

    3. Males over age 50 with typical angina pectoris.

    4. Males receiving digitalis with typical angina pectoris.

26. When palpating for the apical impulse of a 46-year-old female, the nurse practitioner feels a hyperkinetic impulse. The nurse would auscultate for which additional finding?

    1. Pericardial friction rub.

    2. Pansystolic murmur.

    3. Pulsus paradoxus.

    4. Decreased intensity of heart sounds.

27. While assessing a patient with a history of recent myocardial infarction, the nurse practitioner notes pulsus alternans. The nurse would assess for other assessment changes caused by:

    1. Unstable angina.

    2. Cardiogenic shock.

    3. Recurrent myocardial infarction.

    4. Left-sided congestive failure.

Disorders

28. A 70-year-old woman comes to the clinic with the complaint of severe aching of her legs after standing for 10 minutes. What other assessment finding of the lower extremities would support the nurse practitioner's tentative diagnosis of chronic venous insufficiency?

    1. Pitting edema of 3+ and cyanosis on dependency.

2. Shiny skin and dusky red on dependency. Act.

3. Minimal hair and pallor on elevation. Act

4. Pulses 1+ and ulceration involving the toes. Act.

29. The diagnosis of hypertension (HTN) should be established on the basis of:

    1. At least three hypertensive readings in a week.

    2. At least five readings 1 month apart.

    3. One reading of 140 mm Hg systolic and 90 mm Hg diastolic or above.

    4. One reading taken in three different positions.

30. Congestive heart failure (CHF) is a common clinical presentation occurring in a child with congenital heart disease (CHD). What is another common clinical presentation with CHD?

    1. Hypoglycemia.

    2. Hypertension.

    3. Peripheral edema.

    4. Cyanosis.

31. A client has a 2-year history of hypertensive heart disease. The nurse practitioner expects the major pathophysiologic change to be:

    1. Right ventricular hypertrophy.

    2. Left atrial dilatation.

    3. Left ventricular hypertrophy.

    4. Right atrial dilatation.

32. Of the following descriptions, which data most clearly describe atrial tachycardia?

    1. Heart rate of 96, P waves present on each QRS complex, T wave every other beat.

    2. P waves present on every other beat, heart rate of 100, and irregular.

    3. Heart rate of 110, P waves present befor each QRS complex, and regular.

    4. P waves for every third QRS complex, adequate PR interval, rate of 90.

33. What clinical manifestation of a myocardial infarction (MI) is frequently **not** present in the geriatric cardiac client?

    1. Prolonged severe chest pain.

2. Diaphoresis, pallor, syncope.

3. Dyspnea, increasing anxiety.

4. Gastrointestinal distress, orthopnea.

34. The nurse practitioner is performing an assessment on a client who is having difficulty controlling his left-sided CHF. The nurse practitioner understands that the primary symptoms associated with this type of failure are:

    1. Systemic venous congestion. RAF

    2. Dyspnea and pulmonary congestion.

    3. Increased peripheral edema and anorexia.

    4. Atrial fibrillation with a rate around 110.

35. The nurse practitioner is concerned that a post-MI client is developing a problem of constrictive pericarditis. What is a characteristic finding with constrictive pericarditis, and how is it evaluated?

    1. Cardiac tamponade, identified by muffled heart sounds and a paradoxical pulse.

    2. Pericardial triphasic friction rub, best heard at apical area of the heart.

    3. Mitral valve prolapse, characterized by late systolic murmur at apex and left sternal borders.

    4. Altered waves on jugular venous pulse, as determined with a light directed tangentially to illuminate the shadows of the pulsations.

36. A geriatric client has a diagnosis of left-sided CHF. The nurse practitioner would identify what common condition associated with CHF?

    1. Peripheral vascular disease.

    2. Untreated hypertension.

    3. Ventricular dysrhythmias.

    4. Chronic obstructive pulmonary disease.

37. In evaluating the effectiveness of cardiopulmonary resuscitation (CPR) on the adult client, the nurse practitioner would note:

    1. Dilated pupils.

    2. Palpable carotid pulse.

    3. Capillary refill.

    4. Pink and warm skin.

38. The nurse practitioner is evaluating an electro-cardiogram (ECG) of a client who presented at the clinic with complaints of weakness and fainting. His ECG reveals a cardiac rate of 68, absent P waves, regular QRS complex, and T waves present after each QRS complex. What is the best interpretation of this information?

    1. Normal ECG; need to further evaluate client's complaints of weakness.

    2. Third-degree block with junctional rhythm; transfer client to emergency room for cardiology consult.

    3. First-degree block; need to further evaluate client related to cardiac medications.

    4. Administer sublingual nitroglycerin and refer client for a cardiology consult.

39. The nurse practitioner is conducting a follow-up examination on a client with coronary artery disease and a history of pericarditis. Which is one of the characteristic physical findings in pericarditis, and how is it evaluated?

    1. Paradoxical pulse, identified by evaluating the changes in the amplitude of arterial pulse pressure associated with the respiratory cycle.

    2. Pulse deficit, as determined by counting the radial pulse and apical pulse at the same time and evaluating the difference.

    3. Pericardial friction rub, best heard with diaphragm of the stethoscope and loudest to the left of the sternum at the fourth or fifth intercostal space.

    4. An S_4 present, usually heard at the apex with bell of the stethoscope and client in a left lateral position.

40. The symptoms of myocardial infarction (MI) usually experienced by the elderly client include:

    1. Dyspnea and diaphoresis.

    2. Back pain and muscle cramping.

    3. Numbness and tingling of the left arm.

    4. Epigastric pain and nausea.

41. What are the cardiovascular risk factors predisposing females to cardiovascular disease?

    1. Absence of estrogen adversely affects lipoprotein metabolism.

    2. Fat deposited on the hips mobilizes, raising serum cholesterol.

    3. Coronary arteries are longer and wider in diameter.

    4. Resting ejection fraction is lower.

42. The nurse practitioner is planning the treatment of a geriatric client newly diagnosed with hypertension. What parameters are most important in determining the appropriate pharmacologic therapy?

    1. Determine medications and dosage based on the client's weight, age, and drug availability.

    2. Begin step method utilizing diuretics and beta-adrenergic blockers.

    3. Initiate lifestyle changes before beginning medications.

    4. Determine other medical conditions for which the client is being treated.

43. Which statement accurately describes coronary artery disease (CAD) in geriatric clients?

    1. Cardiovascular disease is increased in the female client receiving estrogen replacement.

    2. A major risk factor for cardiovascular disease in females and males is chronic hypertension.

    3. The majority of geriatric clients with CAD also have type 2 diabetes.

    4. Males over 60 years old continue to experience the highest level of CAD.

44. A client with a history of chronic obstructive pulmonary disease (COPD) comes to the clinic for his annual checkup with complaints of increasing difficulty breathing. Assessment findings include S_3 gallop, early systolic ejection click, and increased P-wave amplitude in leads II, III, and aV_F of the ECG. The nurse practitioner would expect to observe which change on the chest x-ray film?

    1. Hypertrophy of the left ventricle.

    2. Hypertrophy of the right ventricle.

    3. Hypertrophy of the left atrium and ventricle.

    4. Hypertrophy of the right atrium and ventricle.

45. When cardiac output falls in CHF, the body attempts to compensate. What electrolyte imbalances result from this response?

    1. Hypernatremia and hyperkalemia.

    2. Hyponatremia and hypokalemia.

    3. Hypophosphatemia and hypercalcemia.

    4. Hyperphosphatemia and hypocalcemia.

46. When assessing the carotid pulse of a 72-year-old client at a community-based clinic, the nurse practitioner notes a bounding pulse with rapid rise and sudden collapse. The nurse practitioner would include which additional assessment to support this finding?

    1. Auscultation for a diastolic murmur.

    2. Auscultation for paradoxical pulse.

    3. BP in both arms lying, sitting, and standing.

    4. BP for an auscultatory gap.

47. Clinical manifestations of congestive heart failure (CHF) in an infant are:

    1. Easily fatigued, central cyanosis, tachycardia, tachypnea, splenomegaly.

    2. Coughing, diaphoresis, peripheral edema, hepatomegaly.

    3. Tachycardia, tachypnea, easily fatigued, paleness, hepatomegaly.

    4. Peripheral edema, coughing, splenomegaly, hepatomegaly, tachycardia.

48. The nurse practitioner understands that the pain experienced with angina pectoris or MI is caused by irritation of the myocardial nerve fibers by the increase in:

    1. Blood glucose.

    2. Lactic acid.

    3. Serum potassium.

    4. Serum magnesium.

49. New York Heart Functional Class III for clients with cardiac disease is characterized by:

    1. Symptoms present at rest, with any activity leading to increased discomfort.

    2. Slight limitation in ordinary activity, resulting in fatigue, palpitations, dyspnea, or angina.

    3. No physical limitation in activity.

    4. Marked limitation in activity, comfortable at rest, but ordinary activity leads to symptoms.

50. During the history and physical examination of a client with suspected early CHF, which is the most prominent finding?

    1. Moist crackles in the lung bases bilaterally.

    2. Anorexia with weight loss of 3 lb in 1 week.

    3. Increased urine output and peripheral edema.

    4. Facial edema and distended neck veins.

51. Chest pain that is sudden and severe, described as "tearing," and accompanied by a decrease in peripheral pulses may indicate a diagnosis of:

    1. Angina.

    2. Acute MI.

    3. Aortic dissection.

    4. Pericarditis.

52. Dietary therapy for hyperlipidemia occurs in two steps, a Step I diet and a Step II diet. A Step I diet includes, as daily intake:

    1. Total fat ≤30% of total calories, <300 mg cholesterol, 8%–10% saturated fat.

    2. Total fat ≤30% of total calories, <200 mg cholesterol, <7% saturated fat.

    3. Total fat ≤40% of total calories, <400 mg cholesterol, <15% saturated fat.

    4. Total fat ≤30% of total calories, <2000 total calories, <3 gm sodium.

53. The most frequent life-threatening dysrhythmia experienced by a client with an acute MI is:

    1. Atrial fibrillation.

    2. Ventricular tachycardia.

    3. Third-degree heart block.

    4. Ventricular fibrillation.

54. A young child is scheduled for surgical repair of tetralogy of Fallot. What does the nurse practitioner expect the child's hemoglobin (Hgb) values to show, and what kind of lesion does the child have?

   1. Hgb 18 gm/dl, cyanotic.

   2. Hgb 3 gm/dl, cyanotic.

   3. Hgb 10 gm/dl, acyanotic.

   4. Hgb 18 gm/dl, acyanotic.

55. In an overweight older female client with an elevated cholesterol level and abnormal lipoprotein profile, the first step in treatment includes:

   1. Prescribing a bile acid sequestrant agent.

   2. Initiation of a diet and exercise program.

   3. Estrogen replacement therapy.

   4. Referral to a cardiologist.

56. Clients with chronic atrial fibrillation are at risk for which condition?

   1. Sudden cardiac death.

   2. Cerebrovascular accident.

   3. Ventricular tachycardia.

   4. Acute myocardial infarction.

57. The nurse practitioner understands that the most common symptom of CHF in adults is:

   1. Anorexia.

   2. Dependent edema.

   3. Dyspnea.

   4. Weakness.

58. The nurse practitioner teaches the cardiac client to avoid foods high in saturated fats, which include:

   1. Nuts, legumes, and seeds.

   2. Fish, shellfish, and mussels.

   3. Palm oil, coconut oil, and butter.

   4. Peanut oil, soybean oil, and olive oil.

59. An elderly male client is complaining of chest pain. A parameter to assist the nurse practitioner to differentiate the chest pain of angina from that of an infarction is:

   1. Myocardial pain with an infarction is more severe.

2. Anginal pain is more substernal and does not radiate to other areas.

3. Anginal pain is frequently relieved by nitroglycerin.

4. Pain from an infarction is always associated with other symptoms.

60. The nurse practitioner is evaluating a client in the office who is complaining of chest pain with BP of 86/52. The ECG shows some signs of ischemia, and the client is to be transferred to the emergency department. What drug might the nurse practitioner give the client while awaiting transfer?

   1. Furosemide (Lasix) 40 mg IV.

   2. Morphine sulfate 25 mg IV.

   3. Nitroglycerin SL.

   4. Acetylsalicylic acid (ASA; aspirin) 81 mg PO.

61. Which would not be considered as contributing to the development of thrombophlebitis?

   1. Excessive use of oral anticoagulants.

   2. Blow to the leg or arm.

   3. Recent IV therapy.

   4. Secondary to pregnancy.

62. An elderly client is being evaluated for a complaint of dizziness. What symptom/observation will make the nurse practitioner consider that this is a life-threatening event?

   1. The dizziness occurs in certain positions.

   2. It is accompanied by tinnitus.

   3. The symptoms worsen when standing.

   4. It is preceded by rapid breathing.

63. A 28-year-old male presents to the nurse practitioner with a history of chest pain that has been increasing over the past several days. The client states that the pain worsens on lying down. He denies any shortness of breath, cough, or radiation of the pain. He does give a history of a recent infection with coxsackievirus. Examination shows that the client has a cardiac friction rub. One probable diagnosis considered by the nurse practitioner is:

   1. Acute myocardial infarction.

   2. Pleural effusion.

3. Pericarditis.

4. Esophageal reflux.

64. The nurse practitioner would most likely suspect which differential diagnosis for an elderly client presenting with atrial fibrillation and functional decline?

1. Hyperthyroidism.

2. Hypothyroidism.

3. Sick sinus syndrome.

4. Congestive heart failure.

65. Which assessment made by the nurse practitioner for an older client would be a deviation from the normal changes of aging?

1. Decreased exercise tolerance.

2. Grade II/VI systolic ejection murmur.

3. Prolongation of PR intervals on ECG.

4. Jugular venous pressure (JVP) of 4 cm H_2O

66. Cardiac auscultation of an older client reveals a grade II/VI murmur heard best at the second right intercostal space. The murmur is louder with squatting. There is a small carotid pulse with a delayed upstroke. The client's history is benign, and his activity tolerance is within normal limits for his age. The nurse practitioner would interpret this murmur to be indicative of:

1. Aortic regurgitation.

2. Aortic stenosis.

3. Mitral valve prolapse.

4. Mitral regurgitation.

67. What is the most frequently diagnosed valvular heart problem in elderly clients?

1. Aortic stenosis.

2. Mitral stenosis.

3. Mitral regurgitation.

4. Aortic regurgitation.

68. A middle-aged man with no known risk factors for coronary artery disease presents with a cholesterol level of 255 mg/dl. The nurse practitioner would:

1. Start him on an HMG CoA reductase inhibitor.

2. Start him on a Step I diet.

3. Repeat cholesterol and obtain HDL and calculated LDL levels.

4. Do nothing, since he has no coronary risks other than male gender.

69. The nurse practitioner understands that the most likely cause of hypertension in a young child is:

1. Glomerulonephritis.

2. Pheochromocytoma.

3. Rheumatic fever.

4. Hyperthyroidism.

70. Which of the following would be pertinent in the past medical history of a child who is being evaluated for cardiovascular disease?

1. Kawasaki disease.

2. Hypothyroidism.

3. Osteogenic sarcoma.

4. Tourette's syndrome.

71. The nurse practitioner would refer a child with the following findings to a pediatric cardiologist for workup and evaluation within 1–2 weeks:

1. Signs of exercise intolerance, dyspnea, and elevated pulse.

2. Poor feeding, increased cyanosis with crying, and dizziness.

3. Nonfunctional heart murmur, respiratory crackles, and retarded growth and development.

4. Systolic ejection murmur, grade II, which disappears on sitting.

72. Infective endocarditis prophylaxis may be required for children with congenital heart defects in which of the following conditions?

1. Dental procedures such as simple adjustment of orthodontic appliances.

2. Cardiac catheterization.

3. Tonsillectomy and/or adenoidectomy.

4. Insertion of tympanostomy tubes.

73. For the congenital heart disease (CHD) child with a permanent pacemaker, electrical safety precautions include avoidance of:

    1. Cellular phones.

    2. Microwave ovens.

    3. Household electrical appliances.

    4. Metal detectors.

74. A child is having a workup for rheumatic fever. His physical findings are 103.6°F temperature, migratory joint pain, increased erythrocyte sedimentation rate (ESR). According to the Jones Criteria, what is essential for the diagnosis of rheumatic fever?

    1. History of group A streptococcal throat infection.

    2. Carditis.

    3. Sydenham's chorea.

    4. History of erythema marginatum for past 3 days.

Pharmacology

75. A 75-year-old client presents to the office complaining of "not feeling well." He has a history of chronic lung disease and CHF. His vital signs are pulse 78 and irregular, respirations 26, and BP 158/100. An ECG indicates sinus rhythm and confirms the rate. The PR interval is 0.28 second, P waves are present, and each is followed by a QRS complex. There are frequent premature atrial beats. The client is taking digitalis, potassium, theophylline, hydrochlorothiazide, and a calcium channel blocker. What is the next best action to take?

    1. Obtain serum theophylline, digitalis, and potassium levels.

    2. Increase dosage of calcium blocker and diuretic.

    3. Order pulmonary function studies.

    4. Refer the client to a cardiologist.

76. A 49-year-old female was started on a thiazide diuretic for hypertension 1 month ago. She arrives in the clinic complaining of muscle cramps and dizziness. Physical exam findings are:

- BP 132/88 (previous 186/112)
- Pulse 112
- Respirations 24
- Tenting positive
- Skin turgor decreased
- Neck veins flat
- STAT serum electrolytes:
    - —Sodium 114 mEq/L
    - —Chloride 92 mEq/L
    - —Potassium 3.0 mEq/L
- STAT blood glucose 201 mg/dl

Initial treatment for this client should include fluid replacement:

1. Orally with free water and a potassium supplement.

2. Intravenously with normal saline and regular insulin subcutaneously.

3. Intravenously with 1000 ml of normal saline with 40 mEq KCl at 50 ml/hr.

4. Intravenously with 1000 ml of lactated Ringer's solution at 250 ml/hr.

77. A client is recovering from an acute episode of thrombophlebitis and is being treated with warfarin (Coumadin) 5 mg PO daily. In reviewing medication information, the nurse practitioner would include what information in her teaching?

    1. Do not take a multivitamin supplement.

    2. Limit dairy products.

    3. Aerobic exercises are the most effective.

    4. Maintain a daily record of intake and output.

78. The nurse practitioner is evaluating a client who is "not feeling good." He has a history of CAD and CHF. Vital signs are pulse 72, respirations 20, BP 130/88, and temperature normal. He has no complaints of chest pain or difficulty breathing. He had some nausea but no vomiting over the past 2 days. Lower extremities are negative for edema. The client states he has been able to take his medications. His current medications are digoxin (Lanoxin) 0.25 bid, hydrochlorothiazide (HydroDiuril) 100 mg bid, potassium (Micro-K) 10 mEq daily, and nitroglycerin transdermal patches. What is the priority of care for this client?

    1. STAT ECG and white blood cell count (WBC).

    2. Arterial blood gases and oxygen at 4 L/min.

3. Serum digoxin and potassium levels.

4. Serial cardiac enzymes now and q6h ×2.

79. The nurse practitioner has prescribed losartan (Cozaar) 50 mg PO qd. This medication promotes vasodilatation by:

    1. Inhibiting conversion of angiotensin I to angiotensin II.

    2. Promoting release of aldosterone.

    3. Promoting synthesis of prostaglandin.

    4. Inhibiting calcium influx into smooth muscle cells.

80. A client with a history of hypertension is started on Aldactone 50 mg PO qd. The nurse practitioner instructs the client to call the clinic if which symptoms are experienced?

    1. Increased irritability, abdominal cramping, and lower extremity weakness.

    2. Decreased reflex response, nausea, and vomiting.

    3. Muscle twitching, numbness of the limbs, and depression.

    4. Weight gain, excessive thirst, and fever.

81. A client with a history of unstable angina is seen in the cardiac clinic for a checkup. The assessment reveals increased weight of 10 lb, distended jugular neck veins, and an S_3. What changes in the pharmacologic treatment should be initiated?

    1. Discontinue beta-blockers and calcium channel blockers.

    2. Initiate thrombolytic therapy.

    3. Discontinue nitrate and aspirin therapy.

    4. Initiate diuretic and vasoconstrictor therapy.

82. A client arrives at the emergency room of a small rural hospital complaining that he "feels like my heart is racing." He is connected to a cardiac monitor, which reveals supraventricular tachycardia at a rate of 184 beats/min, QRS complex <0.10 second, and BP 112/62. Which treatment modality is indicated?

    1. Synchronized cardioversion with 50 joules.

    2. Defibrillation with 100 joules.

    3. Adenosine 6 mg IV push.

    4. Lidocaine 1 mg/kg IV push.

83. An 80-year-old client with a history of glaucoma develops unstable angina. He is started on diltiazem (Cardizem) 30 mg PO qid and aspirin 324 mg PO qd in addition to timolol ophthalmic solution (Timoptic) 1 gtt OD bid. This client would have an increased risk for:

    1. Bleeding episodes.

    2. Fainting episodes and falls.

    3. Rebound supraventricular tachycardia.

    4. Blurred vision.

84. A client with a serum cholesterol level of 256 mg/dl, HDL of 38 mg/dl, and LDL of 172 mg/dl is instructed on dietary modifications and niacin (nicotinic acid) 1 gm PO tid. Specific instructions include:

    1. Limiting daily fluid intake.

    2. Taking measures to minimize orthostatic hypotension.

    3. Administering the drug an hour after eating.

    4. Avoid exposure to direct sunlight.

85. When monitoring for the therapeutic effects of verapamil (Calan SR), the nurse practitioner would assess for:

    1. Increase in heart rate.

    2. Decrease in systemic vascular resistance.

    3. Increase in blood pressure.

    4. Decrease in ventricular premature beats.

86. An adult male client with essential hypertension is treated by the nurse practitioner with sodium restriction and hydrochlorothiazide (Diuril) 25 mg PO daily. After 3 months of therapy, the client's blood pressure is measured at 160/110 mm Hg. At this point, the nurse practitioner would:

    1. Begin enalapril (Vasotec) 5 mg qd.

    2. Begin with 50 mg of metoprolol (Toprol XL) qd.

    3. Add 25 mg of hydrochlorothiazide (Diuril) daily.

    4. Discontinue Diuril and change to captopril (Capoten) 50 mg tid.

87. When prescribing antihypertensive drug therapy for elderly clients, the nurse practitioner recognizes that which class of antihypertensive agents should be avoided with elderly persons?

    1. Calcium entry antagonists.

    2. Diuretics.

    3. Beta-blockers.

    4. Angiotensin-converting enzyme (ACE) inhibitors.

88. Medications used in managing ischemic heart disease include:

    1. Beta-blockers, sedatives, aspirin.

    2. Nitrates, beta-blockers, calcium channel blockers, aspirin.

    3. Vasoconstrictors, aspirin, anxiolytics.

    4. Nitrates, ACE inhibitors, aspirin, lipid-lowering drugs.

89. The nurse practitioner initiates antihypertensive therapy for a middle-aged nonsmoking male. One week later the client returns for a follow-up visit and complains of a recurrent dry cough since initiating the medications. This is most likely a side effect of:

    1. Beta-blocker.

    2. Thiazide diuretic.

    3. ACE inhibitor.

    4. Calcium channel blocker.

90. The role of digoxin in the management of CHF is indicated:

    1. With atrial fibrillation.

    2. With mitral stenosis.

    3. With normal ejection fraction.

    4. Due to acute pericardial disease.

91. The nurse practitioner should monitor the elderly client for which of the most common adverse reactions of digoxin?

    1. Blurred vision.

    2. Confusion.

    3. Diarrhea.

    4. Eating disorder.

92. The nurse practitioner has been successfully treating an older client's hypertension with diet, exercise, and HydroDiuril 25 mg PO qd for 5 months. During today's clinic visit, the client's BP was 154/90 and temperature 99.9°F. The physical examination revealed clear breath sounds, S_1 and S_2 with no murmurs, gallops, or rubs; and no JVD. The client denied syncope, headaches, or visual changes; there was a tender and edematous right ankle. Which laboratory values would be most appropriate for evaluation?

    1. Blood urea nitrogen and sodium.

    2. Serum cholesterol and serum calcium.

    3. Serum potassium and blood count.

    4. Serum uric acid and complete blood count.

93. An elderly white male with a long history of COPD has recently developed hypertension. Which class of antihypertensive agents should the nurse practitioner avoid for this client?

    1. ACE inhibitors.

    2. Beta-blockers.

    3. Calcium channel blockers.

    4. Diuretics.

94. Which class of pharmacologic agents would the nurse practitioner select for a hypertensive elderly client with a new diagnosis of CHF?

    1. ACE inhibitors.

    2. Beta-blockers.

    3. Calcium channel blockers.

    4. Diuretics.

95. A mildly hypertensive male client presents with red, painful swelling of the great toe. In addition to treating the gout, the nurse practitioner also knows he/she must:

    1. Order laboratory studies for diabetes.

    2. Explore for possible alcohol abuse.

    3. Advise him to lose weight.

    4. Change his thiazide antihypertensive.

96. An elderly male with a diagnosis of systolic hypertension 3 months ago presents for follow-up care. He is on a no-added-salt diet and has lost 8 lb in 3 months. Weekly BP checks at a senior center average 180s/70s. The health history

includes benign prostatic hyperplasia, diet-controlled type 2 diabetes, and CAD with an MI 8 years ago. His chief complaint includes periodic angina, occasional heartburn, slowed urine stream with some dribbling, and decreasing energy level. The BP today is 188/78. Current medications are cimetidine (Tagamet) 200 mg prn, ASA 325 mg qd, nitroglycerin, and Maalox prn. The client is married and sexually active. Which medication would the nurse practitioner initiate after a complete physical, including ECG, and all indicated blood work?

1. ACE inhibitor.

2. Diuretic.

3. α_1-Adrenergic blocker.

4. β-Adrenergic blocker.

97. A geriatric client has been on procainamide (Pronestyl) for 4 years to control his cardiac dysrhythmias. The nurse practitioner would evaluate for what side effect in the chronic use of this medication?

1. Elevated liver function tests.

2. Appearance of antinuclear antibodies.

3. Shortened AV interval.

4. Tachycardia.

98. Secondary prophylaxis for acute rheumatic fever (ARF) in a 25-year-old schoolteacher includes:

1. Penicillin V 125–250 mg PO bid indefinitely.

2. Erythromycin 800 mg PO bid.

3. One-time dose of 2.0 million units benzathine penicillin G combined with penicillin G procaine (Bicillin C-R) IM.

4. No medication prophylaxis is needed after client reaches the early 20s.

99. A client has been prescribed lisinopril (Prinivil) 5 mg PO qd for hypertension. He has developed an intractable cough that is unrelated to heart failure. Which of the following medications can be substituted for this ACE inhibitor?

1. Calcium channel blocker.

2. Digoxin.

3. Another ACE inhibitor (hydralazine/nitrate).

4. Angiotensin receptor blockers (ARB).

100. A 60-year-old male with a history of unstable angina comes to the clinic complaining of increased pain that is not relieved by his nitroglycerin. During the assessment, the nurse practitioner notes elevation of the ST segment on the ECG. Oxygen therapy is administered and an IV line inserted. What other therapy should be initiated while arranging transfer to an acute care facility?

1. Lidocaine drip at 2 mg/min.

2. Metoprolol (Toprol) 100 mg PO.

3. Morphine 2 mg IV push.

4. Aspirin 160 mg PO.

101. A 54-year-old client with type 2 diabetes has been diagnosed with hypertension. Which antihypertensive drug is the recommended choice to treat hypertension in clients with diabetes?

1. Beta-blocker.

2. Diuretic.

3. Calcium channel blocker.

4. ACE inhibitor.

102. A 68-year-old with a history of MI who has experienced atrial fibrillation for 2 years comes to the clinic with a complaint of "increasing difficulty breathing and occasionally awakening at night with feeling of smothering." Which pharmacologic therapy would be appropriate?

1. Digitalis and ACE inhibitor.

2. Loop diuretic and beta-blocker.

3. Thiazide diuretic and calcium channel blocker.

4. Alpha-1-blocker and nitrate.

103. A client with coronary artery disease has cholesterol count of 278 mg/dl and triglyceride level of 300 mg/dl. The nurse practitioner initiates therapy with lovastatin (Mevacor) 20 mg daily. The client is instructed to take the Mevacor daily:

1. In the morning with breakfast.

2. 30 minutes before eating breakfast.

3. In the evening.

4. Around noon.

104. A toddler has ingested some of his grandfather's pills. The toddler is vomiting, feels weak, and has a first-degree atrioventricular (AV) block pattern on the ECG. The grandfather brings in four medication bottles. Which is the most likely medication the toddler ingested?

    1. Amitriptyline (Elavil).

    2. Digoxin (Lanoxin).

    3. Furosemide (Lasix).

    4. Aspirin.

105. A 70-year-old white female is a resident of a long-term care facility where the nurse practitioner makes rounds on a weekly basis. The nurse is reviewing recent laboratory results and notices the following: serum potassium 5.9, serum sodium 144, serum chloride 111, BUN 28, and creatinine 1.8. Her current medications include furosemide (Lasix) 20 mg PO qd, potassium chloride (K-Dur) 16 mEq PO qd, captopril (Capoten) 25 mg PO qd, and citalopram (Celexa) 10 mg PO qd. There have been no changes in her medications. What is the likely cause of the elevated serum potassium?

    1. Furosemide.

    2. Potassium chloride.

    3. Captopril.

    4. Citalopram.

Answers & Rationales

Physical Examination & Diagnostic Tests

1. **(1)** S₁ is heard loudest at the apex, S₂ at the base. Each sound should be carefully assessed as to the intensity of the sound in each area.

2. **(3)** The PMI represents the thrust and contraction of the left ventricle (LV). The LV lies behind the right ventricle (RV) and extends to the left, forming the left border of the heart.

3. **(2)** The correct procedure is to listen for carotid bruits with the bell of the stethoscope, which brings out low-frequency sounds and filters out high-frequency sound. The bell should be placed very lightly on the neck with just enough pressure to seal the edge.

4. **(2)** The purpose of inspection and palpation of the precordium is to determine the presence and extent of normal and abnormal pulsations. A slight retraction of the chest wall just medial to the midclavicular line in the fifth interspace is a normal finding, whereas marked or active retraction of the rib is abnormal and may indicate pericardial disease. Pericardial friction rubs are heard by auscultation.

5. **(1)** The splitting during inspiration refers to S₁ and S₂. The S₃ is normal in children, young adults, and pregnant women. In the older adult with heart disease, this often signifies myocardial failure.

6. **(3)** The right side of the chest close to the sternal border at the second intercostal space is the correct area to auscultate the aortic valve. The mitral valve is auscultated at the fifth left intercostal space at the midclavicular line. The tricuspid value is auscultated at the fourth left intercostal space at the sternal border. The pulmonic valve is auscultated at the second left intercostal space at the sternal border.

7. **(2)** A 12-hour fast is recommended because of the influence of intake on cholesterol levels, which may increase. A normal diet for the 7 days prior to the exam is recommended so that an accurate picture of the client's normal life is obtained. Alcohol should not be consumed for 48 hours before the test because it may increase cholesterol, HDL, LDL, and triglyceride levels. If possible, all medication should be withheld until the test is over, especially corticosteroids, diuretics, beta-blockers, oral contraceptives, and estrogens.

8. **(1)** An S₄ is a normal variant in people 65 years and older and may result from increased resistance to ventricular filling during atrial contraction.

9. **(1)** According to the classification of hypertension, a BP of 168/100 is within the moderate range.

10. **(2)** The fifth intercostal space at the midclavicular line on the left side is the best place to auscultate the closure sounds of the mitral valve. Option #1 describes the area of the tricuspid valve, Option #3 the pulmonic valve area, and Option #4 the aortic valve area.

11. **(3)** It is important to determine if the coolness extends proximally from the hand, for which palpation of pulses would be appropriate.

12. **(1)** Closure of the AV valves, which allows the filling of both ventricles simultaneously, produces the first heart sound (S_1); closure of the aortic and pulmonic valves produces the second heart sound (S_2).

13. **(4)** The apical and peripheral (radial) pulses must be evaluated simultaneously to determine if all the apical beats are being reflected in the radial pulse. If there is an apical rate of 100 and a radial rate of 94, the client is said to have a pulse deficit of 6 points. This is usually done with two people counting over the same period.

14. **(3)** A grade V heart murmur is very loud and can be heard with the stethoscope partly off the chest wall. A grade VI murmur is the loudest, is audible with the stethoscope just removed from contact with the chest wall, and is accompanied by a thrill. A grade I murmur is barely audible or very faint with the bell of the stethoscope.

15. **(4)** The normal aging process impairs automaticity, conductivity, and contractility. Ischemic changes and degeneration decrease sinus node automaticity and conduction velocity, resulting in bradycardic rhythms or atrial fibrillation. The poor myocardial contractility, usually related to hypertension or valvular disease, causes decreased ventricular emptying and increased filling pressures. These changes predispose the elderly client to congestive heart failure.

16. **(4)** The most sensitive area on the examiner's hand is the back of the fingers.

17. **(3)** Desired levels for a lipid profile are total cholesterol <200 mg/dl, HDL >35 mg/dl, LDL <130 mg/dl, and triglycerides <250 mg/dl. A high total cholesterol coupled with a low HDL is a positive risk factor for coronary heart disease, the greatest concern for this client, who also has an elevated LDL level. These parameters together would mandate intervention.

18. **(2)** Weak or absent pulses are associated with coarctation of the aorta and are not indicative of the other cardiovascular diseases.

19. **(3)** Dressler's syndrome (post-MI syndrome) may develop 1–4 weeks post-MI and is characterized by pericarditis with effusion and fever. Dressler's syndrome is caused by antigen-antibody reactions. Laboratory findings include elevated white blood count and erythrocyte sedimentation rate. Treatment includes corticosteroids.

20. **(2)** A machinery-like murmur is consistent with patent ductus arteriosus (PDA). The turbulent flow of blood from the aorta through the PDA to the pulmonary artery results in this characteristic murmur. Coarctation presents with upper extremity hypertension, systolic murmur, and weak or absent femoral pulses. Ventricular septal defect is characterized by a loud, harsh, pansystolic murmur heard best at the lower left sternal border. Aortic stenosis has a systolic murmur.

21. **(1)** Jugular vein distention (JVD) is common in geriatric clients. If JVD is present when the client's head is elevated 45 degrees, further examination is necessary regarding the venous pressure, which reflects pressure in the right-sided heart chambers. The supine position will increase venous pressure and does not provide valid information in this situation. Auscultation for carotid bruits is an important part of assessment but is not significant in evaluating JVD.

22. **(1)** Mitral valve stenosis is a diastolic murmur of low intensity heard at the apex of the heart. Option #2 describes characteristics of a murmur with aortic stenosis. Option #3, a holosystolic murmur, is characteristic of mitral regurgitation, which allows for backflow of blood from ventricles into the atrium. Option #4 best describes aortic regurgitation.

23. **(3)** The client had a left ventricular MI. One of the most common complications is left-sided failure resulting in congestive heart failure. This would manifest first as pulmonary congestion and difficulty breathing.

24. **(4)** Classically, intermittent claudication is described as pain in the lower extremity on activity that is relieved by stopping the activity.

25. **(3)** A positive result on stress testing indicates the likelihood of CAD with 98% accuracy in males over age 50. Results are progressively lower in asymptomatic persons, with false-positive results increased in asymptomatic men under age 40, premenopausal women without risk factors, and clients taking digitalis.

26. **(2)** A hyperkinetic impulse (increased amplitude) is caused by pressure overload of the left ventricle. Causes include hyperthyroidism, severe anemia, or mitral regurgitation. A pansystolic murmur is a classic finding of mitral regurgitation.

27. **(4)** Pulsus alternans (weak pulse alternating with strong pulse) is caused by left ventricular failure and is usually accompanied by an S_3 heart sound.

Disorders

28. **(1)** This assessment reflects changes caused by chronic venous insufficiency. The other assessment findings reflect chronic arterial insufficiency.

29. **(1)** A diagnosis of HTN from a single measurement of blood pressure (BP) elevation should not be done. A minimum of three readings with an average systolic BP of 140 mm Hg and diastolic of 90 mm Hg establishes the diagnosis. An average of two or more readings taken at each of two or more visits should follow an initial screening. The client should be seated with the arm at heart level. No caffeine or nicotine ingestion should be allowed for 30 minutes before the reading. The room should be quiet at least 5 minutes, and an appropriate cuff should be used. Another high reading should be confirmed within 2 months.

30. **(4)** Most cases of CHF in children result from congenital heart disease, and most occur during the first year of life. Although the clinical presentation of a child with CHD will vary with the specific defect, the clinical manifestations usually relate to the degree of CHF or cyanosis.

31. **(3)** In the early stages of hypertensive heart disease, when there is an increased peripheral resistance to blood flow, the most significant change occurring in the heart is left ventricular hypertrophy. This is associated with an increase in the size of the myocardial cells without a corresponding increase in cell number (hyperplasia). Over time, all the other options listed occur in the heart.

32. **(3)** Sinus or atrial tachycardia is characterized by a rate of 100 beats/min or higher, P waves present for each QRS complex, PR interval below 0.20, T wave after each QRS complex, and regular rhythm.

33. **(1)** The classic chest pain of MI may not be present in the geriatric client due to altered pain perception and diminished pain sensation.

34. **(2)** Respiratory symptoms are predominant in clients with left-sided heart failure. Venous congestion and peripheral edema are associated with right-sided failure.

35. **(1)** Cardiac tamponade occurs as a complication of pericarditis. An excessive accumulation of fluids between the pericardium and the myocardium interferes with effective cardiac contraction and produces a paradoxical pulse. The triphasic friction rub is common to pericarditis but is not indicative of a complication of constrictive pericarditis. Jugular venous pressure is used to determine levels of venous distention.

36. **(2)** Untreated hypertension causes significant increased work of the left ventricle, eventually causing CHF.

37. **(2)** Palpable carotid pulse with each compression is the best sign of effective CPR. The other answers are appropriate but not the best indicators of effective resuscitation efforts.

38. **(2)** This is a description of complete block with hemodynamic consequences. The client should be seen immediately by a cardiologist for possible pacemaker insertion. First-degree block has characteristic P waves and a long PR interval. In addition to referral for follow-up, the client should be seen by a cardiologist as soon as possible.

39. **(3)** A triphasic friction rub or a pericardial rub occurs in the majority of clients with pericarditis. Paradoxical pulse may occur if constrictive pericarditis and cardiac tamponade are present. Pulse deficits and presence of S_4 are not characteristic of problems with pericarditis.

40. **(1)** Elderly individuals experience atypical symptoms of MI, including dyspnea, diaphoresis, vomiting, syncope, confusion, and weakness.

41. **(1)** Cardiovascular risk factors predisposing women to cardiovascular disease include smaller body size, declining estrogen level, heart and thoracic cavity smaller and lighter, coronary arteries smaller in diameter, shorter PR interval, higher resting ejection fraction. Increased body fat percentage and fat distributed in the abdomen may be mobilized more easily in response to stress. This may raise serum cholesterol and blood glucose levels.

42. **(4)** The nurse practitioner must consider the geriatric client's other medical problems and treatment before prescribing medications for hypertension. Frequently, geriatric clients cannot take beta-blockers due to chronic pulmonary conditions; the client may already be taking diuretics for problems of fluid retention. Step therapy is appropriate if there is no other significant medical history. Lifestyle changes should be initiated and medications adjusted as changes are made.

43. **(2)** Hypertension is considered a major factor in the development of CAD in the geriatric client. Female clients have an increased incidence of CAD after menopause; estrogen replacement appears to have cardioprotective effects on the heart, thus decreasing the incidence of CAD. Although diabetic clients have an increased incidence of CAD, most CAD clients are not diabetic.

44. **(4)** Cor pulmonale is characterized by hypertrophy of the right ventricle secondary to pulmonary hypertension (resistance). The increased P-wave amplitude (P pulmonale) occurs as the right atrium enlarges.

45. **(2)** Excess secretion of aldosterone predisposes to potassium excretion. Total body sodium content will be above normal, but the excessive secretion of antidiuretic hormone causes greater retention of water, diluting the serum level.

46. **(1)** Water-hammer pulse (bounding pulse with a rapid rise and sudden collapse) results from an increase in pulse pressure and may be caused by increased stroke volume, decreased peripheral vascular resistance, or both. Because the nurse practitioner suspects either aortic regurgitation or patent ductus arteriosus (primarily in children), auscultation for a diastolic murmur is indicated.

47. **(3)** Most cases of CHF in infants result from congenital heart disease during the first 12 months of life. Symptoms result from the decreased cardiac output and the infant's compensatory mechanisms. Symptoms include tachypnea, dyspnea, tachycardia, paleness, and easy fatigability. Additional symptoms include periorbital edema, hepatomegaly, difficult feeding, and persistent cough. Diaphoresis, central cyanosis, and peripheral edema are not necessarily associated with CHF but may be manifestations of the underlying congenital heart defect.

48. **(2)** Occlusion of the coronary arteries deprives the myocardial cells of glucose needed for aerobic metabolism. Anaerobic metabolism occurs, which causes the accumulation of lactic acid. Lactic acid irritates the myocardial nerve fibers, sending pain messages to the cardiac nerves and upper thoracic posterior roots located in the left shoulder and arm.

49. **(4)** Option #1 is Functional Class IV. Option #2 is Functional Class II. Option #3 is Class I. Option #4, the correct response, is Functional Class III.

50. **(1)** The moist crackles (rales) heard in the bases of the lung are the most prominent physical examination findings of early CHF. They are caused from transudation of fluid into the alveoli and into the airways. Later findings include distended neck veins, peripheral edema, hepatomegaly, and ascites (rather than weight loss).

51. **(3)** Aortic dissection almost invariably begins with sudden onset of severe chest pain that is tearing or ripping in quality and is accompanied by absent or decreased peripheral pulses and neurologic deficits. The pain of angina and acute MI is usually described as "pressure." Pericarditis produces pain that is more gradual in onset.

52. **(1)** A Step I diet involves daily intake of ≤30% total calorie intake made up of fat, <300 mg/day cholesterol intake, and 8%–10% daily saturated fat intake. A decrease to <200 mg/day of cholesterol and 7% saturated fat is a Step II diet, prescribed if Step I is ineffective. The third selection is closer to the current average American's diet. Although important for weight and BP control, watching calorie and sodium intake is not part of a Step I diet plan for hyperlipidemia.

53. **(4)** Although the other dysrhythmias may occur after MI, the most life-threatening is ventricular fibrillation. The vast majority of deaths due to ventricular fibrillation occur within the first 24 hours, and more than half of these occur in the first hour. The majority of out-of-hospital deaths from MI are caused by ventricular fibrillation.

54. **(1)** Congenital heart disease is usually classified as acyanotic or cyanotic. Cyanotic heart defects (right-to-left shunts) include tetralogy of Fallot, severe pulmonary stenosis, pulmonary atresia, tricuspid atresia, and transposition of the great vessels. Children with cyanotic heart disease develop polycythemia to increase the oxygen-carrying capacity of the blood. Additionally, the child with a cyanotic heart defect should have hemoglobin of at least 16 gm/dl.

55. **(2)** Diet and exercise are the mainstay of any treatment program and would be used initially in all cases. A bile acid sequestrant agent or estrogen replacement therapy may eventually be necessary if no improvement is seen with diet/exercise therapy. Referral to a cardiologist is not necessary, unless the client develops symptoms or shows resistance to treatment.

56. **(2)** A cerebrovascular accident (CVA) is often the outcome of chronic atrial fibrillation due to the blood pooling in the quivering atria. For this reason, warfarin (Coumadin) should be maintained at an international normalized ratio (INR) of 2–3. Some trials suggest aspirin may provide adequate anticoagulation in doses of 160–325 mg/day.

57. **(3)** Dyspnea is the most common symptom of CHF. Initially it is present only with moderate exertion, but as severity of CHF increases, dyspnea may occur with mild exertion or at rest. Fatigue is another common complaint. Right-sided heart failure is associated with weakness, anorexia, nausea, and dependent edema. Chronic left ventricular failure usually leads to right ventricular failure.

58. **(3)** Palm and coconut oils, along with butter, are very high in saturated fats and should be avoided. The other selections are moderately high in fat content but are mainly unsaturated fats.

59. **(3)** Anginal pain is difficult to differentiate from pain of an infarction. One of the most characteristic symptoms is the relief of the anginal pain with the administration of sublingual nitroglycerin.

60. **(4)** Aspirin helps prevent the formation of platelet-aggregating substances and may help the occlusion of narrowed coronary arteries. Although furosemide and morphine have a role in treating acute MI, ASA can be readily given in the typical primary care office. Nitroglycerin should not be given because the client's systolic BP is less than 90 mm Hg.

61. **(1)** Superficial inflammation of a vein may be caused by trauma (e.g., blow to the arm or leg), or recent IV therapy with irritating fluids or may occur secondary to pregnancy, especially during the postpartum period, due to the increase in clotting factors (thromboplastin). Excessive use of oral anticoagulants can lead to bleeding, but not to thrombophlebitis. Deep vein thrombosis (DVT) associated with thrombophlebitis results from prolonged bed rest, major surgical procedures, injury to the blood vessel wall, and hypercoagulable states, such as use of oral contraceptives, especially in women who smoke or have cancer, and polycythemia vera.

62. **(3)** Dizziness that improves when lying down and worsens when standing is symptomatic of cardiac involvement and may indicate serious cardiac dysrhythmias. If it occurs in certain positions, the dizziness suggests benign positional vertigo, which is common in elderly persons. Dizziness accompanied by tinnitus is common in acute labyrinthitis and, if preceded by rapid breathing, may be caused by hyperventilation.

63. **(3)** The stated history of a recent coxsackievirus infection, pain that worsens when supine, and a friction rub is classic for viral pericarditis. The client's age makes an acute MI unlikely, and the pain is not typical for pleural effusion or reflux.

64. **(1)** Signs and symptoms of hyperthyroidism in the older adult include progressive functional decline, atrial fibrillation, MI, tachycardia, weakness, fatigue, weight loss, anorexia, diarrhea, nervousness, tremor, pruritus, memory loss, and heat intolerance. Symptoms of hypothyroidism include arthralgia, weakness, decreased mental function, depression, constipation, weight loss, dry coarse skin with yellowish cast, dry sparse hair, and masklike puffy face with periorbital

edema. Bradycardia would be assessed with both sick sinus syndrome and CHF. Sick sinus syndrome is often associated with the "bradycardia-tachycardia" syndrome.

65. **(4)** A jugular venous pressure of 4 cm H_2O is a sign of CHF. Option #1 is a normal sign of aging. Option #2 is a result of sclerosing of the aorta, which occurs with aging. Option #3 is expected with the aging process.

66. **(2)** This assessment is consistent with aortic stenosis. Aortic regurgitation is a diastolic murmur secondary to rheumatic heart disease, for which no history is given. Mitral valve disease is one of the most common valvular disorders. A small percentage of mitral valve prolapse clients do experience autonomic dysfunction and complain of palpitations, atypical chest pain, orthostatic dizziness, near-syncope, cold extremities, throbbing headaches, and neurasthenia and manifest tachydysrhythmias. Mitral regurgitation clients may remain asymptomatic for many years because the left ventricle dilates and adjusts well to the increase in volume load. Onset of dyspnea and fatigue may not occur for decades.

67. **(1)** Aortic stenosis is most common and is caused by calcification. The symptoms would include syncope, angina, and dyspnea on exertion.

68. **(3)** The nurse practitioner needs to repeat the cholesterol and obtain HDL and LDL values before initiating any treatment. The HDL and LDL will help stratify risks and guide aggressiveness of intervention.

69. **(1)** Although all these conditions can lead to hypertension, the most common in infants and young children is secondary hypertension due to renal disease (e.g., glomerulonephritis, polycystic kidneys, nephrosis). Endocrine-induced hypertension is the second most common cause.

70. **(1)** The two major conditions known to play a causative role in the development of cardiovascular disease in children are untreated streptococcal infections involving group A beta-hemolytic streptococci (leads to cardiac valve problems) and Kawasaki disease (leads to coronary artery aneurysm).

71. **(4)** Options #1, #2, and #3 are considered unstable and acute, and these clients should be immediately referred to a pediatric cardiologist. Children with a murmur need to be evaluated further, but it is not considered emergency as long as they are asymptomatic, have normal activity and exercise, and are growing normally.

72. **(3)** Procedures for which endocarditis prophylaxis is recommended include dental procedures known to induce gingival bleeding. It is also recommended for surgical procedures that involve the respiratory mucosa such as tonsillectomy/adenoidectomy. Endocarditis prophylaxis is not recommended for insertion of tympanostomy tubes, cardiac catheterization, simple dental procedures, or endotracheal intubation.

73. **(4)** For the child with a pacemaker, an electric shock may irreparably damage the pacemaker, and immediate surgical replacement would be necessary. There is no risk of electromagnetic interference between the permanent pacemaker and household items such as electrical appliances, radios, electronic equipment, cellular phones, or microwave ovens. Ovens and pacemakers have filtering systems that prevent interference with the pacemaker's function. Metal detectors have an electromagnetic field that could alter the pacemaker's function temporarily. In addition, the alarm will be set off as a result of the metal in the pacemaker.

74. **(1)** According to the Jones Criteria, in addition to two major manifestations (carditis, polyarthritis, Sydenham's chorea, erythema marginatum, subcutaneous nodules) or one major and two minor manifestations (arthralgia, fever, elevated erythrocyte sedimentation rate, C-reactive protein, prolonged PR interval), a diagnosis of rheumatic fever is highly likely if there is evidence of a previous group A streptococcal infection.

Pharmacology

75. **(1)** This client is presenting with symptoms of digitalis toxicity—first-degree block and increasing cardiac irritability. If the potassium level is low, it may be precipitating the toxicity.

Also, it is important to determine that serum theophylline levels remain within the therapeutic range. No evidence indicates that the pulmonary disease is progressing. The blood pressure may be adequately controlled for this client; further information should be obtained before adjusting the medications. Based on the information presented, referral to a cardiologist is not appropriate at this time.

76. **(3)** Thiazide diuretics inhibit sodium reabsorption, promoting the excretion of sodium, chloride, and water. As the extracellular fluid volume decreases, plasma renin activity and aldosterone levels increase, resulting in potassium loss. Treatment is to restore the volume with normal saline and correct the potassium depletion. If the sodium is increased too rapidly, irreversible neurologic damage can occur.

77. **(1)** Vitamin K is an antidote for warfarin. Increased intake of green leafy vegetables could cause an increase in vitamin K levels and decrease the effectiveness of the medication. Also, multivitamin supplements may contain additional vitamin K.

78. **(3)** The client presents with the classic profile of digitalis toxicity, which is frequently related to hypokalemia, especially since the potassium replacement is rather low for an adult and there is a history of poor eating and nausea. The actions listed in the other options may be taken, but it is important to determine the presence of hypokalemia and digitalis toxicity so that these may be addressed immediately.

79. **(1)** ACE inhibitors such as losartan (Cozaar) decrease the conversion of angiotensin I to angiotensin II, a potent vasoconstrictor, and inhibit the release of aldosterone.

80. **(1)** Aldactone is a potassium-sparing diuretic. Clients should be instructed on signs of hyperkalemia.

81. **(1)** Beta-blockers are myocardial depressants that suppress heart rate and contraction (negative inotropic). Calcium channel blockers decrease atrioventricular conduction, which suppresses heart rate. Both drugs are contraindicated with the onset of left ventricular dysfunction. The increase in JVD and 10-lb gain are associated with the right side. The presence, of an S_3 indicates left venticular dysfunction, especially when associated with signs and symptoms of right sided failure.

82. **(3)** The American Heart Association's Advanced Cardiac Life Support (ACLS) guidelines recommend adenosine as the drug of choice for emergency treatment of supraventricular tachycardia when a client is hemodynamically stable.

83. **(2)** The combination of calcium channel blockers and β-adrenergic blocking agents, systemic or ophthalmic, may result in bradycardia and/or hypotension.

84. **(2)** Niacin can cause vasodilatation, leading to orthostatic hypotension. Antihyperlipidemic drugs may cause constipation. Antihyperlipidemic effectiveness is enhanced when taken before or with meals.

85. **(2)** Calcium channel blockers (a) depress the rate of discharge from the sinoatrial node and conduction velocity through the atrioventricular node, causing a decrease in heart rate; (b) relax the coronary and systemic arteries, producing vasodilatation (decrease in afterload and blood pressure); and (c) decrease myocardial contractility (negative inotropic effect).

86. **(2)** If lifestyle modifications (low-salt diet, weight loss, stopping smoking, exercise, etc.) fail to reduce the client's blood pressure, then it is recommended to continue the lifestyle modifications and start drug therapy. The preferred drugs (unless contraindicated) for uncomplicated hypertension are diuretics or beta-blockers. Depending on co-morbid conditions, other drugs might be preferable. For example, for diabetes type 1 with proteinuria, you would use ACE inhibitors rather than a beta blocker. It is important to start with a low dose of a long-acting, once daily drug and slowly titrate the dose. In this situation, a diuretic was started first with the next logical progression to a beta blocker because there were no co-morbid conditions listed.

87. **(3)** Blood pressure should be lowered cautiously using smaller doses of calcium entry antagonists, ACE inhibitors, or diuretics in elderly clients. Beta-blockers are not appropriate in normal doses for elderly persons because of decreased beta-receptor sensitivity in these clients. Larger doses also result in depression, impotence, fatigue, and declining

mental function. Elderly clients are especially likely to experience CHF and peripheral vascular insufficiency from β-adrenergic blocker toxicity.

88. **(2)** Nitrates are venous and arterial dilators that decrease myocardial oxygen demand. Beta-blockers have an antianginal effect and reduce myocardial oxygen demand. Calcium channel blockers relieve myocardial ischemic by reducing myocardial oxygen demand and dilate coronary arteries. Aspirin is effective for primary and secondary prevention of MI. Unless contraindicated, small doses of ASA (162–325 mg daily) should be prescribed for clients with angina. Clients remaining symptomatic when treated with nitrates, beta-blockers, or calcium channel blockers should be treated with a beta-blocker plus another agent. Appropriate combinations are a nitrate or beta-blocker plus a calcium channel blocker other than verapamil. Combination therapy does not include sedatives, vasoconstrictors, ACE inhibitors, or lipid-lowering drugs.

89. **(3)** Adverse side effects of ACE inhibitors include cough (1%–30%), headache, and dizziness. Adverse effects of calcium channel blockers include peripheral edema, dizziness, headache, nausea, and tachycardia. Adverse effects of thiazide diuretics include nausea, vomiting, diarrhea, dizziness, and headache. Side effects of beta-blockers include fatigue, impotence, depression, and shortness of breath.

90. **(1)** Digoxin, once a first-line drug for all clients with CHF, is now used in clients with atrial fibrillation, other tachycardias, and left ventricular dysfunction. By controlling the ventricular rate in the client with atrial fibrillation or tachycardias, cardiac output increases. In cases of diastolic dysfunction with a sinus rhythm, digitalis is of no benefit. Digoxin is of relatively little value in most forms of cardiomyopathy, myocarditis, mitral stenosis, and chronic constrictive pericarditis.

91. **(2)** Noncardiac adverse reactions include a change in the mental status. Although visual disturbances, diarrhea, anorexia, nausea, or vomiting are also adverse reactions, they are not the most common in elderly clients.

92. **(4)** The assessments indicate gout. A side effect of hydrochlorothiazide is hyperuricemia. Blood for a CBC should be drawn before therapy. The other distracters are not addressing the assessment of a tender and edematous right ankle. The cardiac assessments were benign. No evidence indicates a concern for hypo/hypernatremia or hypo/hyperkalemia.

93. **(2)** Beta-blockers increase peripheral vascular resistance, a phenomenon that already occurs with normal aging, so these drugs can precipitate or worsen symptoms of asthma, COPD, peripheral vascular disease, sexual dysfunction, or CHF. The other classes have no effect or decrease the effect on peripheral resistance.

94. **(1)** ACE inhibitors have been shown to prolong life in clients with CHF by improving overall cardiac function. Options #2 and #3 should be contraindicated in CHF. Although Option #4 may be correct, it is not a priority to Option #1.

95. **(4)** The most likely precipitating cause of this client's gout is the thiazide diuretic used to control his hypertension, since it blocks the excretion of uric acid. Although gout may be more common in obese, alcoholic, and diabetic clients, these conditions are not indicated here.

96. **(1)** The ACE inhibitor will preserve renal function and have less impact on sexual functioning. The nurse practitioner must monitor potassium and carefully follow renal status for change. The ACE inhibitor has fewer negative side effects or interactions with this client's other medical conditions.

97. **(2)** Of clients receiving long-term procainamide therapy, 80% develop antinuclear antibodies, and 23% of these develop a lupus-like syndrome.

98. **(1)** Secondary prevention or preventing the recurrent attacks of ARF is controversial. Some authorities identify (a) reaching the early 20s and (b) 5 years since the last ARF attack as the criteria to stop the use of prophylactic penicillin, unless the client is at increased risk of exposure to streptococcal infections, as are schoolteachers or health professionals. Other authorities recommend lifelong prophylactic drug therapy. Although erythromycin is an alternative medication for penicillin-sensitive individuals, the dose in Option #2 is for a client having a dental or surgical procedure. The secondary prophylactic dose for erythromycin is 250 mg PO bid.

99. **(4)** An annoying untoward effect of ACE inhibitors is an intractable cough. Angiotensin receptor blockers can be substituted as long as the cough is not related to heart failure. A hydralazine/nitrate combination can be substituted if there is significant renal insufficiency or angioedema present. Antidysrhythmic agents, calcium channel blockers, and nonsteroidal antiinflammatory drugs (NSAIDs) should be avoided.

100. **(4)** The American Heart Association recommends that ASA be administered ASAP whenever a client is suspected of having an MI. The decreased platelet aggregation effect of ASA helps limit the size of the myocardial damage.

101. **(4)** ACE inhibitors enhance renal function with patients with diabetes

102. **(1)** The client with atrial fibrillation is exhibiting symptoms of left ventricular (LV) failure. Treatment recommendations include enhancing contractility with a positive inotropic agent, and ACE inhibitors have been shown to slow LV dilatation.

103. **(3)** Because most cholesterol is synthesized between midnight and 3 AM, HMG CoA reductase inhibitors are best taken in the evening.

104. **(2)** Nausea, vomiting, and anorexia are common side effects of many medications. The first-degree AV block confirms the ingestion of digoxin in this situation. Tricyclic antidepressant toxicity is characterized by agitation and anticholingeric symptoms; furosemide toxicity by hypokalemia, weakness, and cardiac dysrhythmias; and aspirin toxicity by tinnitus, confusion, gastrointestinal symptoms, and rapid, deep respirations.

105. **(2)** The likely cause of the elevated serum potassium is the potassium chloride. The nurse practitioner should hold the K-Dur and order daily serum potassium monitoring until levels return to normal. The client is taking furosemide, which is a potassium-wasting diuretic, and the amount of potassium given to compensate for the anticipated losses apparently was too much. This often occurs as a result of the changes of aging. Once serum potassium returns to normal, the level is monitored again at 1 week. With the low dose of furosemide and with captopril (an ACE inhibitor that may retain potassium), the client may not need potassium chloride restarted.

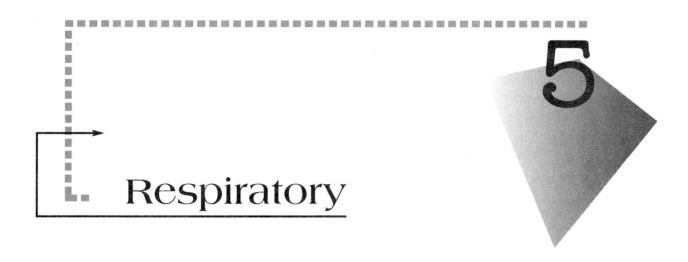

Respiratory

Physical Examination & Diagnostic Tests

1. The nurse practitioner knows that normal breath sounds that have a low pitch and soft intensity and that are heard better on inspiration are called:

   1. Bronchial. ✓
   2. Vesicular.
   3. Bronchovesicular.
   4. Rhonchi.

2. When auscultating for vocal resonance in a client with possible consolidation of lung tissue, the nurse practitioner hears "a-a-a" when the client says "e-e-e." This is called:

   1. Tactile fremitus.
   2. Bronchophony.
   3. Whispered pectoriloquy.
   4. Egophony. ✓

3. The nurse practitioner understands that in percussion of the lungs, hyperresonance is:

   1. A normal finding in the adult client.
   2. Common in pediatric clients.
   3. Characterized by soft intensity, high pitch, short duration, and extremely dull quality.
   4. Characterized by loud intensity, high pitch, medium duration, and dull quality.

4. What is the correct procedure when percussing the chest?

   1. Percuss the entire right side of the anterior chest and move to the left side.
   2. Begin at the upper left side of the posterior chest and compare to the respective anterior side, moving from front to back.
   3. Percuss systematically and symmetrically the anterior chest, moving from left to right side, then percuss the posterior chest.
   4. Percuss the posterior chest, then measure for diaphragmatic excursion on the anterior chest.

5. The nurse practitioner understands that pleural friction rubs are:

   1. Auscultated in the lower anterolateral chest. ✓

   2. Heard best at the end of expiration.

   3. Characterized by a continuous, low-pitched, snoring sound heard early in inspiration.

   4. Noted when the client says "e-e-e" and the examiner hears through the stethoscope "a-a-a."

6. Normal physiologic changes in the respiratory system of the geriatric client include:

   1. Increased rigidity of rib cage and increase in anteroposterior (AP) diameter of chest. ✓

   2. Increased ciliary action resulting in more forceful and recurrent cough.

   3. Increase in number of smaller alveoli with decreased residual capacity.

   4. Decrease in AP diameter of rib cage with decreased lung expansion.

7. When assessing for tactile fremitus, the nurse practitioner would place the hands over what area of the client's chest?

   1. On the anterior chest at level of sixth intercostal space.

   2. At level of bifurcation of the bronchi on posterior chest wall.

   3. On the scapula and sternum.

   4. At level of the diaphragm on posterior chest wall. ✓

8. On assessment of the client's respiratory status, crepitation is felt over the third rib at the midaxillary line on the left side. What is the interpretation of this finding?

   1. There is consolidation of fluid in the left lower lobe of the lung.

   2. Severe inflammation is present on the visceral pleural surfaces of the left lung.

   3. An increase in pressure has occurred in the pleural cavity on the right lung.

   4. Air is present in the subcutaneous tissue from an air leak in the respiratory system. ✓

9. An important anatomic landmark on the anterior thoracic wall is the angle of Louis. Where on the thorax is this landmark present?

   1. The midnipple line on either side of the manubrium.

   2. Bilaterally at the manubriosternal junction. ✓

   3. Midline at the base of the suprasternal notch.

   4. Just below the clavicle but above the manubrium.

10. During the assessment of a geriatric client's respiratory status, the nurse practitioner determines the presence of coarse tactile fremitus posteriorly at the second intercostal space. The best interpretation of this finding is:

    1. Increased air trapping in the alveoli on the affected side.

    2. Presence of fluid or solid mass within the lungs.

    3. Increased pressure in the bronchial tree.

    4. Presence of hyperactive airway disease.

11. When the lateral diameter of the chest is the same size as the AP diameter, the nurse practitioner correctly documents this finding as a:

    1. Biot's deviated chest.

    2. Pigeon chest.

    3. Funnel chest.

    4. Barrel chest. ✓

12. Cystic fibrosis (CF) is the preliminary diagnosis for a young girl who was brought to the clinic for evaluation. The test that will be used to rule out CF is:

    1. Hemoccult test.

    2. Sweat chloride test. ✓

    3. Sputum culture and sensitivity.

    4. Glucose tolerance test.

13. The nurse practitioner is planning a community screening program for lung cancer in geriatric clients. The current evidence-based practice suggests that:

    1. Bronchoscopy with biopsy for cytology should be done every 2–3 years for smokers.

    2. Primary prevention (through discouraging tobacco use) is more effective than screening.

3. Routine screening for lung cancer decreases mortality.

4. Chest x-ray and comparison with previous x-ray is a sensitive test for lung cancer. ✓

14. An adult male client comes to the clinic with the chief complaint of "coughing up blood" and night sweats. He has no history of respiratory or cardiac problems. His vital signs are pulse 96, respirations 28, blood pressure (BP) 140/92, and temperature 99°F orally. The initial diagnostic evaluation of this client includes:

    1. Electrocardiogram, pulmonary function studies, sputum cytology.

    2. PPD skin test, chest x-ray, sputum smear for acid-fast bacillus. ✓

    3. ABG studies, complete blood count, chest x-ray.

    4. Direct bronchoscopy with biopsy and complement fixation antibody titer.

15. A male client comes into the clinic complaining of increased fatigue, irritability, and depression. He reports having difficulty sleeping and wakes up frequently during the night. Based on these symptoms, what else should be determined?

    1. Presence of ongoing daytime sleepiness. osk

    2. History of depression.

    3. Fluctuations in blood pressure.

    4. Recent changes in medications. ✓

16. When assessing the pulmonary function studies of a client, which assessment finding is seen in chronic airflow limitation such as emphysema?

    1. Decreased forced vital capacity (FVC) and forced expiratory volume in 1 second (FEV_1). ✓

    2. Increased functional residual capacity (FRC) and residual volume (RV).

    3. Decreased RV and increased total lung capacity (TLC).

    4. Increased FEV_1 and TLC.

17. When interpreting purified protein derivative (PPD) skin tests in clients at a long-term care facility, the nurse practitioner identifies positive results in individuals with:

    1. Redness or erythema at the site.

    2. Induration reaction ≥5 mm.

    3. Induration reaction ≥10 mm.

    4. Induration reaction up to 15 mm.

Disorders

18. A client has received a blunt trauma injury to his chest. Which assessment finding would be most indicative of further respiratory complications?

    1. Complaints of increased pain over the affected area.

    2. Oximetry readings consistently about 90%.

    3. Decreased breath sounds on the affected side.

    4. Fever of 102°F and increased sputum production.

19. The nurse understands that the following characteristic is more likely to occur when the adult client has pneumonia (due to *Streptococcus pneumoniae*) rather than bronchitis:

    1. Rusty sputum.

    2. Cough. ✓

    3. Dyspnea.

    4. Wheezing.

20. A child is recovering from tuberculosis. What information should be included in a teaching plan for her home care?

    1. It is critical for the child to take medications at the prescribed time; do not skip doses or allow the supply to run out.

    2. Respiratory isolation procedures need to be carried out at home; the child should avoid contact with immediate family members.

    3. It will be necessary for the parent to return to the clinic every week to have the child's sputum checked for viable bacteria.

    4. The child may experience a rash along with nausea and vomiting from the medications; the parent should decrease the dosage if this occurs.

21. What would be a priority intervention for a client experiencing a respiratory arrest?

    1. Start chest compressions at 15 compressions and two breaths.

    2. Open the airway with a head tilt and chin lift.

    3. Give oxygen using rebreathing mask at 10 L/min.

    4. Pinch the nose and give two breaths.

22. A client comes to the emergency department (ED) complaining of difficulty breathing. What is most important to establish initially in this client?

    1. Type of activity that produces the dyspnea. ✓

    2. Presence of consolidation on chest x-ray.

    3. ABG levels with respect to oxygen pressures.

    4. Presence of bilateral breath sounds over the lower lobes.

23. A client is severely dyspneic, and the history strongly suggests the possibility of a foreign body in the bronchi. What observation would contribute to the documentation of this problem?

    1. Unilateral retraction of the right chest wall.

    2. Presence of crepitation on the anterior chest wall.

    3. Retraction of the lower chest wall.

    4. A friction rub heard over the area of the bronchi.

24. The nurse practitioner is assessing a client who is complaining of shortness of breath and chest discomfort. His respirations are shallow at 26 breaths/min. When evaluating the diaphragmatic excursion, it is determined that the diaphragm on the right is slightly higher than on the left side. The best interpretation of these findings is:

    1. This is normal due to the liver on the right side.

    2. There may be atelectasis in the right lower lobe.

    3. Consolidation is present in the right lower lobe. ✓

    4. This indicates the presence of early stages of chronic obstructive lung disease.

25. A 22-year-old male comes to the office complaining of chest pain and shortness of breath. He states the problems started suddenly after running sprints in basketball practice. He states he has no past history of pulmonary problems. He is about 72 inches tall and 145 lb, with pulse rate 118, respiratory rate 30, decreased breath sounds, and hyperresonance over left lung. Based on the findings, what is the best diagnosis for this client?

    1. Spontaneous pneumothorax. ✓

    2. Exercise-induced asthma.

    3. Pulmonary edema.

    4. Acute bronchiectasis.

26. A young woman presents at the clinic with complaints of tingling in her face and hands, sudden shortness of breath, and vague chest discomfort. She appears very anxious and denies any history of respiratory problems. On examination her hands are cool to touch; her vital signs are respirations 34, pulse regular at 100, BP 110/76, and normal temperature. Respiratory examination reveals bilateral breath sounds with tachypnea, no adventitious sounds, and normal percussion and visual examination of the chest. What is the best immediate treatment?

    1. Rebreathing into paper bag and encouraging controlled diaphragmatic breathing. ✓

    2. Two puffs of short-acting bronchdilator (albuterol) with metered-dose inhaler (MDI).

    3. Oxygen at 4 L and arterial blood gases (ABGs) after 30 minutes.

    4. Establish intravenous (IV) line; infuse 500 ml normal saline for volume depletion.

27. An 18-month-old infant brought to the ED is awake, lethargic, and in severe respiratory distress. His mother states that he has not been sick and was playing on the floor when he suddenly began coughing, choking, and gagging. He has expiratory wheezes, with decreased breath sounds over right lower lobes; respirations 36, pulse 130, temperature normal. Portable chest x-ray shows hyperinflation on expiratory views. The best treatment for this infant is:

    1. Bronchoscopy as soon as possible.

    2. Cool-mist therapy with racemic epinephrine.

    3. Antibiotics with chest physiotherapy.

    4. Immediate endotracheal intubation and ventilation.

28. A 4-month-old client presents to the office with a history of several days of rhinorrhea, cough, low-grade fever, and increased respiratory rate. What is the most likely diagnosis?

    1. Croup.

    2. Epiglottitis.

    3. Tracheitis.

    4. Bronchiolitis.

29. A client with newly diagnosed chronic obstructive pulmonary disease (COPD) is being discharged from the hospital. The nurse practitioner is discussing home care with the client. What information is important for the practitioner to include in the home care teaching?

    1. Use the bronchodilator before exercising.

    2. Maintain bed rest for the first few days at home.

    3. Decrease amount of fluid intake to prevent fluid overload.

    4. Maintain oxygen flow rate of about 5–7 L.

30. A client is admitted to a rural ED by ambulance. Primary assessment reveals:

    - Respirations: 38/min with use of accessory muscles, prolonged expiration, and wheezes
    - ECG: Sinus tachycardia of 140 beats/min
    - BP: 192/98 mm Hg
    - Lethargic: Responds to name only by opening eye
    - Cyanosis of lips

    Therapeutic interventions initiated by emergency medical technicians include:

    - IV therapy with D_5W at 30 ml/hr
    - O_2 therapy at 48% by Venturi mask

    STAT arterial blood gases (ABGs) indicate:

    - pH of 7.24.
    - $Paco_2$ of 82 mm Hg.
    - Pao_2 of 76 mm Hg.
    - HCO_3^- of 36 mEq/L.

    Before obtaining a second set of ABGs, the nurse practitioner would:

    1. Assist respirations using bag-valve mask with 100% oxygen.

    2. Administer 1 ampule of sodium bicarbonate.

    3. Change oxygen delivery to nasal cannula at 2 L.

    4. Disconnect the supplemental oxygen.

31. Instructions on nutritional therapy for the elderly COPD client would include foods that are:

    1. High caloric, high protein, low carbohydrate.

    2. High caloric, low protein, high carbohydrate.

    3. Low caloric, high protein, low carbohydrate.

    4. Low caloric, low protein, high carbohydrate.

32. Age-associated changes that increase the risk for pneumonia in the elderly client include an increase in:

    1. Compliance of the chest wall.

    2. Diameter of the trachea and bronchi.

    3. Lung parenchyma.

    4. Cough forcefulness.

33. An adult client arrives at the clinic complaining of difficulty breathing, a cough, and chest pain. History indicates that she was discharged from the hospital 2 days ago after a cesarean section and has a 15-pack-year smoking history. Diagnostic studies should include:

    1. Sputum for culture and sensitivity.

    2. Cardiac troponin proteins.

    3. Pulse oximetry.

    4. Arterial blood gases.

34. The nurse practitioner is aware that the flu or influenza:

    1. Can be caused by receiving a flu vaccine when one's resistance is low.

    2. Is characterized by a slow, insidious onset of chills, fever, and muscle aches.

    3. In older adults may persist for several weeks with symptoms of lack of energy and extreme tiredness.

    4. Is primarily contagious in the early autumn and spring, with children at greatest risk.

35. During physical examination of a 2-year-old diagnosed with possible cystic fibrosis, the child passes a stool. The nurse practitioner would expect the stool's appearance to be:

    1. Yellow and loose.

    2. Small and constipated.

    3. Green and odorous.

    4. Large and bulky.

36. An adult client with a history of asthma calls to tell the nurse practitioner that she is "blowing 55%" on the peak flowmeter. What advice would the nurse practitioner give this client?

    1. Call an ambulance immediately.

    2. Use a bronchodilator now and come in for evaluation in the office today. ✓

    3. Come in for office evaluation this week.

    4. Refer to a pulmonary physician.

37. An elderly client is evaluated by the nurse practitioner for a complaint of cough, fever, chest pain, and sputum production. In gathering a history on this client, it is important to know if the client has:

    1. Received the pneumococcal vaccine.

    2. Traveled out of the country.

    3. Pets in the household.

    4. Recently started new medications.

38. An elderly client presents with signs and symptoms that make the nurse practitioner suspect the diagnosis of pneumonia. Which assessment would the nurse practitioner most likely evaluate during the examination?

    1. Chest pain with inspiration.

    2. Confusion with a low-grade temperature.

    3. Congested, productive cough.

    4. Fever with leukocytosis.

39. In developing a plan for an older client with pneumonia, the nurse practitioner understands that 30%–40% of community-acquired pneumonia is caused by which organism?

    1. *Haemophilus influenzae.*

    2. *Klebsiella pneumoniae.*

    3. *Mycobacterium tuberculosis.*

    4. *Streptococcus pneumoniae.*

40. What would be most appropriate to include in the health promotion plan for an older client who is at risk for developing pneumonia?

    1. Administer the pneumococcal vaccination annually.

    2. Administer the pneumococcal vaccination and yearly influenza immunization.

    3. Sputum culture annually along with a chest x-ray.

    4. Purified protein derivative (PPD) every 3–5 years.

41. The nurse practitioner evaluates an older client with a current history of alcoholism. The client presents with an elevated temperature, congested cough producing rusty sputum, and occasional chills. The suspected diagnosis is bacterial pneumonia. The Gram-stained sputum smear would most likely reveal which organism?

    1. *Haemophilus influenzae.*

    2. *Klebsiella pneumoniae.*

    3. *Staphylococcus aureus.*

    4. *Streptococcus pneumoniae.*

42. An elderly client residing in a nursing home has recently been exposed to tuberculosis (TB). The nurse practitioner interprets the initial PPD test to be negative. Which plan would be most appropriate at this time?

    1. Evaluate client in another year.

    2. Repeat PPD test in 1 week.

    3. Ignore results and immediately begin ethambutol.

    4. Evaluate client in 6 months, since he is asymptomatic at this time.

43. The nurse practitioner knows that Horner's syndrome is often associated with:

    1. Chronic bronchitis.

    2. Pulmonary tuberculosis.

    3. Pancoast's syndrome of lung cancer.

    4. Pulmonary embolism.

44. An adult client who smokes presents with complaints of breathlessness. The nurse practitioner notes on examination dilated blood vessels on the chest and mild edema of the head and supraclavicular area. She recognizes this condition as:

    1. Thyroid abnormality.

    2. Chronic bronchitis with mild congestive failure.

    3. Asthma with fluid retention.

    4. Superior vena cava obstruction.

45. A 3-year-old client with a history of asthma presents to the office for evaluation by the nurse practitioner. The child has never used a peak flowmeter. What quick tool can the nurse practitioner use to assess the severity of this child's distress?

    1. ABG study.

    2. Child's inability to complete a sentence.

    3. Chest x-ray.

    4. Presence of runny nose.

46. An elderly client presents with postural hypotension, and laboratory studies reveal hyponatremia. Which is the most likely cause of these findings?

    1. Diabetic ketoacidosis.

    2. Severe trauma.

    3. Bronchogenic carcinoma.

    4. Antacid overuse.

47. The nurse practitioner knows the following about asthma in elderly clients:

    1. Subcutaneous epinephrine is standard therapy.

    2. It is usually of the allergic type.

    3. Attacks are usually preceded by viral infections.

    4. Clinical presentation is usually dyspnea, costal retraction, and fever.

48. Clinical signs and symptoms of late-phase asthma include:

    1. Bronchoconstriction refractory to bronchodilator therapy.

    2. Sneezing, watery eyes, and cough.

    3. Wheezing and increased sputum production.

    4. Bronchodilatation secondary to release of histamine.

49. The nurse practitioner is assessing a client for asthma. What is a common clinical manifestation of asthma?

    1. Pruritus.

    2. Diffuse crackles.

    3. Nocturnal exacerbation.

    4. Chronic hypoxemia.

50. During a routine follow-up visit for a client with asthma, she states that she has been doing fine except that, when she goes out for dinner, she has increased bronchospasm and wheezing. Which of the following would be an appropriate response by the nurse practitioner?

    1. "Have you been taking your medication?"

    2. "Do you usually have wine with dinner?"

    3. "I recommend you do not go out for dinner."

    4. "Does going out to dinner make you stressed?"

51. A mother tells the nurse practitioner that her child has nocturnal asthma attacks. The nurse practitioner would expect the mother to explain that the attacks are the worst:

    1. At midnight.

    2. Two hours after going to bed.

    3. Immediately after falling asleep.

    4. At 4 AM.

52. The nurse practitioner understands the following about tuberculosis (TB):

    1. Infants are more likely than children to present with wheezing and rales.

    2. Older children develop disseminated disease and meningitis more often than infants.

    3. Affected infants and young children are more likely to have a PPD skin test ≥ 15 mm.

    4. Adults are rarely the source of the disease when a child develops TB.

53. During a triannual visit to the clinic for routine care, the mother reports that her infant diagnosed with bronchopulmonary dysplasia (BPD) has been vomiting after each gastrostomy feeding. The nurse practitioner notes that the infant's weight gain is adequate and would recommend:

    1. Referral to the pediatrician for follow-up.

    2. Reduction in amount of formula for the gastrostomy feeding.

    3. Addition of 3 oz of Pedialyte for the next two feedings.

    4. Positioning of the infant in a prone position after feedings with head and trunk elevated.

54. A 3-year-old child with up-to-date immunizations is brought to the office by his mother with a fairly rapid onset of stridor and a high-pitched wheeze. In view of this information, what would be the **least** important condition to consider for the differential diagnosis?

    1. Croup.

    2. Foreign body aspiration.

    3. Epiglottitis.

    4. Bacterial tracheitis.

55. The practitioner is evaluating a 60-year-old man with symptoms characteristic of obstructive sleep apnea. An overnight polysmnogram (PSG) is ordered. What is the characteristic result of this study that would confirm sleep apnea?

    1. Loud snoring all night long.

    2. Oxygen desaturation and 10-second periods of apnea.

    3. Frequent periods of brief arousal during sleep.

    4. Periods of 5-second apnea with brief arousal.

56. The practitioner is screening geriatric clients for problems related to sleep apnea. What risk factors are typically associated with this condition?

    1. Male, obese, over 55 years old.

    2. Female, obese, over 35 years old.

    3. Female, history of respiratory problems, loud snoring.

    4. Male, history of chronic respiratory disease, increased daytime sleeping.

57. A client comes to the clinic complaining of difficulty breathing, lethargy, and coughing up blood in his sputum. He has no history of chronic illness or major health problems. The nurse practitioner orders diagnostic tests to determine the problem. What diagnostic test results would require immediate treatment of this client?

    1. Positive sputum smear for acid-fast bacillus.

    2. Sputum culture positive for *Pneumocystis carinii*.

    3. Presence of hemolysis on complement fixation test.

    4. Oxygen saturation 94%, leukocyte count >5000 WBCs/mm^3.

Pharmacology

58. The nurse practitioner is following up on a client who is experiencing acute asthmatic problems. Albuterol (Proventil) by metered-dose inhaler (MDI) has been ordered as treatment. Which client response would indicate to the nurse practitioner that the client understands how to take his medication?

    1. "I will take 1 puff of the medication, then wait a minute before taking the second puff."

    2. "I will take 2 puffs of the medication every 4 hours, even if I am not short of breath."

    3. "It is important for me to take this medication on a regular cycle to prevent future attacks."

    4. "I will take 2 puffs, one right after the other, whenever I begin to get short of breath."

59. A client who was recently diagnosed with tuberculosis calls the clinic because her urine is reddish orange. She is taking isoniazid (INH), rifampin (Rifadin), and pyrazinamide. What would be an appropriate response for the nurse practitioner to make?

    1. "This is a urinary tract infection symptom; drink plenty of fluids."

    2. "This is a normal response to the rifampin."

    3. "Often this is an indication of liver toxicity. Stop the medications."

    4. "This is probably bleeding, and you should see a physician immediately."

60. A 15-year-old girl comes to the ED with complaints of extreme shortness of breath. She is confused, and her past medical history is not available. Her vital signs are pulse 124, respirations 32, BP 124/80, and temperature normal. Physical examination reveals diffuse expiratory wheezes, hyperresonance on percussion, and prolonged expiratory phase. The best treatment for this client includes:

1. Aminophylline by mouth.

2. Beclomethasone (Beclovent) inhaler.

3. Epinephrine by injection.

4. Albuterol (Proventil) by MDI.

61. A client with a history of bronchial asthma is seen in the clinic for increased episodes of difficulty breathing. He has been taking theophylline 100 mg PO tid. He is 40 years old and obese with an 18-pack-year history of cigarette smoking and excessive intake of coffee daily. He eats a low-carbohydrate, high-protein diet. Which identified factors decrease the therapeutic effects of the theophylline?

1. Age and gender.

2. Coffee intake and weight.

3. Age and weight.

4. Smoking history and diet.

62. A 70-year-old man comes to the clinic with complaints that he is experiencing increased difficulty breathing over the past few days. He has a history of COPD and coronary artery disease. He was recently diagnosed with hypertension. Examination reveals no jugular vein distention, a slight increase in AP diameter of the chest, and no productive cough. Breath sounds are present, but expiratory wheezes are noted bilaterally, and he denies any chest pain. His vital signs are pulse 72, respirations 34, and BP 170/100. His current medications are ipratropium (Atrovent) inhaler 2 puffs q6h, nitroglycerin transdermal patches, and propranolol (Inderal) 60 mg PO bid. What is the best treatment for this client?

1. Discontinue propranolol and begin verapamil (Calan) 80 mg PO tid qd.

2. Begin theophylline (Theo-24; methylxanthine) 200 mg q12h PO.

3. Discontinue propranolol (Inderal) and begin atenolol (Tenormin) 50 mg PO qd.

4. Start beclomethasone (Beclovent) inhaler 2 puffs 3–4 times daily.

63. The recommended range for maintaining serum theophylline levels is:

1. 0.05–2 µg/ml.

2. 10–20 µg/ml

3. 20–25 µg/ml.

4. 30–40 µg/ml.

64. A client in a long-term facility whose roommate has been diagnosed with active tuberculosis should be started on chemoprophylaxis:

1. As soon as possible and initiated at the time of screening skin testing.

2. In 72 hours after PPD skin test results are obtained.

3. Only if PPD skin test results are positive.

4. In 3 months if the repeated skin test is positive.

65. In adults with asthma, the most common reason outpatient treatment fails, resulting in hospitalization, is:

1. Exposure to allergens.

2. Increased use of steroids.

3. Improper inhaler technique.

4. Use of cromolyn inhalers.

66. Which can elevate theophylline levels?

1. Concomitant treatment with cimetidine (Tagamet).

2. Intravenous ampicillin.

3. Heavy smoking.

4. History of seizure disorder.

67. A client with a long history of chronic airflow limitation has noticed a change in sputum over the past few days, with increased amount of thick yellow-green mucus and congestion. What would be the appropriate therapy?

1. Hismanal 10 mg PO qd.

2. Augmentin 500 mg PO tid for 10 days.

3. Tylenol with codeine.

4. Vancenase MDI 2 puffs prn.

68. Which medication is most effective in promoting a decrease in airway inflammation as well as providing long-term medication coverage in a client with asthma?

    1. Montelukast (Singulair).

    2. Beclomethasone (Vanceril, Beclovent).

    3. Albuterol (Proventil, Ventolin).

    4. Salmeterol (Serevent).

69. The nurse practitioner is planning prophylactic treatment for a client with asthma. Which is the best medication for the asthmatic client who is not currently experiencing an exacerbation?

    1. Antibiotic.

    2. Inhaled glucocorticoid.

    3. β_2-Agonist.

    4. Methacholine challenge.

70. Clients with asthma need to be instructed to:

    1. Begin inhaled steroids as soon as symptoms appear.

    2. Take 2 puffs of β_2-agonist prn using MDI.

    3. Use inhaled steroids when they experience bronchospasm.

    4. Start antibiotic regimen when they experience bronchospasm.

71. The nurse practitioner understands that an appropriate medication regimen for a child with drug-susceptible pulmonary tuberculosis (TB) is:

    1. Montelukast (Singulair) therapy with rifampin (Rifadin).

    2. Streptomycin, pyrazinamide, and rimantadine (Flumadine).

    3. Isoniazid (INH), pyrazinamide, and rifampin.

    4. Montelukast therapy with pyrimethamine (Fansidar).

72. During a routine well-child examination of a 4-year-old, the nurse practitioner learns that the paternal grandmother has just been diagnosed with active TB. The mother states that the grandmother had stayed in their home for a week during the summer. The child has no signs

of TB and has a negative PPD. What action should the nurse practitioner take?

    1. Prescribe no medications, but schedule a repeat PPD in 2 months.

    2. Administer 1 ml gamma globulin IM.

    3. Start combination therapy with isoniazid (INH) and rifampin (Rifadin) for 15 months.

    4. Start isoniazid (INH) therapy for 3 months and then reevaluate.

73. A client presents in the clinic with a dry, hacking, nonproductive cough that is interfering with her sleep. The nurse practitioner would encourage the client to purchase an over-the-counter preparation that contains:

    1. Pseudoephedrine.

    2. Diphenhydramine.

    3. Guaifenesin.

    4. Dextromethorphan.

74. Indications for antibiotic use in a child with asthmatic bronchitis would include:

    1. History of two episodes in 4 months.

    2. Rhinitis and a productive cough.

    3. High fever and rales.

    4. Low-grade fever and sibilant wheezes.

75. A 10-year-old taking INH prophylactically for exposure to TB complains of headache, palpitations, rash, and diarrhea. Management would be based on:

    1. Avoidance of foods containing tyramine and histamine.

    2. Addition of pyridoxine to the diet.

    3. Change in therapy from INH to rifampin.

    4. Evaluation for for hepatic impairment.

76. What is the initial treatment of choice for children diagnosed with bronchiolitis?

    1. Increase fluids; albuterol (Ventolin) in saline inhalation every 4–6 hours.

    2. Prednisolone (Pediapred) immediately and continue over 3–5 days.

3. Diphenhydramine HCl (Benadryl) as long as symptoms persist.

4. Amoxicillin over 10–14 days; aerosol humidification.

77. A 10-year-old boy is experiencing problems with wheezing, coughing, and shortness of breath about 4 hours after basketball practice. He has normal respirations and only experiences the problems after exercise. He is experiencing no other respiratory problems, and the physical findings are within normal limits. What is the treatment of choice for this child?

1. Albuterol (Ventolin) 2 puffs MDI 20–30 minutes before exercise.

2. Cromolyn sodium (Intal) 2 puffs each morning.

3. Theophylline (Theo-24; methylxanthine) 100 mg PO bid.

4. Beclomethasone (Beclovent) 2 puffs 3–4 times daily.

78. A client with chronic asthma is seen in the clinic complaining of vomiting and stomach cramps. He is confused and is unsure what medications he is currently taking. His vital signs are BP 158/92, pulse 152 and irregular, and respirations 28 and shallow. What STAT diagnostic study should be obtained?

1. Serum electrolytes.

2. Digoxin level.

3. Theophylline level.

4. Arterial blood gases.

79. A client is seen in the clinic complaining of increased difficulty breathing and an intermittent productive cough that worsens in the evening. The history revels that the client has a 20-pack-year history of smoking. Breath sounds are clear to auscultation, there is no evidence of fever, and chest radiography is within normal limits. The nurse practitioner instructs the client concerning the importance of smoking cessation and fluid therapy and prescribes:

1. Erythromycin 500 mg PO qid × 14 days.

2. Albuterol 2 mg PO tid. ✓

3. Mucomyst 10 ml 10% solution q4h prn.

4. Tetracycline 100 mg q12h × 14 days.

80. When initiating preventive care to decrease the incidence of pneumonia in clients in an extended-care facility, the nurse practitioner would identify clients receiving immunosuppressive therapy, repeated antibiotic use, sedation, and:

1. β_1-Adrenergic blockers.

2. Calcium channel blockers.

3. Diuretics.

4. Histamine (H_2) antagonists.

81. An older adult client presents with complaints of dyspnea, cough, fatigue, and dependent edema that has been worsening over the past few days. In planning treatment, the nurse practitioner considers:

1. Streptokinase therapy.

2. Referral for hospitalization for evaluation of heart function.

> depends on severity

3. Prescription for furosemide (Lasix) 40 mg PO qd.

4. Addition of a calcium channel blocker to the client's medications.

82. A client with a history of Parkinson's disease has a positive TB skin test, and INH is ordered as a prophylactic medication. Before beginning INH, it is important for the nurse practitioner to determine:

1. If the client's Parkinson's condition is being treated with levodopa (Larodopa). ✓

2. How long the client has been diagnosed with Parkinson's disease.

3. How much respiratory compromise the client is currently experiencing.

4. The adequacy of urine output and renal function.

3 b/c INH to ↓ results

83. A geriatric client with a history of COPD is seen for an upper respiratory infection, and the nurse practitioner decides to have the physician prescribe erythromycin. On review of the client's history, what current medication would be a contraindication to the administration of erythromycin?

1. Theophylline (Theo-24). ✓

2. Lisinopril (Zestril).

3. Moexipril (Univasc).

4. Atenolol (Tenormin).

84. A 50-year-old white male with a history of COPD presents to the clinic with increased dyspnea, temperature 39°C (102°F), pulse 104, respirations 44, and O_2 saturation of 84%. Physical examination reveals diffuse rales and rhonchi bilaterally. Medications include atenolol (Tenormin) 25 mg PO qd, prednisone (Deltasone) 10 mg PO qd, ipratropium (Atrovent) 1–2 puffs 18 μg qid prn, and fluticasone propionate (Advair), 2 puffs 100/50 bid. The nurse practitioner's preliminary diagnosis is pneumonia, pending chest x-ray results. Which medication puts this patient at risk to become immunocompromised?

1. Atenolol.

2. Prednisone.

3. Ipratropium.

4. Fluticasone.

Answers & Rationales

Physical Examination & Diagnostic Tests

1. **(2)** Vesicular breath sounds are heard over normal lung tissue. The inspiratory phase of these low-pitched soft sounds is heard better and is about 2.5 times longer than the expiratory phase. Bronchial breath sounds, normally heard over the trachea, are high-pitched loud sounds with a shortened inspiratory and lengthened expiratory phase. Bronchovesicular breath sounds, heard mainly over the second interspace anteriorly and between the scapulae posteriorly, have an intermediate pitch and intensity with equal duration of expiratory and inspiratory sounds. Rhonchi are abnormal breath sounds that are low pitched with a snoring quality.

2. **(4)** Tactile fremitus is a palpable vibration of the thoracic wall that is produced when the client speaks. Bronchophony is the increase in loudness and clarity of vocal resonance. Whispered pectoriloquy is exaggerated bronchophony and is heard through a stethoscope when the client whispers a series of words (e.g., "ninety-nine"). In egophony, the spoken voice has a nasal or bleating quality when heard through a stethoscope, and the spoken "e-e-e" sounds like "a-a-a."

3. **(2)** Hyperresonance is an abnormal percussion tone in adults but occurs normally in a child's lung. It is characterized by very loud intensity, very low pitch, long duration, and a booming quality.

4. **(3)** Both the anterior and the posterior chest should be percussed systematically and symmetrically, moving from left to right. Diaphragmatic excursion is usually only measured on the posterior chest.

5. **(1)** Pleural friction rubs are loud, dry, creaking or grating sounds produced by the rubbing together of inflamed and roughened pleural surfaces. Rubs are heard best during the latter part of inspiration and the beginning of expiration and in the lower anterolateral chest. Option #3 is characteristic of sonorous rhonchi. Option #4 is characteristic of egophony.

6. **(1)** With aging the number of alveoli decreases. The alveoli become rigid and lose their recoil and elasticity, which affects the client's ability to exhale effectively. Residual volume increases, whereas basilar inflation and ability to expel foreign matter decrease. The AP diameter of the chest increases, as seen in clients with kyphosis.

7. **(2)** The bifurcation of the trachea or bronchi on the posterior chest wall is the best area for assessment of tactile fremitus. Care should be taken to avoid the area over the scapula and sternum because bone dampens vibrations.

8. **(4)** Crepitation or crepitus (also called subcutaneous emphysema) usually results from air bubbles under the skin caused by a rupture in the respiratory system. Infection by a gas-producing organism is a less common cause. Crepitation always requires attention.

9. **(2)** This landmark can be used to determine the position of the second rib and intercostal space and corresponding spaces below that level. The angle of Louis is a visible and palpable angle of the sternum at the point where the second rib attaches to the sternum.

10. **(2)** Fluid or a solid mass transmits the vibrations, so tactile fremitus may be felt on the exterior chest wall. Increased air trapping decreases or masks fremitus. A reactive airway results in wheezing due to an edematous airway.

11. **(4)** The adult chest is somewhat asymmetric, and the AP diameter is often half the transverse diameter. Pigeon chest (pectus carinatum) is a forward protrusion of the sternum with the ribs sloping back. Funnel chest (pectus excavatum) is a depression of the sternum. Barrel chest occurs when the AP diameter equals the transverse diameter.

12. **(2)** Sweat chloride test is positive for CF due to the abnormal amount of sodium chloride in the sweat. Hemoccult is a test for blood in the stool. Sputum culture and sensitivity help determine which medication is effective against an organism. Glucose tolerance test is performed to diagnose diabetes.

13. **(2)** "Primary prevention is more effective than screening in reducing the lung cancer morbidity and mortality" (*Guide to Clinical Preventive Services*, 1996, p. 137). Current evidence-based research does not support routine screening for lung cancer. There is insufficient evidence that lung cancer screening by x-ray or sputum cytology reduces mortality. Bronchoscopy with biopsy is a diagnostic test, not a screening test.

14. **(2)** The client should be initially evaluated for tuberculosis. Pulmonary function studies, arterial blood gas (ABG) studies, and bronchoscopy are not indicated at this time. Complement fixation studies are done to diagnose atypical pneumonia.

15. **(1)** Ongoing daytime sleepiness is the hallmark of obstructive sleep apnea (OSA). Options #3 and 4 should be evaluated, but symptoms reported are classic with OSA.

16. **(2)** Hyperinflation due to air trapping causes an increase in FRC, RV, and TLC (which may be twice normal). A corresponding decrease in FVC and FEV$_1$ occurs. This causes a flattening of the diaphragm, decreased inspiratory efficiency, and increased work of breathing.

17. **(3)** Positive interpretation of PPD skin test results are as follows:

Induration	Positive Test Result
≥5 mm	Individuals with human immunodeficiency virus (HIV) infection
	Individuals in recent close contact with persons who have active tuberculosis (TB)
	Individuals with chest x-ray indicating healed TB
≥10 mm	Medically underserved individuals
	Intravenous drug users
	Residents in long-term care facilities and health care workers
≥15 mm	All individuals

Disorders

18. **(3)** The most common respiratory complication after a traumatic injury to the chest is pneumothorax caused from a fractured rib. Oximetry readings at 90% and increased pain are expected at this point and may not be indicative of a problem.

19. **(1)** Pneumococcal pneumonia due to *Streptococcus pneumoniae* often presents abruptly with high fever, shaking chills (rigor), cough productive of purulent or rusty sputum, headache, and pleuritic chest pain. In acute bronchitis, cough is the primary symptom and initially is dry and nonproductive. Fever, dyspnea, wheezing, and possible mucoid sputum production are also characteristic of acute bronchitis.

20. **(1)** On discharge a client must understand the importance of taking medications as prescribed. Missed doses increase mutation of the tubercle bacillus and decrease the medication's effectiveness. Respiratory isolation at home is not necessary, and if she experiences problems of rash, nausea, and vomiting, she should contact her health care provider. Weekly sputum checks are not necessary.

21. **(2)** According to the American Heart Association, the protocol for cardiopulmonary resuscitation (CPR; rescue breathing) due to respiratory arrest would be to open the airway by tilting the head and lifting the chin.

22. **(1)** It is most important to determine what precipitates the dyspnea. Is it present during rest, or does it occur with activity? What level of activity precipitates dyspnea? This information is necessary to determine the severity of the client's complaint.

23. **(1)** The most common area for a foreign body obstruction is the right bronchi, which produces a unilateral retraction of the right chest wall. Retraction of the lower chest occurs with lower respiratory problems such as asthma. A pleural friction rub is heard when there is inflammation between the visceral and parietal pleura. Crepitation is present when air is leaking into the subcutaneous tissue.

24. **(1)** This is a normal finding due to the bulk of the liver. Atelectasis and consolidation present with normal diaphragmatic movement but with dullness to percussion over the affected area. Obstructive lung disease results in hyperresonance and limited diaphragmatic excursion but is bilateral.

25. **(1)** Spontaneous pneumothorax occurs in healthy, thin young adults, especially after strenuous exercise; predominant symptoms include sudden pain and dyspnea. The clinical hallmark of asthma is wheezing; with pulmonary edema there is frequently coughing, frothy sputum, and crackles heard on auscultation. Bronchiectasis is most often chronic and is characterized by moist crackles and wheezing on ausculation; cough is usually present.

26. **(1)** The situation described is hyperventilation; by slowing breathing and breathing into a paper bag, the carbon dioxide levels will be restored and the acid-base problem resolved. Albuterol, oxygen, ABGs, and IV fluids are not appropriate initial treatment.

27. **(1)** The child has the symptoms and history that are consistent with a partial airway obstruction from aspiration of a foreign body. Direct laryngoscopy or bronchoscopy is necessary to remove the foreign body. Chest physiotherapy may dislodge the object and force it farther into the airway. Antibiotics and epinephrine will not be effective. There is no need to intubate the infant if the foreign body can be removed.

28. **(4)** Croup, epiglottitis, and tracheitis are all middle respiratory tract infections with a rapid onset. Bronchiolitis is a lower respiratory tract infection that has a more gradual onset and no "barking" sound to the cough.

29. **(1)** To prevent dyspnea on activity, the bronchodilator should be used before walking or increased physical activity. The client should not stay in bed and should be encouraged to increase activity gradually. Fluid intake of 2–3 L/day should be encouraged, unless there are cardiac problems. The oxygen level should not exceed a 3- to 4-L flow.

30. **(3)** Elevated serum bicarbonate (HCO_3^-) levels are expected in clients with chronic hypercapnia. Hypoventilation and acidemia can result when too much oxygen is delivered. Supplemental oxygen should not be discontinued because arterial oxygen partial pressure (PaO_2) levels decrease faster than the stimulus to breathe returns to eliminate the accumulated store of carbon dioxide (CO_2). Discontinuing supplemental oxygen, even for a short time, could cause serious complications.

31. **(1)** Nutritional needs are meet by high-caloric, high-protein foods. High-carbohydrate foods need to be avoided in clients who retain CO_2 because carbohydrates metabolize into CO_2 as a waste product.

32. **(2)** Age-associated physiologic changes include:

    - Decreased compliance of chest wall, making deep inspiration difficult.
    - Trachea and bronchi increase in diameter, increasing dead space and resulting in a decreased volume of air reaching the alveoli. Increase in small airway closure results in decreased vital capacity and increased residual volume.
    - Lung parenchyma become less elastic, which decreases function of the alveoli.
    - Breathing becomes shallower and cough less forceful because respiratory muscles weaken.

33. **(4)** The client is at risk for a pulmonary embolism as a result of hypercoagulation related to giving birth, smoking, and vascular injury (recent surgery). Assessment reveals common symptoms of pulmonary embolism: dyspnea, cough, and pleuritic pain. Diagnostic tests include ABGs, 12-lead

electrocardiogram (ECG), chest x-ray, and echocardiogram.

34. **(3)** The flu or influenza is a highly contagious respiratory infection that occurs epidemically during the winter cold months. It is characterized by a sudden onset of chills, elevated temperature (101°–104°F), headache, fatigue, muscle pain, dry cough, laryngitis, rhinorrhea, and red eyes occurring 24–48 hours after exposure directly through respiratory droplets from an infected person or indirectly by drinking from a contaminated glass. Flu vaccines do not cause the flu; they are made with a killed virus.

35. **(4)** In CF the stools are large, bulky, and foul smelling (steatorrhea). Yellow stools are indicative of liver or gallbladder problems. Green stools often indicate a rapid transit time and may be associated with an infection.

36. **(2)** This client is considered to be in the "yellow" zone of personal best peak flow but is close to the "red" zone (50% or less of personal best). The client should use her bronchodilator immediately and if not improved may need emergency intervention by the nurse practitioner.

37. **(1)** The pneumococcal vaccine is recommended for elderly clients because their immune system is less efficient. The symptoms of fever, chest pain, and sputum production suggest pneumonia.

38. **(2)** Confusion may be the first sign that the elderly client is septic. The client may not have a temperature or leukocytosis. The client may not experience any discomfort or a cough.

39. **(4)** *Streptococcus pneumoniae* is the most common cause of community-acquired and nursing home–acquired pneumonia and the most common bacterial pathogen (30%–40% of pneumonia cases). *Haemophilus influenzae* is common in elderly clients with underlying chronic diseases (e.g., COPD, diabetes). *Klebsiella pneumoniae* and other gram-negative bacteria are pathogens in alcoholics, immunocompromised hosts, and hospitalized clients. *Mycobacterium tuberculosis* is an infrequent cause of pneumonia.

40. **(2)** Pneumococcal vaccination and yearly influenza immunization will decrease complications and hospitalizations for the older client. The pneumococcal vaccination is not administered annually. Options #3 and #4 are not recommended. The PPD should be done annually for high-risk clients.

41. **(2)** *Klebsiella pneumoniae* is an important pathogen in alcoholic clients. *Staphylococcus aureus* generally affects elderly clients recovering from influenza and is also common in hospitalized and diabetic clients. (See rationale for answer to Question 39.)

42. **(2)** Up to 25% of elderly clients with newly diagnosed TB have a negative tuberculin skin test due to waning cellular immunity with senescence. If the initial PPD test is negative, a repeat PPD test 1 week later is recommended in elderly clients. The repeat test is useful to stimulate a booster phenomenon in clients whose initial infection occurred many years earlier. The other options contain incorrect information.

43. **(3)** Horner's syndrome, which is paralysis of the cervical sympathetic nerves resulting in ptosis, loss of sweating, constriction of the pupil, and sinking of the eyeball on one side, is often associated with malignant tumors in the upper lung leading to nerve compression.

44. **(4)** Superior vena cava obstruction is a complication of malignancy involving the mediastinum and rapidly progresses into an oncologic emergency.

45. **(2)** In children too young to use a peak flowmeter properly, the inability to cry or complete a sentence may indicate an acute asthma attack. An ABG study is usually not performed in office settings, and a chest x-ray will most likely agitate the child and take too long to process.

46. **(3)** Hyponatremia results from an overproduction of antidiuretic hormone caused by ectopic production from the bronchogenic tumor. Ketoacidosis and trauma result in fluid loss causing hypernatremia, as does overuse of sodium-containing antacids.

47. **(3)** In older individuals the asthma is usually accompanied by infection. It is rarely allergic, and costal retraction and fever are not usually seen. Subcutaneous epinephrine is not standard treatment but may be indicated in emergency situations.

48. **(1)** Late-phase asthma occurs at 6–12 hours after the initial or acute bronchoconstrictive phase. The inflammatory response is the result of mast cell degranulation and release of histamine. Histamine acts on the lung by causing bronchoconstriction, vascular permeability, and vasodilatation. In late-phase asthma, bronchoconstriction is refractory to most bronchodilator therapy.

49. **(3)** Nocturnal exacerbation of asthma is a common clinical sign. It is linked to the variation in circulating catecholamines and vagal tone. Chronic hypoxemia and diffuse crackles are seen in the client with chronic bronchitis. Pruritus is often seen in contact allergic reactions.

50. **(2)** Asking the client about the consumption of wine with dinner is the most appropriate response. Many wines, especially white wines, contain sulfites that can trigger a mild allergic response.

51. **(4)** Nocturnal asthma attacks are generally the worse at 4 AM, when bronchial constriction occurs due to changes in the circadian rhythm that affect bronchial reactivity.

52. **(1)** In addition to more symptoms of wheezing and rales, infants with TB are more likely to develop disseminated disease such as meningitis and to have a negative PPD skin test. Usually, the transmission of the disease can be traced to an affected adult living in the household.

53. **(4)** Maintaining a high caloric intake is important in the care of infants with BPD to promote growth and nourishment of developing lung tissue. Infants may have gastroesophageal reflux (GER) after feedings. Initially, positioning should be tried, then feedings may be thickened or given in smaller amounts more frequently. If the problem persists or weight gain is inadequate, referral to a pediatrican is indicated.

54. **(3)** If this child is up-to-date on immunizations, he should have had his vaccine for *Haemophilus influenzae* type b (Hb), the most common cause of epiglottitis. A dramatic decline in the incidence of epiglottis and *H. influenzae* type b infections is associated closely with the history of Hb vaccines. Considering the age of this child and the suddenness of the onset, the most likely diagnosis is foreign body aspiration.

55. **(2)** Desaturation and 10-second periods of apnea are diagnostic of sleep apnea. Loud snoring at night, frequent arousals during the night, and sleeping during the day are characteristic of the problem, but not diagnostic.

56. **(1)** Male, over 55–60 years old, obese, nasal allergies, and polyps are common factors associated with obstructive sleep apnea. Snoring, daytime sleeping, and general feeling of fatigue are frequently reported symptoms.

57. **(1)** The positive sputum for acid-fast bacillus is indicative of active tuberculosis. *Pneumocystis carinii* is a common organism in healthy respiratory tracts; it becomes a problem if the client is immunocompromised. Hemolysis on a complement fixation test is a negative finding. When oxygen saturation is low and white blood cell (WBC) count is within normal range, treatment is not as important as it is with tuberculosis.

Pharmacology

58. **(1)** A 1-minute lapse between the two puffs is necessary for the medication to be most effective. The first puff opens the upper airways, allowing more effective penetration of the lower tract with the second puff.

59. **(2)** The client would not stop taking the medications because this is a common side effect of rifampin. Also, soft contact lenses may become discolored.

60. **(4)** Beta-agonist (albuterol) by MDI is the first line of treatment to decrease airflow obstruction. Aminophylline by mouth would take too long to be effective. Epinephrine is used predominantly for anaphylactic reaction. Beclovent is a steroid inhaler that is most effective when used prophylactically rather than in acute episodes.

61. **(4)** Because tobacco increases metabolism of theophylline, a higher dosage is required in smokers than in nonsmokers. A high-protein low-carbohydrate diet increases the metabolism of theophylline and decreases serum concentrations. Coffee (and other

xanthine-containing beverages) may increase the central nervous system effects of xanthine derivatives.

62. **(1)** Beta-blockers (propranolol, atenolol) are known to exacerbate chronic respiratory problems. Another antihypertensive, such as a calcium channel blocker, should be considered. The client's pulse is 74 and blood pressure remains elevated, which indicates the beta-blocker is probably not effective in decreasing BP in this client. Theophylline derivatives are not indicated unless other medications are not effective. Drug interactions and increased levels of toxicity present problems in the elderly client.

63. **(2)** Therapeutic plasma levels range from 10–20 µg/ml. Drug levels ≥20 µg/ml are associated with toxicity.

64. **(1)** Chemoprophylaxis is initiated at the time of the screening skin testing. Skin testing should be repeated in 3 months if initial test results are negative. If the second skin testing is negative, chemoprophylaxis can be stopped.

65. **(3)** One of the most common causes of outpatient treatment failure is improper inhaler technique. Exposure to allergens may trigger an asthma attack, but proper use of inhalers will control the attacks. Use of both steroids and cromolyn inhalers has decreased the severity of asthma attacks.

66. **(1)** Theophylline is used in the treatment of chronic lung disease and can accumulate in toxic levels. Cimetidine decreases the hepatic clearance of theophylline. Nicotine and some antiseizure drugs may actually increase clearance, and ampicillin does not change the clearance.

67. **(2)** Antibiotic therapy is indicated when there is a change in color, consistency, or amount of sputum. Cough suppressants and antihistamines should be avoided.

68. **(2)** Beclomethasone is a long-acting corticosteroid that stabilizes mast cells and greatly reduces mast cell degranulation when exposed to allergens. Albuterol is short-acting bronchodilator used as a rescue medication. Salmeterol is a long-acting bronchodilator most useful in controlling nocturnal asthma symptoms. Montelukast, a leukotriene receptor antagonist, inhibits bronchoconstriction and is used as an adjunct to bronchodilators and corticosteroids.

69. **(2)** Treatment of the client with asthma includes inhaled glucocorticoids for their antiinflammatory effects. Antibiotics are indicated if there is a concurrent infection, such as acute bronchitis. β_2-Agonists are used for their bronchodilator effects and rapid onset of action. Methacholine challenge is used in the diagnosis of asthma.

70. **(2)** Clients with asthma should be instructed to keep their inhaled β_2-agonists with them at all times in case of bronchospasm and use them as necessary (prn). The β_2-agonists are effective in reversing bronchospasm. Inhaled steroids are long acting and will not give immediate relief, so the client should be instructed to use them as prescribed. Beginning antibiotics is not indicated for acute bronchospasm.

71. **(3)** These are the common drugs used for combination therapy for the treatment of tuberculosis in children. Rimantadine is an antiviral; pyrimethamine is an antimalarial. Montelukast therapy is not indicated due to the virulence of the tubercle bacillus.

72. **(4)** Close contacts of clients with an active case of TB should be placed on isoniazid single-drug therapy, even if the tuberculin skin test is negative. This early treatment will destroy the tubercle bacilli before hypersensitivity develops. The isoniazid should be continued for 3 months for those whose skin test remains negative and who show no evidence of disease. If there is a positive skin test conversion, isoniazid (10–20 mg/kg) should be continued for 1 year. If the child develops TB symptoms, he should be given isoniazid and rifampin (10 mg/kg) for 1 year.

73. **(4)** Dextromethorphan is specific for control of coughing. Guaifenesin is an expectorant, pseudoephedrine a decongestant, and diphenhydramine an antihistamime.

74. **(3)** Rhinitis and a productive cough are common and are not cause for concern unless the mucus begins to change color and is accompanied by a high fever. The wheezes are also common, if the mucus is loose. A high fever and rales indicate further deterioration and possible bacterial infection.

75. **(2)** Pyridoxine (vitamin B_6) is added to prevent peripheral neuropathy. Foods containing tyramine and histamine (e.g., tuna, aged cheese, yeast vitamin supplements) cause interaction with monoamine oxidase inhibitors (MAOIs). Anorexia, jaundice, malaise, and fatigue would be signs of hepatic involvement.

76. **(1)** Bronchodilators are frequently effective for acute episodes. Antibiotics and antihistamines are not effective and should not be used. The condition is usually treated symptomatically. If the child does not improve, consult a physician.

77. **(1)** Medications should be taken only when the child is planning to exercise and anticipates respiratory difficulty. Cromolyn and beclomethasone are steroids and do not provide immediate relief. Theophylline should be avoided unless symptoms progressively worsen and cannot be controlled with inhalation therapy.

78. **(3)** The drug therapy regimen for chronic asthma may included theophylline. Symptoms of toxicity include anorexia, nausea, vomiting, confusion, restlessness, tachycardia, dysrhythmias, and seizures.

79. **(2)** The hallmark clinical presentation of acute bronchitis is a productive cough. The nurse practitioner should rule out pneumonia, as done with this client through the normal chest x-ray and breath sounds. Bronchodilators (albuterol) have been found to eliminate the cough of acute bronchitis. Antibiotic therapy (erythromycin and tetracycline) is not recommended. Research has demonstrated that antibiotic-susceptible organisms rarely cause acute bronchitis.

80. **(4)** Histamine H_2 antagonists neutralize the normal gastric acid barrier, allowing for an increased colonization of gram-negative bacilli and *Staphylococcus aureus*.

81. **(2)** Worsening dyspnea and fatigue with increasing cough may indicate early pulmonary edema. Clients with pulmonary edema require hospitalization with oxygen therapy, IV furosemide (Lasix), and morphine. Clients suspected of having pulmonary edema **should not** be treated as outpatients. Calcium channel blockers are of little benefit in heart failure.

82. **(1)** INH requires concurrent administration of vitamin B_6 to prevent problems of optic neuritis. Vitamin B_6 will decrease the effectiveness of levodopa. If the client is to receive INH, his antiparkinson medication needs to be reevaluated.

83. **(1)** Combination of theophylline and erythromycin-based antibiotics may result in decreased metabolism of theophylline. Another antibiotic should be considered. (*Testing tip: Three of the distracters are antihypertensive medications; only one is different, and it is the correct answer.*)

84. **(2)** Prednisone is a corticosteroid that suppresses immune response and puts the client in an immunocompromised state, making him more susceptible to infections. Clients on prednisone therapy should be educated about the risk for developing infections and the need to seek medical attention if they suspect illness. Atenolol is a beta-blocker used as an antihypertensive. Ipratropium is a bronchodilator used as a rescue inhaler. Fluticasone propionate is a bronchodilator used twice daily (bid).

Immune & Allergy

6

Physical Examination & Diagnostic Tests

1. When taking the history of a client with known allergies, what is the most important information to determine?

   1. Reaction associated with each allergen.

   2. Drug allergies.

   3. Food allergies.

   4. Environmental exposure.

2. Which test is used to determine the concentration of gamma globulins that contain most of the immunoglobulins?

   1. Immunofixation electrophoresis.

   2. Complement fixation.

   3. Protein electrophoresis.

   4. Antinuclear antibody (ANA).

3. Which diagnostic studies are used in the differential diagnosis of systemic lupus erythematosus (SLE)?

   1. CBC, SMA-12, ESR.

   2. Chest radiograph, and coagulation profile.

   3. ANA, ESR, and C-reactive protein.

   4. CBC, urinalysis, and chest radiograph.

4. Which tests are appropriate for the nurse practitioner to order in an initial workup for asymptomatic clients at risk for human immunodeficiency virus (HIV) infection?

   1. CD4 count and HIV enzyme-linked immunosorbent assay (ELISA).

   2. Serology for cytomegalovirus, herpes simplex, and Epstein-Barr virus.

   3. HIV ELISA and Western blot.

   4. Hepatitis screen and Western blot.

5. The nurse practitioner would identify which laboratory finding as most significant in a client with joint pain, "butterfly rash," photosensitivity, weight loss, and fever?

   1. Presence of antinuclear antibodies (ANAs).

   2. Negative serum complement level.

   3. Decreased red blood cells (RBCs).

   4. Glycosuria.

6. When assessing a client for angioedema, the nurse practitioner would examine the:

   1. Neck and ears.

   2. Heart sounds.

   3. Abdomen.

   4. Eyes and mouth.

7. Clients who believe they have been exposed to HIV should have an HIV antibody test how soon after the exposure?

   1. The next day and 2 months later.

   2. 6 months after exposure and again at 12 months.

   3. 6–12 weeks after exposure and again at 6 months.

   4. 4 weeks and 12 weeks.

8. The most reliable test for the presence of specific immunoglobulin E (IgE) antibody is:

   1. Skin testing.

   2. Radioallergosorbent testing (RAST).

   3. Smears for eosinophils.

   4. Complete blood count (CBC).

9. To diagnose allergic rhinitis in the primary care office setting, the nurse practitioner would consider performing:

   1. Nasal smear for eosinophils.

   2. Total serum IgE.

   3. Skin testing.

   4. RAST.

10. The nurse practitioner is evaluating the tuberculosis (TB) skin test on an immunocompetent 6-year-old child who has no risk factors for TB.

The purified protein derivative (PPD) is considered positive for this client when it measures:

   1. 5 mm.

   2. 10 mm.

   3. 15 mm.

   4. 20 mm.

Disorders

11. A young adult presents to the clinic with a 10-day history of fever, myalgia, sore throat, and measles-like rash. The client is not taking any medications. Which of the following viral syndromes is characterized by a measles-like rash?

   1. Influenza.

   2. Varicella.

   3. HIV.

   4. Mononucleosis.

12. A young woman presents to the urgent care center reporting that a male "date" vaginally raped her last night. She is treated today for *Chlamydia* infection, gonorrhea, and syphilis and started on a 1-month course of medications to prevent HIV (as well as pregnancy prevention drugs). She wants to know why she needs the HIV therapy since no one she knows has "AIDS." The nurse practitioner's counseling is based on the knowledge that:

   1. The client could ask the "date" if he has "AIDS."

   2. She probably does not need the therapy, but it is a good idea to take the medications.

   3. More than 30% of HIV-infected individuals are unaware that they are infected.

   4. HIV is not easily transmitted.

13. A client tells the nurse practitioner that her husband's sister has HIV but now she is "cured." She takes medications, and "her doctor cannot find the virus in her blood." Which response would be appropriate?

   1. "Oh, I'm so sorry, but she must be mistaken; AIDS is not curable."

   2. "That is wonderful news, but are you sure?"

3. "You must be very happy; I didn't know that was possible."

4. "I've heard that the new medications are very good at lowering the virus counts.

14. A co-worker has just stuck herself with a needle while performing a phlebotomy. She asks the nurse practitioner for help and asks that the nurse manager not be told. What should be the nurse practitioner's initial response?

   1. Send the co-worker to the nurse manager.

   2. Sit with her and calm her down.

   3. Put on gloves, run water, and make her "bleed" the site under running water for several minutes.

   4. Put on gloves and pour povidone-iodine (Betadine) on the area.

15. An adult client presents to the clinic with fatigue, sore throat, and myalgia. On examination the nurse practitioner finds lymphadenopathy and a slightly enlarged spleen. Based on the history, the nurse adds acute HIV infection to the differential diagnosis. Which STAT laboratory result increases concern about HIV infection?

   1. Normochromic, normocytic (NC/NC) anemia.

   2. Leukopenia and thrombocytopenia.

   3. Lymphocytosis.

   4. Proteinuria.

16. A woman comes to clinic for the first time in the seventh month of her pregnancy. She knows that she has HIV disease but has not been receiving care. Physical examination includes Doppler ultrasound of the fetal heart, prenatal panel, and urine specimen. The nurse practitioner discusses the client's urgent need for obstetric and prenatal care and is making calls to arrange those services. The client refuses, saying that it is too late and that she "knows" her baby is infected. The nurse practitioner's response is based on the following information:

   1. All infants contract HIV from their mother unless she takes medications.

   2. It is not too late to begin antiviral medications to decrease the risk to the baby.

3. Her viral load is probably high, and the baby does already have HIV.

4. HIV is fatal to infants who contract it.

17. A new mother tells the clinic nurse that her infant was born HIV positive. She asks the nurse practitioner how long her baby has to live. The nurse's response would be based on the knowledge that:

   1. The antibodies present in the infant's blood may reflect the antibodies received from the mother at birth.

   2. If antibodies are present at birth, the infant has acquired immunodeficiency syndrome (AIDS) in an active form.

   3. Because the infant is HIV positive, the child will develop full-blown AIDS within 3 years.

   4. The antibodies detected at birth indicate presence of the HIV; the test does not indicate when the child will develop AIDS.

18. Client education regarding common antigens of anaphylaxis includes:

   1. Extreme weather.

   2. Egg albumin.

   3. Pungent odors.

   4. Animal dandruff.

19. The nurse practitioner understands that an HIV infection results in a reduction of:

   1. Helper T cells.

   2. Suppressor T cells.

   3. Killer T cells.

   4. Suppressor B cells.

20. Which assessment findings are typically associated with a diagnosis of SLE?

   1. Excitability, diarrhea, and vomiting.

   2. High fever, measles-like rash on limbs, and weight gain.

   3. Joint pain, malar rash, and photosensitivity.

   4. Weight loss, diarrhea, and epigastric pain.

21. After a repeat HIV antibody test, a client continues to test positive but is asymptomatic. Which of the following is important for the nurse practitioner to understand regarding the transmission of the virus by this client?

    1. The client is infectious when symptoms are active.

    2. The client is infectious for life.

    3. The dormant virus is not infectious while the client is asymptomatic and the T-cell count is high.

    4. Laboratory tests should be done monthly to identify the infectious periods of the disease process.

22. A young woman has just received news of a positive HIV test. She does not want her sexual partner to be informed. What is the nurse practitioner's most appropriate response?

    1. Respect for her decision, since she is the client.

    2. Informing her now that the nurse has a legal responsibility to inform her partner.

    3. Counseling her about the nurse's ethical responsibility to inform all sexual partners.

    4. Noting her decision in the record for future reference.

23. The nurse practitioner has been assigned a new client. The problem list indicates this client has CREST syndrome. The nurse practitioner will be following this client for what condition?

    1. Scleroderma.

    2. Dental caries.

    3. Systemic lupus erythematosus.

    4. Rheumatoid arthritis.

24. A client presenting with complaints of fatigue, malaise, arthralgias, oral ulcers, malar rash, and positive ANA test would most likely be diagnosed as having:

    1. Rheumatoid arthritis.

    2. Fibromyalgia.

    3. Scleroderma.

    4. Systemic lupus erythematosus.

25. What are the most common clinical manifestations of Sjögren's syndrome?

    1. Corneal dryness and lack of saliva.

    2. Increased urination and hunger.

    3. Abdominal discomfort and headaches.

    4. Joint destruction and alopecia.

26. An elderly female client presents to the nurse practitioner with low-grade temperature and unilateral throbbing headache. She also reports scalp sensitivity and some visual disturbances. Laboratory results show a greatly elevated ESR and anemia. She has been relatively healthy except for a recent history of polymyalgia rheumatica (PMR). Symptoms indicate a clinical presentation of:

    1. Bacterial meningitis.

    2. Acute migraine headache.

    3. Temporal (giant cell) arteritis.

    4. Subdural hematoma.

27. A middle-aged female client presents with weight loss, heartburn, dysphagia, dry cough, pain, stiffness of the fingers and knees, and Raynaud's phenomenon. The nurse practitioner recognizes these as the symptoms of:

    1. Rheumatoid arthritis.

    2. Lupus erythematosus.

    3. Graft-versus-host disease (GVHD).

    4. Scleroderma.

28. The erythematous confluent macular eruption of the face known as the "butterfly rash" is characteristic of:

    1. Allergic drug eruption.

    2. Systemic lupus erythematosus.

    3. Rosacea.

    4. Seborrheic dermatitis.

29. The nurse practitioner is discussing general health care with a female client with SLE who is in remission. What are important points to include in the teaching?

    1. Avoid becoming pregnant.

    2. Decrease physical and psychological stress.

3. Avoid isometric and aerobic exercise.

4. Maintain diet low in fat and carbohydrates.

30. A 50-year-old male client presents with complaints of frequent sinus infections, decrease in ability to hear, and arthralgias. Laboratory findings are mild normochromic/normocytic anemia, elevated ESR, mild hypergammaglobulinemia (elevated IgA), proteinuria, and hematuria with granular or cellular casts. Physical findings include mild conjunctivitis, vasculitic dermatitis, chronic cough, chest pain, dyspnea, paranasal sinus pain, occasional epistaxis, and imbalance of intake and output. What would be a tentative diagnosis?

    1. Connective tissue disease.

    2. Wegener's granulomatosis.

    3. Pulmonary neoplasm.

    4. Infectious granulomatous disease.

31. A client presents with sneezing, watery eyes, postnasal drip, and sore throat. What diagnosis does the symptoms suggest?

    1. Acute bronchitis.

    2. Allergic rhinitis.

    3. Asthma exacerbation.

    4. Influenza.

32. A 70-year-old woman presents with complaints of morning headache, malaise, and anorexia. What condition would the nurse practitioner suspect?

    1. Pneumonia.

    2. Temporal arteritis.

    3. Herpes zoster.

    4. Postmenopausal symptoms.

33. When teaching a client about risk factors and prevention of transmission of HIV, which statement is most appropriate?

    1. HIV can be transmitted by casual kissing.

    2. Unprotected oral sex with an infected partner is not advised. *true*

    3. Sharing an office with an HIV-positive person increases the risk of HIV exposure.

    4. Using the same bathroom as an infected family member puts one at risk of HIV exposure.

34. Signs and symptoms that alert the nurse practitioner to identify a client who is at an increased risk for HIV infection include:

    1. Night sweats.

    2. Malaise and fatigue.

    3. Frequent sexually transmitted diseases (STDs).

    4. Swollen glands and diarrhea.

35. HIV is classified as a:

    1. Cytomegalovirus.

    2. Herpetic virus.

    3. Papillomavirus.

    4. Retrovirus.

36. What are the most frequently occurring symptoms of SLE?

    1. Splenomegaly and Raynaud's syndrome.

    2. Pulmonary effusions and hepatomegaly.

    3. Butterfly rash on face and lymphadenopathy.

    4. Fever, arthritis, arthralgia, and weight loss.

37. A systemic IgE-mediated antigen-antibody response resulting in a life-threatening massive release of mediators is:

    1. Generalized seizures.

    2. Allergic rhinitis.

    3. Anaphylaxis.

    4. Status asthmaticus.

38. The release of histamine results in:

    1. Bronchospasm, vasodilatation, and vascular permeability.

    2. Bronchodilatation, vasodilatation, and vascular permeability.

    3. Smooth muscle contraction, decreased vascular permeability, and vasoconstriction.

    4. Pain, increased vascular permeability, and bronchodilatation.

39. After a bone marrow transplant (BMT) the nurse practitioner can expect the peak onset of an acute graft-versus-host disease (GVHD) to occur:

    1. Between 10 and 15 days posttransplant.

    2. Between 30 and 50 days posttransplant.

    3. Between 1 and 5 days posttransplant.

    4. At 100 days posttransplant.

40. A client has a history of recent BMT. The nurse practitioner identifies signs and symptoms of GVHD to include:

    1. Fever, headache, and mental status changes.

    2. Chills, fever, and urticaria over flank area.

    3. Increased serum bilirubin, maculopapular rash, and green watery diarrhea.

    4. Decreased RBCs, hematocrit, and hemoglobin; petechiae; and increased bleeding tendencies.

41. The pathogenesis of systemic lupus erythematosus (SLE) is characterized by autoantibody development. This results in:

    1. Increased T suppressor cell.

    2. B-cell decrease.

    3. Polyclonal hypogammaglobulinemia.

    4. Decreased T suppressor cells and inhibited cell activity.

42. What cell is responsible for the activation of the immune response?

    1. Band neutrophil.

    2. T4 lymphocyte.

    3. Segmented neutrophil.

    4. B lymphocytes.

43. A 22-year-old male presents with breathlessness, weight loss, nonproductive cough, temperature 38°C (100.4°F), pulse 124, respirations 36, blood pressure 120/78, and history of positive HIV serum test. Based on this information, which is the most accurate diagnosis?

    1. *Klebsiella pneumoniae* infection.

    2. Kaposi's sarcoma.

    3. *Pneumocystis carinii* pneumonia.

    4. Lymphoma.

44. An adult client presents at the clinic, and his family states he has a history of anaphylactic reactions. What signs and symptoms indicate to the nurse practitioner that the client is experiencing another reaction?

    1. Cough, wheezing, and hives.

    2. Severe malaise, pallor, stridor, and dyspnea.

    3. Anxiety, nasal congestion, and tachycardia.

    4. Rhinorrhea, nausea, and gastrointestinal cramping.

45. A nurse at the clinic experiences a needle stick from a client with known hepatitis. What immunoglobulin (Ig) should be administered to provide passive immunity?

    1. IgE.

    2. IgA.

    3. IgG.

    4. IgC.

46. Which sign/symptom is indicative of a type I hypersensitivity reaction?

    1. Contact dermatitis.

    2. Immediate wheal-and-flare reaction.

    3. Hematuria.

    4. High fever.

47. Which clients are at risk for developing HIV/AIDS?

    1. Immunocompromised clients.

    2. Sexually active teenagers.

    3. Elderly adults.

    4. Marijuana users.

48. What are the cardiovascular effects of anaphylaxis?

    1. ST-segment and T-wave changes.

    2. Hypertension.

    3. Prolonged PR intervals with elevated QT segment.

    4. Elevated serum enzymes.

49. When assessing a client for SLE, what ophthalmologic findings would the nurse practitioner determine to be consistent with this condition?

    1. Retinal hemorrhages.
    2. Conjunctivitis.
    3. Cotton-wool spots.
    4. Arteriovenous (AV) nicking.

50. What information does the nurse practitioner include in the education for the client with allergic rhinitis?

    1. Monitor air quality and the allergy index.
    2. Use a surgical-type mask when going outdoors.
    3. Remain inside during allergy season.
    4. Avoid working in the garden or yard.

51. A nurse from the operating room (OR) comes into the clinic with complaints of shortness of breath, itching, reddened hands, and wheezing. He says that he does not seem to have the symptoms when he is not working. Based on the history and symptoms, the nurse practitioner would evaluate for:

    1. Sick building syndrome.
    2. Bronchitis.
    3. Latex allergy.
    4. Contact dermatitis.

52. Which statement is true regarding latex allergy?

    1. It usually only produces symptoms of contact dermatitis and allergic rhinorrhea.
    2. It is a progressive disease that worsens with continued exposure.
    3. It affects less than 5% of the health care population.
    4. It is an autoimmune response.

53. Children who have chronic allergic rhinitis often present with clinical symptoms that include:

    1. Mouth breathing and nasal polyps.
    2. Allergic "shiners" and Dennie's sign (Morgan's line).

    3. Thick nasal discharge and sneezing.
    4. Flushed face and fever.

54. What are common sites for adolescent atopic dermatitis?

    1. Cheeks, forehead, and scalp.
    2. Wrists, ankles, and antecubital fossae.
    3. Antecubital fossae, face, neck, and back.
    4. Palmar creases and extensor surface of legs.

Pharmacology

55. An adult patient comes to the urgent care clinic with nausea, vomiting, and acute abdominal pain. His history is significant for HIV disease, and for the last month he has been taking didanosine (Videx) 400 mg qd, lopinavir 3 pills bid, and lamivudine (Epivir) 150 mg bid. After the examination, the nurse practitioner determines that didanosine can cause pancreatitis and lactic acidosis. What laboratory tests would be ordered?

    1. CBC, CD4 count, viral load
    2. CBC, differential, lipase, lactic acid, electrolytes, BUN, creatinine, LFTs
    3. Amylase, lipase, lactic acid
    4. Lipase, amylase, liver function tests (LFTs).

56. Which drugs have been associated with a lupus-like syndrome?

    1. Sulfonamides (Septra DS), penicillin (Pen-Vee K, Penicillin G).
    2. Progestin/estrogen oral contraceptives.
    3. Nonsteroidal antiinflammatory drugs (NSAIDs; Motrin).
    4. Procainamide (Pronestyl), hydralazine (Apresoline).

57. A client is diagnosed with temporal (giant cell) arteritis. What is the medication of choice?

    1. Prednisone (Deltasone).
    2. Ibuprofen (Motrin).
    3. Indomethacin (Indocin).
    4. Azathioprine (Imuran).

58. The clinic is notified that a child is being brought in with a bee sting and that the child is having difficulty breathing. Which medication should the nurse practitioner have available for the child's initial care?

    1. Lidocaine topical ointment.

    2. Epinephrine.

    3. Prednisone.

    4. Benadryl elixir.

59. What is the standard drug used for malaria prophylaxis?

    1. Ampicillin (Omnipen).

    2. Doxycycline (Vibramycin).

    3. Ceftriaxone (Rocephin).

    4. Chloroquine phosphate (Aralen).

60. Which medications are used in the treatment of allergic rhinitis?

    1. Antihistamines, corticosteroids, and environmental control.

    2. Antihistamines, analgesics, and allergen control.

    3. Cholinergics, antibiotics, and analgesics.

    4. Nasal saline, corticosteroids, and antibiotics.

61. Development of an adverse drug reaction depends on which factors?

    1. Client age, prior drug reactions, genetic factors, and degree of exposure.

    2. Client gender, oral route of administration, and history of atrophic disease.

    3. Client age, gender, and genetic factors.

    4. Genetic factors, prior drug reactions, and client gender.

62. A medication frequently used for the prophylaxis as well as initial treatment of *Pneumocystis carinii* pneumonia (PCP) is

    1. Fluconazole (Diflucan).

    2. Amphotericin B (Fungizone).

    3. Trimethoprim-sulfamethoxazole (TMP-SMX; Septra).

    4. Acyclovir (Zovirax).

63. When instructing clients with allergic rhinitis about the use of nasal decongestants, it is important for them to understand:

    1. The condition is self-limiting and will resolve in a matter of weeks whether or not the client is re-exposed to the allergen.

    2. A nasal decongestant used continuously for greater than 3 days can result in a worsening of the symptoms.

    3. It is not necessary to avoid exposure to the allergen once therapy has been initiated.

    4. Allergic rhinitis is only seen in the spring and fall; the condition requires treatment during these seasons only.

64. What is the major advantage of using second-generation antihistamines, such as astemizole (Hismanal) and loratadine (Claritin)?

    1. Decreased cost.

    2. Increased anticholinergic activity.

    3. Delayed absorption.

    4. Do not cross the blood-brain barrier.

65. What is the desired action of sympathomimetics (adrenergics) when used in the treatment of allergic rhinitis?

    1. Promote vasoconstriction in nasal mucosa.

    2. Block mast cell degranulation.

    3. Decrease the effect of histamines.

    4. Increase degranulation and end-organ response.

66. The nurse practitioner is prescribing astemizole (Hismanal) for a geriatric client's allergy problems. When considering the client's current medications, which medication would be a contraindication to the administration of astemizole?

    1. Erythromycin ethylsuccinate (E.E.S.).

    2. Verapamil (Calan).

    3. Propranolol (Inderal).

    4. Captopril (Capoten).

67. Cromolyn sodium (Intal) is used to:

    1. Reduce the histamine load.

    2. Antagonize the effects of histamine.

3. Stabilize the mast cell membrane.

4. Reduce antiemetic activity.

68. In the elderly client, histamine H_1 blockers may cause which side effects?

1. Ataxia.

2. Nausea.

3. Diarrhea.

4. Gastrointestinal upset.

69. What information is important for the nurse practitioner to include when teaching a client about the use of antihistamines?

1. Use of topical antihistamines is safe and has relatively few side effects.

2. Do not use over-the-counter (OTC) medications without consulting the health care provider.

3. Constipation and urinary retention are expected side effects and do not need to be reported.

4. Once antihistamine therapy has been taken for 3 days, avoidance of allergens is not necessary.

70. A primary advantage of using loratadine (Claritin) in treating a client with seasonal allergies is that it:

1. Is supplied as an enteric-coated pill.

2. May be prescribed for once-a-day (qd) dosing.

3. Costs considerably less than other medications.

4. Effectively decreases nasal secretions.

71. What medications are drugs of choice for treatment in secondary therapy for the client with an anaphylactic reaction?

1. Antibiotics and anticholinergics.

2. NSAIDs.

3. Decongestants and expectorants.

4. Antihistamines and corticosteroids.

72. What is an appropriate antihistamine to recommend for a child with allergic rhinitis?

1. Diphenhydramine (Benadryl).

2. Dextromethorphan (Benylin).

3. Guaifenesin (Robitussin).

4. Brompheniramine (Dimetane).

73. A child who weighs 30 lb (13.6 kg) arrives in the office. The mother is concerned that the child is having an allergic reaction to peanuts. The child has hives on most of her body and is beginning to wheeze; she is in acute distress. The nurse practitioner administers:

1. Diphenhydramine (Benadryl) 50 mg PO.

2. Diphenhydramine (Benadryl) 25 mg PO.

3. Epinephrine (Adrenalin) 0.14 ml of a 1:1000 solution.

4. Epinephrine (Adrenalin) 0.3 ml of a 1:1000 solution.

74. During a well-child visit the nurse practitioner notes that the 8-year-old male client is taking 50 mg of grapeseed extract three times a day for allergies. The practitioner bases teaching on the knowledge that:

1. Grapeseed extract is not safe in children under age 12.

2. The client may need loratadine (Claritin) for breakthrough episodes.

3. Grapeseed extract can be toxic for children.

4. The client will need to be monitored for seizures.

75. Children on long-term antihistamine therapy will need supplements due to decreased absorption of:

1. Calcium.

2. Iron.

3. Magnesium.

4. Niacin.

76. Clients newly presenting with signs and symptoms of SLE would have their medication profile reviewed to determine if they are taking any medication that may have caused a drug-induced lupus. Which drug would be most suspect?

1. Digoxin (Lanoxin).

2. Procainamide (Pronestyl).

3. TMP-SMX (Septra).

4. Cimetidine (Tagamet).

6 ▶ Answers & Rationales

Physical Examination & Diagnostic Tests

1. **(1)** The reaction to each allergen is most important to know. Often clients state they have an "allergy" to a particular food or medication, such as nausea, stomach pain, or diarrhea, which they regard as an allergy. The signs and symptoms of the reaction, speed of onset, duration, and successful treatments used in the past are also important information. Medication side effects must be distinguished from true allergic reactions to drugs, so client statements of drug or food allergies should be thoroughly explored.

2. **(3)** In protein electrophoresis, proteins are electrically separated on a strip. It is a screening test to measure various proteins in body fluids, usually serum or urine. It assists in screening for diseases characterized by an increase or decrease in immunoglobulins. Complement fixation and ANA are diagnostic studies for rheumatoid problems. Serum protein electrophoresis is also used to identify occult malignancy in a client with failing health when no cause can be found.

3. **(3)** Although all the tests listed may be included in a complete physical examination, laboratory tests specific to the diagnosis of SLE include antinuclear antibody (ANA), erythrocyte sedimentation rate (ESR), and C-reactive protein. During flares, ESR and C-reactive protein are elevated. The ANA titer in a client with SLE is positive at a 1:80 ratio.

4. **(3)** The initial screening test for HIV is ELISA. If the test is positive, antibodies are confirmed with Western blot. Although serology and hepatitis screening with complete blood count (CBC) and tuberculosis skin test are routinely performed, the initial workup starts with an ELISA test. The CD4 count is performed during the active disease process.

5. **(1)** The majority of clients with SLE have ANAs present in their blood, with leukopenia, thrombocytopenia, lymphopenia, and positive LE cell preparation. Proteinuria with cellular casts is often noted.

6. **(4)** Angioedema is edema of the mucous membrane tissue and is most easily seen in the eyes and mouth. It also affects the tongue, feet, hands, and genitalia. Diffuse erythema may be seen in the upper body parts. Gastrointestinal symptoms (e.g., vomiting, cramping, diarrhea) may occur.

7. **(3)** The HIV antibody develops between 6 and 12 weeks after exposure. Because of the variability of antibody development, it is recommended that the test be repeated in 6 months to confirm the findings.

8. **(1)** The most reliable test for the presence of the specific IgE antibody is the skin test. RAST is less sensitive than skin testing and is difficult to standardize and reproduce results. The smear for eosinophils and CBC are not specific for IgE antibody.

9. **(1)** A nasal smear for eosinophils is a simple office procedure. Many clients who have uncomplicated allergic rhinitis have a normal serum IgE. Skin testing should be performed by allergy-trained providers only. RAST testing is higher in cost and lower in sensitivity.

10. **(3)** A positive PPD for an immunocompetent child is 15 mm. A child who is HIV positive, immunocompromised, or exposed to an active case of TB is considered positive at 5 mm. The child (<4 years of age) who has chronic disease or has been exposed to HIV-positive individuals or persons born in a foreign country is considered positive at 10 mm.

Disorders

11. **(3)** Neither influenza nor mononucleosis typically presents with a rash. Varicella (chickenpox) presents with a vesicular skin eruption. Acute HIV infection is characterized by a history of prolonged fever and a red, raised, discrete skin eruption described as morbilliform ("measles-like").

12. **(3)** Treating a woman who has been raped requires time for client education. It is not safe for the client to confront her attacker for medical information. Evidence based on postexposure prophylaxis (PEP) in health care workers and infants supports its effectiveness. Traumatic sex increases the risk of sexually transmitted disease (STD), including HIV.

13. **(4)** Repeating what the client has said along with more information is appropriate.

14. **(3)** Option #1 does not address the medical need. Option #2 is necessary but not until the nurse practitioner addresses the need to wash the site immediately and at length. Bleeding the site under water is more effective than topical antiseptics (Betadine).

15. **(2)** Acute primary HIV infection depletes the CD4 cells, which produces leukopenia and depletes platelets. NC/NC anemia is present more often in advanced HIV; lymphocytosis is more consistent with mononucleosis.

16. **(2)** Not all infants contract HIV from their mother during pregnancy, and HIV may not be fatal in children with access to effective antiretroviral therapy. Without measurement of the viral load, Option #3 cannot be known. The immune system of some individuals with HIV keeps the viral load under control for many years. It is recommended that the woman be placed on antivirals for the pregnancy.

17. **(4)** It is important to give the mother as much hope as possible but still be realistic about the infant's condition. There is no way to tell when or if the infant will convert to active AIDS. Many infants seroconvert to HIV-negative status.

18. **(2)** Egg albumin is one of many identified common antigens that may result in anaphylactic reaction. Others include vaccines, allergen extracts, sulfonamides, penicillins, hormones, legumes (especially peanuts), berries, nuts, seafood, and venom bites (bee, wasp, yellow jacket). Changes in weather and strong scents and odors are triggers that may precipitate an asthma attack, resulting in bronchospasm and wheezing.

19. **(1)** There is a severe, life-threatening reduction of helper T cells, along with an increase in suppressor T cells. The helper T cells help amplify or increase the production of antibody-forming cells from B lymphocytes after an encounter with an antigen. Killer T cells are produced after mature helper T cells interact with an antigen. Suppressor T cells suppress the formation of antibody-forming cells from B lymphocytes, which, when their numbers are increased, have a detrimental effect on the immunity and ability of the HIV client to make antibody-forming cells.

20. **(3)** The symptoms most often experienced are joint pain, fatigue, Raynaud's phenomenon, chronic low-grade or recurrent fever, sun sensitivity, hair loss, weakness, butterfly (malar) facial rash, and weight loss. Typically, the pulmonary, cardiac, renal, and central nervous systems are involved, which may cause multisystem failure and contribute to mortality in clients with SLE.

21. **(2)** HIV infection creates a chronic infectious state in the body that is transmitted through blood or body fluids and transplacentally throughout the client's life.

22. **(3)** Ethical response includes notification of all persons at risk.

23. **(1)** CREST (**C**alcinosis, **R**aynaud's phenomenon, **E**sophageal dysfunction, **S**clerodactyly, **T**elangiectasia) is associated with a slow, progressive form of scleroderma.

24. **(4)** This client is presenting with 4 of the 11 criteria necessary for diagnosing SLE. No single test exists for SLE, but these characteristics plus laboratory results (ANA, ESR, C-reactive protein) can differentiate the diagnosis.

25. **(1)** Corneal dryness and lack of saliva are the most common clinical manifestations of Sjögren's syndrome. Clients may also have joint inflammation, but this rarely leads to joint destruction.

26. **(3)** About 40% of clients with temporal (giant cell) arteritis have a history of PMR. The other diagnoses may have some of these symptoms, but only arteritis has all the symptoms listed in the situation. It is especially crucial to note visual disturbances because these clients can develop sudden blindness. Definitive diagnosis is confirmed by biopsy. Treatment typically consists of increasing the client's prednisone to 60 mg daily in divided doses for 4 weeks, then gradually decreasing ESR monitoring.

27. **(4)** The symptom of Raynaud's phenomenon differentiates this as scleroderma. The esophageal dysfunction is often an initial complaint in scleroderma, which affects women four times more often than men.

28. **(2)** The butterfly rash is one of the characteristic symptoms of SLE.

29. **(2)** Since SLE is considered an autoimmune disorder, psychological and physical stress can exacerbate the condition. A balanced diet helps to limit the side effects of some medications, and regular exercise helps to reduce arthralgia and myalgia associated with SLE. Barrier contraception is recommended for the female client with SLE. Pregnancy is usually allowed during periods of remission. The stress of pregnancy could cause an acute exacerbation of SLE, however, and the client would require close monitoring by both her rheumatologist and her gynecologist.

30. **(2)** Wegener's granulomatosis is a multisystem disorder that occurs equally in both genders. Peak occurrence is between 40 and 60 years of age. The disease usually targets the upper respiratory tract and the kidneys. Connective tissue disease, pulmonary neoplasm, and infectious granulomatous disease would be considered in the differential diagnosis.

31. **(2)** The signs and symptoms presented are classic for allergic rhinitis. Acute bronchitis would present with cough and yellow or green sputum production. An asthma exacerbation would present with wheezing, chest tightness, decreased forced vital capacity, and history of exposure to an allergen. Influenza presents with acute onset, fever, chills, and general malaise.

32. **(2)** The nurse practitioner should suspect temporal arteritis, an inflammatory disorder of unknown etiology affecting large and medium-sized arteries. It occurs two times more frequently in women, most frequently in elderly persons, and rarely in the African American population. The clinical findings would reveal temporal tenderness and temporal bruits. About 40% of the clients who have been diagnosed with PMR also have temporal arteritis, and the elderly client may be relating some of her arthalgia and myalgias to normal changes of aging versus PMR. The nurse practitioner should also check an ESR and consider a referral to a rheumatologist.

33. **(2)** Unprotected oral sex with an HIV-positive person puts one at risk for exposure to the virus. Contact such as casual kissing, or sharing an office or bathroom, does not transmit the virus. The virus is transmitted in body fluids and secretions.

34. **(3)** Frequent STDs would alert the nurse practitioner to the client's lack of protected sex and the possibility of multiple partners. Night sweats, malaise, fatigue, swollen glands, and diarrhea may be associated with many other illnesses.

35. **(4)** HIV is a retrovirus. It contains an enzyme, reverse transcriptase, that copies ribonucleic acid (RNA) into deoxyribonucleic acid (DNA). When it binds to a CD4 receptor, the virus inserts its RNA and enzymes into the cell, where a copy of its RNA is made and enters the cell nucleus. As the infected host cell reproduces, HIV DNA is duplicated and passed on in the infectious cycle.

36. **(4)** Although any of clinical symptoms listed may be present in SLE clients, fever, weight loss, arthritis, and arthralgias occur most often. Butterfly rash of the face and lymphadenopathy occur in less than half the cases. Pulmonary effusion, hepatomegaly, splenomegaly, and Raynaud's syndrome occur in less than a third of SLE clients.

37. **(3)** The massive release of mediators triggers a series of events in target organs. Prior sensitization to the antigen must have occurred to trigger an anaphylactic reaction. Anaphylaxis may result from injection of an antigen, ingested food or drugs, or inhaled antigens.

38. **(1)** The release of histamine results in bronchospasm, vasodilatation, and vascular permeability, leading to wheezing, increased mucus production in the lung, and edema of the airway.

39. **(2)** The onset of acute GVHD occurs between 30 and 50 days after BMT. It results from immunocompetent donor T lymphocytes attacking the host tissues.

40. **(3)** The signs and symptoms of GVHD include maculopapular rash, generalized erythroderma with desquamation, increased bilirubin, increased serum aspartate transaminase (AST, SGOT) and/or increased alkaline phosphatase, abdominal cramping, and diarrhea. Infection is characterized by fever, mental status changes, and headaches. Decreased RBCs, hematocrit, and hemoglobin and petechiae are signs of anemia. Fever, chills, and urticaria are indications of a reaction to white blood cells (WBCs) in the marrow.

41. **(4)** T lymphocytes are the WBCs responsible for control of the immune response. In SLE, T suppressor cells are decreased and cell activity is inhibited, leading to hypergammaglobulinemia and B-cell proliferation.

42. **(2)** The T4 lymphocyte is known as the T helper cell. These cells are responsible for the proliferation of lymphocytes and macrophages, causing activation of the cells in response to an antigen. The B lymphocytes are effector cells that mediate humoral responses by production of antibodies. The band neutrophil and segmented neutrophil are slightly mature and fully mature neutrophils, respectively. Neutrophils are the most abundant cells in the bone marrow and blood.

43. **(3)** Based on the history of an HIV-positive test and the symptoms presented, the client is at risk for *P. carinii* pneumonia. Further examination would include a chest radiograph and pulse oximetry (for oxygen saturation). The lack of purplish lesions is considered in

ruling out Kaposi.s sarcoma. *Klebsiella pneumoniae* is a nosocomial infection, not community acquired. Lymphoma in HIV usually occurs as non-Hodgkin's lymphoma as a primary site in the brain.

44. **(2)** Severe malaise, pallor, stridor, and dyspnea are signs and symptoms associated with a severe anaphylactic reaction. Symptoms may occur immediately or up to 2 hours after exposure to the allergen. Severe reactions require immediate intervention.

45. **(3)** The nurse should be given IgG because it is the major antibody against viruses and bacteria. IgG is the principal mediator of the secondary immune response, which requires repeated response to the same antigen to increase the immune response. There is no IgC antibody. IgA is the secretory immunoglobulin found in tears, saliva, and mucous secretions of the lung and gastrointestinal tract. IgE mediates allergic reactions.

46. **(2)** Type I hypersensitivity reaction causes an immediate wheal-and-flare reaction. Contact dermatitis is seen in type IV (delayed) reaction. Hematuria is seen in type II reaction caused by pre-formed circulating cytotoxic antibodies, as in a blood transfusion reaction or autoimmune hemolytic anemia. High fever may be seen in type III hypersensitivity reaction when large quantities of antigen-antibody complexes are released in the body.

47. **(2)** Sexually active teenagers are the fastest growing group of HIV-positive clients because of unprotected sexual activity. Immunocompromised clients and elderly adults are at no greater risk for developing HIV than any other group. However, an increasing number of elderly males are becoming HIV positive from their association with prostitutes after the loss of their partners. Risk factors for HIV include unprotected sexual contact with persons of unknown HIV status, multiple sexual partners, intravenous drug use, hemophilia, and blood transfusions received before 1985.

48. **(1)** Changes in the electrocardiogram (ECG) are associated with coronary and myocardial ischemia. Although ECG changes suggest myocardial injury, there is no change in the serum enzymes. Other signs and symptoms include hypotension and tachycardia.

49. **(3)** Cotton-wool spots are the most common ophthalmologic problem associated with SLE. Retinal hemorrhages and AV nicking may be seen in the client with hypertension. Conjunctivitis is an infection of the conjunctiva.

50. **(1)** Clients with allergic rhinitis should monitor the air quality and allergy index in their area. A surgical-type mask will not filter out small allergens. Remaining inside during allergy season is an unrealistic expectation and can lead to decreased socialization and increased depression for the client. Clients can enjoy a summer garden if they are careful about the choice of plants and flowers. For example, the client with an allergy to ragweed should avoid daisies, dahlias, and chrysanthemums.

51. **(3)** The OR nurse likely has a latex allergy. The incidence of latex allergies has increased dramatically since the onset of standard precautions and increased use of latex gloves. In an effort to meet the increased demand for gloves, changes in the manufacturing process have resulted in a higher protein count in the gloves. The increased exposure to the protein has led to a proliferation of health care workers being diagnosed with a latex allergy.

52. **(2)** Latex allergy is a progressive disease that worsens with continual exposure. The symptoms range from contact dermatitis to anaphylaxis. Currently, latex allergy affects 17% of health care workers and 39% of dental professionals. Latex allergy is an acquired immune response to the latex protein allergen. No vaccine is available; the only defense is to avoid contact with latex.

53. **(2)** The typical allergic facies consists of allergic "shiners" (black eyes), Morgan's line (Dennie's sign; extra crease below the lower eyelids), and mouth breathing. Nasal polyps are uncommon in childhood allergic rhinitis. The nasal discharge with allergies is usually clear.

54. **(3)** In adolescent and through adult atopic dermatitis, common sites are the popliteal and anticubital fossae, face, neck, upper arms and back, dorsa of the hand, feet, fingers, and toes.

Pharmacology

55. **(2)** Assessment of immune function is unnecessary at this point and would not change management of the acute illness. Options #3 and #4 would assist in the diagnosis of pancreatitis but would not provide information on the client's hydration status, the rest of the biliary tree, or presence of acute infection.

56. **(4)** Procainamide, hydralazine, and isoniazid have been shown to induce a lupus-like syndrome. Discontinuation of the medication results in disappearance of the clinical signs and symptoms. Antibiotics (e.g., sulfonamides, penicillin) have been associated with anaphylactic reactions in some clients. Oral contraceptives may increase blood pressure and the risk for thromboemboli. NSAIDs (e.g., ibuprofen) have been associated with gastrointestinal upset and gastric pain, especially when taken on an empty stomach, and are contraindicated in clients with renal disease.

57. **(1)** Temporal arthritis, seen primarily in elderly clients, can lead to blindness if not treated immediately with corticosteroids. The usual daily dose of prednisone is 60 mg in divided doses initially, then a single morning dose (every-other-day steroids are not used). A **slow** taper is initiated after 4 weeks if the client is asymptomatic and the ESR is decreased. Tapering of the dose is individualized, and the client may be on drug therapy for several months to years. Average time for disease remission is 3–4 years (range 1–10 years).

58. **(2)** Epinephrine would be the first-line drug to be injected for the treatment of the respiratory distress associated with an anaphylactic reaction. The dosage for epinephrine (1:1000, SC) is 0.01 ml/kg for a child and 0.3–0.5 ml/kg for an adult. Benadryl's onset of action is not fast enough. Lidocaine would only topically treat the pain and not the respiratory problem. Antiinflammatory drugs would not be given initially but may be given later if needed for generalized discomfort or pain at the sting site.

59. **(4)** Chloroquine phosphate is the standard drug used for malaria prophylaxis. The dosage is 5 mg/kg body weight up to 300 mg for an adult. Doxycycline is often used to treat

diarrhea associated with traveling to areas where diarrhea is common from drinking the water; it is also used to treat *Chlamydia* infection and pelvic inflammatory disease. Ceftriaxone is used for bacterial septicemia and respiratory and urinary tract infections caused by gram-negative bacilli. Ampicillin is used to treat infections from a variety of organisms and as prophylaxis for bacterial endocarditis.

60. **(1)** Unless there is a secondary bacterial infection, antibiotics are contraindicated. Antihistamines and reduction of exposure to the allergen will help to reduce the symptoms. For continued control and stabilization of the mast cell, corticosteroids are indicated.

61. **(1)** Adults are at greater risk for development of adverse drug reactions, probably due to the increased number of medications used and the amount of exposure and effects of aging on the immune system. Clients with prior drug reactions are more likely to develop reactions to new drugs. The risk of an adverse drug reaction occurs in the first 2–3 weeks of therapy. Prolonged course of therapy, high dosage, and intermittent therapy increase the risk of an adverse reaction. Genetic factors may increase mediator and metabolic pathway activity. Gender has no effect except with muscle relaxants and chymopapain, when women are at greater risk of an adverse drug reaction. Route of drug administration contributes to the risk, with IV, IM, SC, PO, and topical in the order of greatest to least risk.

62. **(3)** TMP-SMX is used to treat as well as prevent *P. carinii* pneumonia, usually with a 21-day course, with up to 7–10 days for a clinical response. Fluconazole and amphotericin B are antifungal drugs. Acyclovir is an antiviral used primarily to treat herpes simplex virus types 1 and 2 and herpes zoster (shingles).

63. **(2)** The chronic use of nasal decongestants for more than 3 days can result in a rebound effect when discontinued, leading to increased nasal congestion from reflex vasodilatation. The condition may take as long as 2–3 weeks to resolve. Allergic rhinitis is not a self-limiting illness associated only with spring and fall. Even though therapy is initiated, the client should be instructed to avoid exposure to the allergen as much as possible.

64. **(4)** The major advantage of the second-generation antihistamines is that they do not cross the blood-brain barrier and therefore do not cause sedation and psychomotor dysfunction. There is little anticholinergic activity and less dry mouth and constipation. The cost of these antihistamines is 15–30 times greater than for the first-generation antihistamines. The medications are rapidly absorbed in 1–2 hours of PO administration on an empty stomach.

65. **(1)** Sympathomimetics (adrenergics) cause vasoconstriction, thereby reducing edema and secretions. Inhaled corticosteroids stabilize mast cells and block degranulation.

66. **(1)** E.E.S. and astemizole should not be administered concurrently. Fatal dysrhythmias may be precipitated by this combination.

67. **(3)** Cromolyn sodium is used to stabilize the mast cell membrane to prevent release of histamine when the cell comes in contact with an antigen. It does not affect the amount of histamine released from the cell, antagonize the effects of histamine, or reduce antiemetic activity.

68. **(1)** The use of H_1 blockers can cause paradoxical central nervous system (CNS) stimulation resulting in ataxia in elderly clients. Antihistamines can cause many simultaneous side effects in older adults, such as impaired vision and gait, which can lead to falls, and impaired thinking, which can interfere with functional skills (cognition) and could necessitate unnecessary hospitalization or nursing home stay. Antihistamines also may interact with the elderly client's numerous medications and exacerbate the side effects (e.g., dry mouth, constipation).

69. **(2)** The client should be instructed not to use OTC medications without consulting the nurse practitioner or pharmacist. The nurse should explain that OTC drugs and herbal supplements are considered medications and that they may interact with prescribed medications. To avoid possible interactions, the client should inform the nurse practitioner of all the OTC drugs and herbals the client is taking. The client should be cautioned on the extended use of topical antihistamines. Antihistamines do not affect circulating histamine, so the client must avoid exposure to a known allergen. Constipation and urinary

retention are adverse effects that should be reported to the nurse practitioner.

70. **(2)** An advantage of using loratadine is the qd dosing, which helps with client compliance. The cost is greater than for some first-generation antihistamines. Loratadine with pseudoephedrine (Claritin D) is an antihistamine/decongestant with bid or extended-release (qd) dosing.

71. **(4)** Medications such as antihistamines and corticosteroids are used to counter mediator release and block release of additional mediators. NSAIDs, antibiotics, and decongestants are contraindicated in the treatment of anaphylatic reaction.

72. **(4)** Although both diphenhydramine and brompheniramine are antihistamines and could be prescribed, brompheniramine would have less CNS sedating effects. Dextromethorphan is an antitussive, and guaifenesin is an expectorant.

73. **(3)** Although diphenhydramine could be administered for itching after the child's distress is relieved, the immediate concern is to prevent respiratory arrest from swelling of the throat's mucosa. The usual epinephrine dose for children is 0.01 ml/kg of the 1:1000 solution.

74. **(2)** Grapeseed extract is a common alternative therapy for allergies with few side effects. It is often not as effective during peak allergy seasons, and an antihistamine (e.g., loratadine) is needed for breakthrough allergy symptoms.

75. **(2)** Antihistamines block the absorption of iron, folate, and vitamin B_{12}.

76. **(2)** Of clients receiving procainamide, 20% develop clinical drug-induced SLE. The other drugs listed have not been associated with SLE.

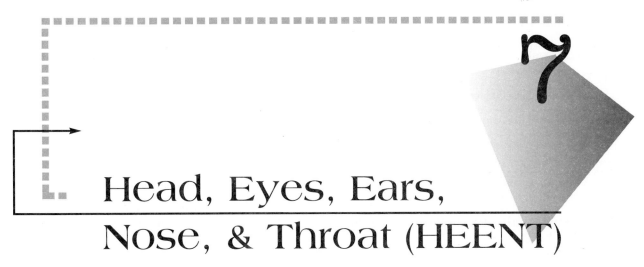

Head, Eyes, Ears, Nose, & Throat (HEENT)

Physical Examination & Diagnostic Tests

Head

1. In examining the mouth of a school-age child, the nurse practitioner notes that the central and lateral permanent incisors have surface pitting and are stained brown. This condition is most suggestive of:

    1. The mother taking tetracycline during pregnancy.

    2. Poor dental hygiene.

    3. Dental fluorosis.

    4. Going to bed with a bottle during infancy.

2. The nurse practitioner is examining lymph nodes in the neck. What is palpated in the anterior triangle of the neck?

    1. Posterior cervical chain.

    2. Anterior superficial chain.

    3. Periauricular lymph nodes.

    4. Supraclavicular lymph nodes.

Eyes

3. When using an ophthalmoscope, the nurse practitioner:

    1. Holds the ophthalmoscope in the right hand (uses right eye) while examining the client's left eye.

    2. Starts the examination with the lens set at zero.

    3. Begins in a position 1 inch from the eye to check the red light reflex.

    4. Examines the anterior chamber in a well-lighted room and asks the client to focus on an object.

4. The visual screening for a 4-year-old boy is recorded as 20/40 in both eyes. The nurse practitioner should now:

    1. Have the child return in 1 month to have his vision rechecked.

    2. Refer the child to an ophthalmologist.

    3. Recheck his vision to make sure that it is accurate.

    4. Record the findings as normal for age.

5. The nurse practitioner checking for strabismus would use which test?

    1. Cover-uncover test.

    2. Bruchner's test.

    3. Ishihara's test.

    4. Snellen's test.

6. The nurse practitioner observes lid lag in a client with:

    1. Myasthenia gravis.

    2. Hyperthyroidism.

    3. Hordeolum.

    4. Chalazion.

7. The nurse practitioner is examining an elderly woman. There is a glossy white circle around the pupils of her eyes, and the pupil has a decreased reaction to the direct light reflex. She has a history of presbyopia. Correct interpretation of these findings is:

    1. Beginning development of cataracts with a significant decrease in visual acuity.

    2. Normal changes in the eyes as a result of the aging process.

    3. Decrease in depth perception and early eye changes associated with glaucoma.

    4. Visual changes secondary to long-term treatment with digitoxin and corticosteroids.

8. The nurse practitioner is preparing to examine the eyes of an adult client. To examine the optic disc and retinal vessels, the practitioner uses which aperture on the ophthalmoscope?

    1. Small aperture.

    2. Red-free filter.

    3. Slit.

    4. Grid.

9. When testing the eyes for the presence of a normal consensual response, the nurse practitioner:

    1. Shines the light into the client's pupil and observes the rate of pupillary constriction.

    2. Directs the light into one pupil and observes for the constriction or response of other pupil.

    3. Holds a card in front of one eye and has the client focus on a fixed object, removes the card, and observes movement of the newly uncovered eye.

    4. Asks the client to focus on an object, then directs a light source to the bridge of the nose while observing for symmetric reflection in both eyes.

10. On ophthalmic examination, there appears to be a narrowing or blocking of the vein at the point where an arteriole crosses over it. The significance of this finding is:

    1. The need to evaluate the client for chronic hypertension.

    2. The possibility of increased ocular pressure associated with glaucoma.

    3. Its association with papilledema, causing decreased venous drainage.

    4. It may represent a small embolus in the retinal vessels.

11. When examining the eyes, the nurse practitioner determines that the pupils change in size when the client focuses from a close object to a distant object. This is interpreted as:

    1. Normal visual accommodation.

    2. Intact extraocular motor nerves.

    3. Appropriate consensual response.

    4. Visual acuity within normal limits.

12. During a preschool screening for visual acuity, the nurse practitioner would also assess for:

    1. Pupils that are equal and reactive.

    2. Intraocular pressure by tonometry.

    3. Diplopia.

    4. Strabismus.

Ears

13. When examining the ears of an adult client, the nurse practitioner determines the tympanic membrane (TM) is gray and translucent. This is interpreted as:

    1. Scarring from previous infections.

    2. Decreased circulation to the membrane.

    3. Presence of serous fluid behind the membrane.

    4. Normal characteristics of the adult ear.

14. The Rinne test is performed to determine conduction of sound through the bone and auditory canal. A normal Rinne test is described as:

    1. Equal conduction through mastoid bone and ear canal.

    2. Air conduction twice as long as bone conduction.

    3. Bone conduction twice as long as air conduction.

    4. Sound is clearer with bone conduction than air conduction.

15. When assessing the tympanic membrane, specific landmarks are determined and described according to the face of a clock. Where are the normal landmarks for the right TM located?

    1. Direct light reflex at 5- to 6-o'clock position, malleus at 1 to 2 o'clock, with umbo in center.

    2. Manubrium slanted to the left, with malleus at 10-o'clock position.

    3. Direct light reflex in center of membrane, with malleus at 9-o'clock position.

    4. Umbo to the left, with anterior malleolar folds at 10-o'clock position.

16. A 4-year-old child's pure-tone audiometry reveals 25 decibels (dB) in the left ear and 43 dB in the right ear. The nurse practitioner would interpret these findings as:

    1. Inconclusive; pure-tone audiometry is not accurate in children less than 5 years of age.

    2. Within normal limits for age.

    3. Normal hearing in the left ear and moderate hearing loss in the right ear.

    4. Mild hearing loss in the left ear and normal hearing in the right ear.

17. The nurse practitioner knows that an infant with low or obliquely set ears also has an increased incidence of:

    1. Cataracts.

    2. Hyaline membrane disease.

    3. Genitourinary defects.

    4. Cardiovascular anomalies.

Nose

18. The nurse practitioner understands that nasal mucosa:

    1. Is redder than oral mucosa.

    2. Is pale and translucent in appearance.

    3. Appears pink and boggy, without exudate.

    4. Appears dark pink, with watery secretion.

Throat

19. Throat cultures are indicated for the following suspected causes of pharyngitis:

    1. Rhinovirus and coronavirus infection.

    2. Group A β-hemolytic streptococci.

    3. Mononucleosis.

    4. *Candida albicans*.

20. Which of the following statement is **true** regarding tonsils?

    1. Children with large tonsils are more prone to tonsillitis than those with small tonsils.

    2. Tonsils enlarge as the child grows older.

    3. Hypertrophied tonsils in children usually represent a normal finding.

    4. Most cases of tonsillitis are caused by a β-hemolytic streptococcal infection.

21. An adolescent arrives at the clinic with a complaint of low-grade fever, sore throat, slight headache, and fatigue. On physical examination the nurse practitioner finds exudative tonsils bilaterally, red pharynx with white patches, and enlarged posterior cervical neck nodes. The nurse practitioner would expect which laboratory test result?

    1. Positive rapid strep test.
    2. Positive monospot test.
    3. Decreased white blood cell (WBC) count.
    4. Positive viral throat cultures.

Disorders

Head

22. An adult client presents to the office with a white plaque near the base of the tongue. The nurse practitioner notes that the plaque does not wipe off and assesses it as:

    1. Hemangioma.
    2. Leukoplakia.
    3. Papilloma.
    4. Erythroplasia.

23. Which of the following are predominant risk factors for oral carcinoma?

    1. History of dental infections and age <40.
    2. Tobacco use and alcohol use.
    3. Herpes simplex virus type 1 and tobacco use.
    4. Alcohol use and history of dental abscess.

24. The hallmark of early oral cancer is:

    1. Tissue retraction.
    2. Thickening oral tissues.
    3. Persistent (>14 days) local inflammation.
    4. Halitosis and cough.

25. An adult male client is being evaluated for a complaint of a sore throat. He states that he has difficulty swallowing and has some mouth pain. On examination the nurse practitioner finds that the client's mouth, tongue, and pharynx are coated with white curdlike plaques that are difficult to remove and leave a red surface when scraped with a tongue blade. What would be the best action for the nurse practitioner to take at this time?

    1. Refer the client to an ear, nose, and throat specialist for evaluation.
    2. Have the physician prescribe amoxicillin 500 mg PO tid × 10 days.
    3. Encourage the client to have human immunodeficiency virus (HIV) screening.
    4. Recommend clear liquids only for the next few days.

26. The nurse practitioner knows that the most common site for head and neck cancer is the:

    1. Sinuses.
    2. Oral cavity.
    3. Larynx.
    4. Nasal cavity.

27. The nurse practitioner taking a preschooler's history learns that the family does not have fluoridated drinking water. With consideration of the concerns about fluorosis, what is the most appropriate nursing intervention?

    1. Prescribe 5 ml of 0.02% fluoride solution (Fluorinse) once daily.
    2. Instruct patients to use a pea-size fluoridated dentrifice and to supervise toothbrushing.
    3. Instruct parents to use bottled drinking water.
    4. Refer to dentist for topical application of fluoride.

Eyes

28. A client who is a sheet metal worker complains of something in his right eye since this morning. Before beginning treatment, the nurse practitioner should:

    1. Instill local anesthetic.
    2. Check the visual acuity.
    3. Flush the eye with tap water for 30 minutes.
    4. Stain the eye with fluorescein.

29. A mother reports that her toddler awoke this morning with eye redness and a swollen eyelid. The nurse practitioner notes that the child is afebrile and the eyelid is nontender and uniformly swollen. The most likely diagnosis is:

    1. Blepharitis.

    2. Hordeolum.

    3. Insect bite.

    4. Dacryocystitis.

30. On examination the nurse practitioner notes that a 2-week-old infant's left eye is watering and crusted material is on the eyelids. No edema or erythema is noted. The nurse practitioner would make the diagnosis of:

    1. Nasolacrimal duct obstruction.

    2. Conjunctivitis.

    3. Congenital dacrocystocele.

    4. Corneal abrasion.

31. A client is being prepared for cataract surgery. What information is important for the nurse practitioner to explain to the client?

    1. The procedure is short, and the client usually goes home the morning after the surgery.

    2. Both eyes will be patched for the first 24 hours, and it is important for the client to stay in bed.

    3. The client may have problems with headache and eye pain for the first 24 hours and should take the pain medication provided.

    4. Clients usually go home 2–3 hours after the surgery; the client will have increased tearing, but it should not be painful.

32. A client works as a welder. He finished work about 8 hours ago and discovered the protective glass on his welding hood was cracked. He is complaining of agonizing pain and photophobia. The correct diagnosis and action are:

    1. Chemical keratitis; dilate with atropine twice daily.

    2. Viral conjunctivitis; sulfonamide drops four times daily.

    3. Corneal abrasion; binocular patching with polymyxin ointment.

    4. Ultraviolet keratitis; antibiotic drops, NSAID topical drops, patching optional.

33. A geriatric client presents at the clinic with complaints of blurred vision that has increasingly worsened over the past 2 years. The client also has a problem with glare but not with pain. The nurse practitioner would first evaluate for the presence of:

    1. Glaucoma.

    2. Retinal detachment.

    3. Degeneration of macula.

    4. Cataracts.

34. An adult client presents to the nurse practitioner for evaluation of a red, itchy eye for 1 day. The client states that when he awoke, the eye was matted shut. The client can recall no trauma to the eye. The pupils are equal and reactive, and the client denies any pain to the eye. The nurse practitioner treats this client for:

    1. Conjunctivitis.

    2. Corneal abrasion.

    3. Glaucoma.

    4. Iritis.

35. Which assessment of the eye is a deviation from common age-related changes?

    1. Arcus senilis.

    2. Presbyopia.

    3. Sensitivity to glare.

    4. Sustained nystagmus.

36. During routine physical examination of a 30-year-old client, the nurse practitioner identifies arcus senilis. What is the significance of this disorder?

    1. High potential for future blindness.

    2. None; normal variant of aging process.

    3. Abnormal lipid metabolism requiring medical management.

    4. Hereditary variant of no consequence.

37. A 70-year-old client comes to the clinic complaining of an increased sensitivity to glare, difficulty adapting to darkness, and altered depth perception. The nurse practitioner should suspect:

    1. Cataract.

    2. Macular degeneration.

    3. Glaucoma.

    4. Normal age-related changes.

38. A mother brings her 6-week-old infant to the clinic because she is concerned that the child's eyes are crossed. What is the nurse practitioner's most appropriate response?

    1. Explain to the mother that this is normal; reevaluate the child at 3 months of age.

    2. Refer the infant to an ophthalmologist.

    3. Provide the mother with normal saline eye drops for the infant.

    4. Have the mother alternate patching one eye then the other every 6 hours.

39. In assessing a child with bacterial conjunctivitis, the nurse practitioner finds:

    1. Minimal tearing, moderate itching, and profuse exudate.

    2. Severe itching, moderate tearing, and minimal discharge.

    3. Minimal itching, moderate tearing, and mucoid exudate.

    4. Minimal itching, moderate tearing, and profuse exudate.

40. The nurse practitioner makes the diagnosis of nasolacrimal obstruction in a 1-week-old infant who presents with "leaking" of the right eye and a yellow discharge in the inner canthus of both eyes. Which of the following interventions would be **contraindicated**?

    1. Neosporin ophthalmic drops.

    2. Massaging the lacrimal duct for 1 minute four times daily.

    3. Cleansing the eye with warm water four times daily.

    4. Dexamethasone (Decadron) ophthalmic drops.

Ears

41. A child is diagnosed by the nurse practitioner with acute otitis media (AOM). During pneumatic otoscopy the nurse practitioner expects the tympanic membrane (TM) to be:

    1. Immobile, painful, with absent or decreased landmarks.

    2. Mobile, painful, with absent or decreased landmarks.

    3. Immobile, not painful, with landmarks visualized.

    4. Mobile, not painful, full and bulging.

42. In teaching clients how to avoid acoustic trauma due to noise in the very loud range, the nurse practitioner knows that noise is loudest from a:

    1. Vacuum cleaner.

    2. Power mower.

    3. Clothes washer.

    4. Food blender.

43. A geriatric client is complaining of difficulty hearing and states that the problem seems to have worsened over the past few years. What finding would support a diagnosis of presbycusis?

    1. Complaint that they can hear voices, but everyone mumbles.

    2. Rinne test indicating air conduction greater than bone conduction.

    3. History of long-term tetracycline therapy for chronic infections.

    4. Long-term family history of chronic hearing loss.

44. A 6-year-old child is seen by the nurse practitioner for ear pain. The child is afebrile. The left ear canal is extremely edematous and moderately inflamed, with thick yellowish drainage at the external meatus. The child denies putting anything in the ear canal, but the nurse practitioner finds that the child swims frequently. The most likely diagnosis is:

    1. Acute otitis media.

    2. Serous otitis media.

    3. Sinusitis.

    4. Otitis externa.

45. Which of the following organisms is **least likely** to cause otitis media?

    1. *Moraxella catarrhalis.*

    2. *Streptococcus pneumoniae.*

    3. *Chlamydia trachomatis.*

    4. *Haemophilus influenzae.*

46. Risk factors for acute otitis media (AOM) include:

    1. Second-hand smoke, attending day care, American Indians and Eskimos.

    2. Chinese race, previous otitis media, many siblings.

    3. Higher socioeconomic level, full-time day care, allergies.

    4. Summer season, full-time day care, premature at birth.

47. Which assessment of the ear would indicate a deviation from the normal aging process?

    1. Dull, retracted, white tympanic membrane.

    2. An elongated lobule.

    3. A sensorineural hearing loss.

    4. Bulging tympanic membrane with a distorted cone of light.

48. Which statement by the nurse practitioner indicates an understanding of conductive hearing loss in the older client?

    1. "This has occurred due to damage of the eighth cranial nerve from gentamicin."

    2. "This is a result of an inner ear infection."

    3. "This is a normal part of aging and is referred to as presbycusis."

    4. "This may be reversible after the cerumen is removed from the ear canal."

49. A 6-year-old child is examined by the nurse practitioner because of fluctuating hearing problems. The child is afebrile and denies otalgia. The mobility of the tympanic membrane (TM) is decreased when the nurse practitioner performs pneumatic otoscopy. The TM is opaque with no visible landmarks. The child denies putting anything in the ear, and the mother states

the child does not swim frequently. The most likely diagnosis is:

    1. Acute otitis media (AOM).

    2. A foreign body.

    3. Otitis media with effusion (OME).

    4. Otitis externa.

50. Sensory hearing loss is common in industrial settings and preventable with the use of adequate hearing protection. This type of hearing loss is usually first noted with changes at what level?

    1. 500 Hz.

    2. 200 Hz.

    3. 3000–4000 Hz.

    4. Above 4000 Hz.

Nose

51. An adult client presents to the nurse practitioner's office with fever and complaints of right facial pain, copious yellow nasal discharge, and acute pain and headache when bending over. The symptoms have been occurring for about 5 days. There is no transillumination of the right maxillary sinus and that area is very tender to palpation. The client's diagnosis is:

    1. Chronic sinusitis.

    2. Acute sinusitis.

    3. Dental abscess.

    4. Temporal arteritis.

52. The nurse practitioner teaches the mother of a school-age child the following as the most effective preventive measure against the common cold:

    1. Judicious use of vitamin C during cold season.

    2. Ensuring adequate sleep and fluids.

    3. Meticulous handwashing, preferably with an antibacterial soap and warm water.

    4. Avoiding contact with children and adults who have a runny nose, cough, and sore throat.

Throat

53. A 20-year-old client presents to the nurse practitioner's office with a chief complaint of "severe sore throat" for 3 days. The client states he also "ran a fever, but does not know how high it got," and he has been very tired. Physical examination reveals enlarged tonsils with large patchy exudate, inflamed pharynx, and nontender posterior cervical lymphadenopathy. The rest of the exam was unremarkable. The nurse practitioner would make the diagnosis of:

    1. Infectious mononucleosis.

    2. Leukemia.

    3. Scarlet fever.

    4. Oral candidiasis.

54. Which of the following clinical findings are associated with bacterial streptococcal pharyngitis?

    1. Rhinorrhea.

    2. Cough.

    3. Enlarged tonsils with exudate.

    4. Small oral vesicles.

Pharmacology

55. The antibiotics of choice for mild cases of acute sinusitis in the adult are:

    1. Amoxicillin (Amoxil) 500 mg PO tid × 14 days; trimethoprim-sulfamethoxazole (Septra) DS PO 1 q12h × 14 days; penicillin V potassium (Pen-Vee K) 500 mg bid PO × 14 days.

    2. Trimethoprim-sulfamethoxazole DS PO 1 q12h × 14 days; penicillin V potassium (Pen-Vee K) 500 mg PO bid × 14 days.

    3. Penicillin G 150,000 U IM single dose; amoxicillin 500 mg PO tid × 14 days.

    4. Amoxicillin 500 mg PO tid × 14 days; trimethoprim-sulfamethoxazole DS 1 q12h PO × 14 days.

56. A geriatric client is diagnosed with chronic open-angle glaucoma. She has a past history of bradycardia and first-degree atrioventricular block. In consideration of her treatment, what medication is to be avoided?

    1. Pilocarpine (Isopto Carpine).

    2. Timolol (Timoptic).

    3. Hydrochlorothiazide (HydroDiuril).

    4. Acetazolamide (Diamox).

57. Which antibiotic would be appropriate for the nurse practitioner to prescribe for beta-lactamase production by strains of *Haemophilus influenzae* and *Moraxella catarrhalis* in a child with acute otitis media?

    1. Amoxicillin (Amoxil).

    2. Erythromycin-sulfisoxazole (Pediazole).

    3. Penicillin V potassium (Pen-Vee K).

    4. Amoxicillin with clavulanic acid (Augmentin)

58. Prophylactic antibiotics are indicated for which of the following clients who have a history of acute otits media (AOM)?

    1. A 3-year-old with two episodes of AOM in the previous winter.

    2. A 2-year-old with three episodes of AOM within the last 6 months.

    3. A 4-year-old with history of prophylactic antibiotics in last 2 years but without evidence of AOM this year.

    4. A 2-year-old with three episodes of AOM over last 9 months.

59. The treatment plan for a client diagnosed with infectious mononucleosis includes which of the following?

    1. Rest during acute phase.

    2. Avoid exercise during acute phase.

    3. Corticosteroids during acute phase.

    4. Ampicillin orally for 10 days.

60. An adolescent client has had yellowish green nasal discharge and frontal headache for a week. The adolescent's temperature has gone up to 38.4°C (101.2°F) on most afternoons and she has a cough that worsens when she lies down. The physical exam is within normal limits except for the drainage and a slightly erythe-

matous pharynx. She does not have any drug allergies and has not been taking any medications in the last few months. Which medication would be best to prescribe for her?

1. Diphenhydramine (Benadryl).

2. Erythromycin (E-Mycin).

3. Pseudoephedrine (Sudafed).

4. Amoxicillin/clavulanate (Augmentin).

61. A 4-year-old boy (weight 18 kg) is diagnosed with bilateral otitis media. His last ear infection was 6 months ago, and he has no known drug allergies. An appropriate medication to prescribe would be:

1. Ampicillin 40–50 mg/kg/day tid × 7 days.

2. Corticosteroid otic solution 3 gtt both ears × 10 days.

3. Amoxicillin 75–90 mg/kg/day bid × 10 days.

4. Doxycycline 250 mg 1 tsp PO tid × 10 days.

Answers & Rationales

Physical Examination & Diagnostic Tests

Head

1. **(3)** Dental fluorosis causes surface pitting and staining, especially to the central and lateral permanent incisors. Tetracycline would have caused staining of all the teeth. Dental caries would be more indicative of poor dental hygiene. "Baby teeth," not the permanent teeth, would be affected by going to bed with a bottle.

2. **(2)** The conceptualization of triangles is useful in determining the location of palpable lymph nodes in the neck. The sternocleidomastoid muscle is the division between the anterior (containing the anterior superficial cervical chain) and the posterior (containing the posterior cervical chain) triangles. The trapezius muscle marks the posterior border of the posterior triangle. The supraclavicular or scale nodes are palpated in the angle formed by the clavicle and the sternocleidomastoid muscle.

Eyes

3. **(2)** The correct use of the ophthalmoscope involves using the right hand and right eye to examine the client's right eye. The room should be semidarkened for best visualization. The examiner initially inspects the lens and vitreous body from a distance of about 12 inches (at zero setting) and moves closer to the eye, usually rotating the lenses to the positive numbers (+15 to +20), which assists in focusing on near objects.

4. **(4)** A 4-year-old's normal acuity is 20/40; therefore, none of the other answers is appropriate.

5. **(1)** Cover-uncover tests for strabismus; Bruchner's tests the red reflex; Ishihara's tests color perception; and Snellen's tests far vision.

6. **(2)** If the lid margin falls above the limbus (junction line where the sclera and cornea meet) so that some sclera is visible, hyperthyroidism may be present. The lid may lag behind the limbus as the gaze moves from an upward to a downward position. Ptosis is a drooping lid margin that falls at the pupil or below and may indicate an oculomotor lesion or myasthenia gravis. A localized infection of the small glands around the eyelashes in the hair follicle at the lid margin is called a hordeolum. A chalazion is an inflammation or cyst of the meibomian glands that lie within the posterior portion of the eyelid.

7. **(2)** With cataracts there is a clouding of the lens, not a circle around the pupil. The circle around the pupil is arcus senilis, which is normal in the geriatric client. The visual acuity of the client cannot be determined from the information provided. There are no observable pupillary changes in the beginning stages of glaucoma, which is identified by checking the intraocular pressure.

8. **(2)** The red-free filter is used to examine the optic disc for pallor and vascular changes as well as to assess for retinal hemorrhages. The small aperture is used for small pupils, the slit is for the anterior eye, and the grid is for estimating the size of lesions found in the fundal area.

9. **(2)** Consensual response is pupillary constriction of one eye when there is a direct light stimulus to the pupil of the other eye.

10. **(1)** Arteriovenous nicking is associated with chronic hypertension. Intraocular pressure cannot be determined from an ophthalmic examination. Papilledema is associated with swelling around the optic disc. Small emboli are represented by an abrupt impediment or severe narrowing of an arteriole not associated with where the retinal veins and arteries cross.

11. **(1)** Changes in pupil size when focusing from near to distant objects is normal accommodation. Extraocular eye movements refer to the ability to move the eye. Consensual response is constriction of the eye in response to light being shined in the opposite eye. The Snellen eye chart is used to determine the visual acuity.

12. **(4)** Strabismus (malaligned eyes) can be a precursor for amblyopia (decreased visual acuity). It is important to detect strabismus as early as possible in preschool children. Options #1 and #3 are components of a neurologic assessment. Tonometry exams are performed to assess for glaucoma.

Ears

13. **(4)** This describes the normal characteristics of the TM. No evidence indicates scarring or fluid.

14. **(2)** The normal Rinne test is air conduction twice as long as bone conduction (AC > BC).

15. **(1)** This describes the correct position for these landmarks on the right ear. In Option #2 the manubrium slants to the right with the malleus at the 1- to 2-o'clock position for the right ear. Option #3 describes the correct position for the left ear. In Option #4 the umbo is in the center with anterior folds at the 1- to 2-o'clock position for the right ear.

16. **(3)** Pure-tone audiometry is appropriate after age 3 years; 0–25 dB = normal, 26–40 dB = mild hearing loss, and 41–55 dB = moderate hearing loss.

17. **(3)** Low-set or obliquely set ears occur more frequently in children who also have genitourinary defects. None of the other defects is associated with low-set ears.

Nose

18. **(1)** Nasal mucosa is redder than oral mucosa. Increased redness of the nasal mucosa usually indicates infection. Pale, boggy turbinates along with watery secretion often occur with allergic rhinitis. The normal secretion is mucoid. Purulent, crusty, or bloody secretions are abnormal.

Throat

19. **(2)** Rapid screening for streptococcal infection can be done from a throat swab with antigen agglutination kits, but there is a 5%–10% false-negative rate; therefore a culture should be obtained. The heterophile antibody test (monospot test), which rapidly detects heterophile antibodies, compares with the sensitivity and specificity (95% specific and 90% sensitive) of older heterophile antibody tests to diagnose mononucleosis. *Candida albicans* and rhinovirus are not diagnosed by bacterial cultures. Oral candidiasis can be diagnosed with a potassium hydroxide smear.

20. **(3)** Enlarged tonsils are common in young children. As the child grows older, the tonsils recede in size. Only about 25%–30% of tonsillitis is caused by the β-hemolytic streptococcus. Option #1 is a false statement.

21. **(2)** The client in this situation had risk factors (age) and symptoms of mononucleosis, so the monospot or heterophile antibody test should be conducted. The classic triad of mononucleosis symptoms includes sore throat, fever, and posterior cervical lymphadenopathy with or without mild tenderness. Rapid screening for streptococcal infection can be done from throat swab with antigen agglutination kits and would be obtained first, but it would probably be negative. WBC count would be ordered for bacterial pharyngitis; an increased WBC is found with bacterial infection and a decreased WBC with viral agents.

Disorders

Head

22. **(2)** Leukoplakia is a white patch present on the oral mucosa that cannot be rubbed off. Hemangiomas are benign blood vessel proliferations of the lips, tongue, and buccal

mucosa. Erythroplasia is an asymptomatic, red, velvety lesion of the mouth that may indicate malignancy. Papillomas are benign verrucous lesions that are manifestations of human papillomavirus (HPV) infection.

23. **(2)** The high-risk factors for oral cancer are tobacco and alcohol use. The risk increases with the number of cigarettes smoked per day. The disease is age related, occurring in those over 40 years of age and increasing with age. The male/female ratio is 3:1. Other risk factors are use of cigars, pipes, and smokeless tobacco. HPV has been considered in the etiology for squamous cell carcinoma in the upper head and neck.

24. **(3)** Erythroplasia is accompanied by an inflammatory reaction in a client with suspected oral cancer. Erythematous lesion persisting over 14 days strongly suggests early oral cancer. Tissue retraction and thickening of the oral tissues are later signs of oral cancer. Halitosis (odor) may be associated with dysfunction within the oral cavity, nasal cavity, sinuses, or esophageal disorders. Cough is the primary symptom of respiratory disorders such as acute bronchitis or pneumonia.

25. **(3)** Adults who present with thrush (oral candidiasis) may be immunologically impaired. It is important to make the diagnosis of HIV early to start treatment modalities. Treatment with amoxicillin may actually worsen the condition.

26. **(2)** The nurse practitioner knows the risk factors for head and neck cancer include tobacco and alcohol use; poor oral hygiene and occupational exposure to asbestos, coke, nickel, wood, or leather are also risk factors. The most common site is in the oral cavity, accounting for 48% of the head and neck cancer diagnoses.

27. **(2)** A fluoridated dentifrice should be used in a small amount (pea-size) and children under 6 should be supervised so that they do not swallow too much toothpaste, which would put them at risk for fluorosis. The dose of fluoride rinse is too high, and it is inappropriate to prescribe to a preschooler. Bottled water does not contain fluoride. Topical application, although appropriate, is not the best answer.

Eyes

28. **(2)** Check the visual acuity before treatment as a basis for comparison in the event of

complications. Local anesthesia is helpful for a detailed exam, after the initial inspection, and during removal, if indicated. Flushing with normal saline may be helpful to remove an object that is visualized. Staining the eye should come later when preparing to examine for abrasion under ultraviolet light.

29. **(3)** Generalized, diffuse swelling and erythema of the eyelid is associated with an insect bite. Blepharitis is a chronic inflammatory condition characterized by erythema and scaling of the lid margins. Hordeolum, or stye, is an acute, purulent inflammation of the sebaceous glands (usually the meibomian or zeisian) of the eyelids and usually does not involve the entire eyelid. It may be painful, especially over the gland. Dacryocystitis is an inflammation of the lacrimal sac characterized by erythema and swelling over the lacrimal duct.

30. **(1)** Nasolacrimal obstruction occurs in up to 6% of infants. Signs and symptoms include a wet eye with mucoid discharge. Irritated skin and conjunctivitis also may be associated with this condition. There is no redness, which would suggest conjunctivitis. Congenital dacrocystocele presents at birth as a bluish subcutaneous mass. There would be more signs of irritation and pain with a corneal abrasion.

31. **(4)** Clients go home almost immediately after the procedure. Eye patches may be worn for the first 24 hours. Care should be taken to protect the operative eye from injury. There is some discomfort, but pain should not be a problem. The client can be mobile and active as tolerated.

32. **(4)** Exposure to a welding arc can cause ultraviolet burns to the cornea. Treatment with ophthalmic antibiotic drops and topical ophthalmic drops of nonsteroidal antiinflammatory drug (NSAID), such as diclofenac (Voltaren), can be done at home, with recovery expected in 2–3 days. Patching is controversial and generally reserved for severe cases for the first 24 hours only.

33. **(4)** Cataracts are characterized by painless loss of visual acuity over time. Retinal detachment most often occurs suddenly, with partial loss of the field of vision. Glaucoma results in the loss of peripheral vision, and macular degeneration primarily involves the central vision field.

34. **(1)** The chief complaint is pain in corneal abrasion, glaucoma, and iritis. Conjunctivitis presents with no pain and with a history of purulent discharge.

35. **(4)** Sustained nystagmus is indicative of a neurologic complication. The other options include normal age-related changes.

36. **(3)** Arcus senilis is the deposit of lipids at the junction of the cornea and sclera that is present in many people over age 50. When identified in younger individuals, it points to a disorder of lipid metabolism.

37. **(4)** These assessments are normal age-related changes. Signs and symptoms of cataracts include reduced visual acuity, painless progressive loss of vision, and sensitivity to light, especially during night driving. Reduced color discrimination and double vision may also be seen. Macular degeneration presents with a loss of the central vision. Primary open-angle glaucoma presents with occasional headaches and occasionally halos around lights and may be asymptomatic in early stages. Primary angle-closure glaucoma presents with episodes of blurred vision, halos around lights at night, and redness with congestion.

38. **(1)** Strabismus is not an uncommon or abnormal occurrence in infants up until 3 months of age.

39. **(4)** Classic signs of bacterial conjunctivitis include those symptoms listed along with complaints of eyelids being "glued shut" on arising in the morning. Option #2 is indicative of allergic conjunctivitis. Option #3 is indicative of viral conjunctivitis.

40. **(4)** Steroid (dexamethasone) medications are not used to treat nasolacrimal obstruction in infancy. Due to the yellow discharge in the eye, it would be appropriate to prescribe an antibiotic to prevent or treat conjunctivitis. Cleansing the eye with warm water and massaging the lacrimal duct are both appropriate interventions.

Ears

41. **(1)** The diagnosis of AOM is clinical, made by otoscopy based on the appearance of the TM. The bony landmarks are absent or decreased. The TM may be full, bulging, or retracted with pus, and the light reflex is distorted.

Pneumatic otoscopy reveals decreased or absent TM mobility. Erythema is an inconclusive finding, especially in children, because the redness may be caused by crying rather than infection.

42. **(2)** Although all these household appliances are noisy, the client should wear ear plugs or muffs when using a power lawn mower regularly for long periods.

43. **(1)** In presbycusis the ability to hear high-frequency sounds is diminished. These patients have difficulty distinguishing consonant sounds, so words such as "shoe" and "true" are heard as "oo." The Rinne test indicates bone conduction is two times greater than air conduction. Tetracyclines are not ototoxic, and the family history may or may not contribute to the problem.

44. **(4)** The client has the clinical findings of otitis externa, an inflammation and infection of the external ear canal predisposed by excessive wetness, such as swimming. Common organisms responsible for otitis externa include *Pseudomonas aeruginosa, Proteus mirabilis*, and *Enterobacter aerogenes* or fungal organisms of the *Aspergillus* or *Candida* species. Sinusitis clinical findings focus on sinus tenderness and a purulent nasal discharge. Clinical findings of otitis media include ear pain, full or bulging tympanic membrane, decreased or negative mobility, and possible erythema. Findings associated with serous otitis media include opaque or translucent tympanic membrane with air bubbles; landmarks may be absent, and the light reflex may be diffuse or absent.

45. **(3)** The key factor that contributes to acute otitis media (AOM) is a dysfunctional eustachian tube that may allow bacteria from the nasopharynx to the middle ear. The most frequent bacterial organisms that infect the middle ear, especially in children, are similar to those of the nasopharynx: *S. pneumoniae, H. influenzae*, and *M. catarrhalis. Escherichia coli* and *Klebsiella* cause about 15% of AOM cases in babies less than 6 weeks old. Viruses may also cause AOM. *Chlamydia trachomatis* is not a frequent causative agent.

46. **(1)** AOM occurs more during the fall, winter, and spring than summer. American Indians and Eskimos have more repetitive and severe otitis media than members of other races. Children who attend day care centers have

more frequent infections than those who do not. Members of lower socioeconomic levels are more at risk than those at higher levels. Other risk factors are children who live with many siblings or in homes with smokers, children who have developmental abnormalities, and male gender.

47. **(4)** This would be indicative of an inflammation of the middle ear (AOM). The other options include normal changes that occur with aging.

48. **(4)** Conductive hearing loss may result from AOM, perforation of the eardrum, and obstruction of the ear canal, as by cerumen. The other distracters result in sensorineural hearing loss.

49. **(3)** The client with otitis externa, "swimmer's ear," or inflammation of the external auditory canal presents with ear pain. The most common clinical findings include redness and swelling of the external ear canal, pain with manipulation of movement of auricle, no swelling or pain over mastoid, and usually no involvement of TM. The TM is involved in AOM. No evidence indicated that the child placed a foreign body in the ear. The most significant distinction between OME and AOM is that clinical findings of acute infection (e.g., fever, otalgia) are lacking in OME. Clinical findings of OME, the most common cause of hearing loss in children, include relatively asymptomatic, decreased mobility, and bulging opaque TM with no visible landmarks.

50. **(4)** This type of hearing loss presents with high-frequency loss, above the 4000-Hz level, then progresses into voice frequencies at 2000–3000 Hz.

Nose

51. **(2)** The client is experiencing the classic characteristics of acute sinusitis. Chronic sinusitis causes nasal discharge, congestion, headache, and cough for more than 30 days. Dental abscess causes constant, severe, tooth-associated pain and jaw tenderness. Temporal arteritis causes pain in the jaw, tongue, and face but no nasal discharge.

52. **(3)** Transmission of cold viruses is indirect (e.g., self-inoculation from virus on surfaces of inanimate objects to mucous membranes of nose and mouth). Virus is less likely to be spread by the aerosol route. Thus the client should avoid touching the nose and mouth unless the hands have been thoroughly washed. It is impractical to avoid contact because cold viruses are found everywhere. Although many individuals believe vitamin C prevents colds, research to support this claim is minimal.

Throat

53. **(1)** Mononucleosis is often seen in adolescents and young adults. It often presents with fever, exudate on the tonsils, generalized lymphadenopathy, malaise, posterior cervical adenopathy, and palatine petechiae. Leukemia presents with anorexia, irritability, lethargy, and bone pain, with peak incidence in 3- to 5-year-olds. Scarlet fever presents in children 2–10 years old with fever, abdominal pain, headache, sore throat, and strawberry tongue. Oral candidiasis presents with white curdlike plaques on an erythematous mucosa. The tongue is red with a white coat.

54. **(3)** Characteristics of bacterial pharyngitis include headache, mild to severe erythema of tonsils with white or yellow exudate, dysphagia, positive anterior cervical nodes, sore throat with dysphagia, fever >101°-102.5°F, and nausea. Viral organisms that cause herpangina present with small oral vesicles. Cough is the primary symptom of acute bronchitis. Rhinorrhea is associated with allergic rhinitis.

Pharmacology

55. **(4)** Amoxicillin is the first-line antibiotic for mild cases of acute uncomplicated sinusitis in the adult because of cost-effectiveness, efficacy, and cure rates ranging from 67%–100%. For moderate severity and in geographic areas with high beta-lactam resistance, amoxicillin/clavulanate is the next choice. Additional choices include trimethoprim-sulfamethoxazole, cefuroxime, azithromycin, and clarithromycin.

56. **(2)** Beta-blockers cause problems with bradycardia. Timolol can be absorbed systemically from the eye and should not be used.

57. **(4)** Amoxicillin with clavulanic acid is effective against beta-lactamase production. Cephalexin, cefuroxime, or cefixime can be used as alternatives. Erythromycin-sulfisoxazole has recently been reported as less effective. Cephalosporins are effective against beta-lactamase production by *H. influenzae* and *M. catarrhalis*. Amoxicillin is ineffective against beta-lactamase production, as is penicillin V.

58. **(2)** The decision to prescribe prophylactic antibiotics is individualized but should be considered for children who have experienced three documented episodes of AOM in a 6-month period. The risks and benefits should be explained to the parents. Antibiotic prophylaxis has been found to be as effective as ventilating tubes in preventing new cases of AOM.

59. **(1)** Treatment of mononucleosis includes bed rest while the client has fever and myalgia (10–14 days), supportive acetaminophen or ibuprofen, warm saline gargles, and throat lozenges or spray. The client must avoid strenuous exercise and contact sports for 2 months because of the risk of splenic rupture, even if no splenomegaly is detected. Corticosteroids are recommended only in clients with impending airway obstruction. Ampicillin is not recommended because of allergic reaction and rash. About 95% of clients with mononucleosis recover uneventfully with supportive treatment.

60. **(4)** The client is experiencing symptoms of moderately severe acute sinusitis based on the symptoms of facial pressure, headache, and postnasal discharge. The first-line antibiotic to prescribe is amoxicillin/clavulanate for its safety and efficacy. Oral antihistamines such as diphenhydramine should not be used unless the client has allergies. Oral decongestants (pseudoephedrine) are not as effective in clients with sinusitis as are topical agents. Erythromycin is not a first-line antibiotic for sinusitis.

61. **(3)** The recommended treatment for otitis media in a child is amoxicillin 75–90 mg/kg/day, or for this child (18 kg), 250 mg/5 ml, 2.75 tsp bid × 10 days. The other drugs and doses listed are not appropriate treatment for AOM.

Integumentary & Childhood Diseases

Physical Examination & Diagnostic Tests

1. The nurse practitioner describes an annular skin lesion as usually arranged in:

    1. Groups of vesicles erupting unilaterally.

    2. A line.

    3. A pattern of merging together, not discrete.

    4. A circle, or ring shaped.

2. A client has pitting of the nails. The nurse practitioner understands this is associated with:

    1. Psoriasis.

    2. Iron deficiency anemia.

    3. Malnutrition.

    4. Hyperthyroidism.

3. The nurse practitioner is inspecting a dark-skinned individual for signs of jaundice. The best place to observe is:

    1. Sclera of the opened eye.

    2. Palms and soles of the hands and feet.

    3. Oral mucosa.

    4. Nail beds.

4. When assessing a client's hydration status, the best place to evaluate skin turgor on an adult is:

    1. Just below the clavicle.

    2. Below the scapula on the back.

    3. On the inside of the forearm.

    4. On the back of the hand.

5. The Wood's lamp is used to evaluate skin lesions. When the light is shone on the client's skin, a green-yellow fluorescence indicates:

   1. Presence of fungi.

   2. Lichenification.

   3. Keratinized cells.

   4. Bacterial colonies.

6. On examination of a client's skin, the nurse practitioner finds a lesion that is about 0.75 cm in diameter, brown, circumscribed, flat, and nonpalpable. What is the correct term for this lesion?

   1. Macule.

   2. Papule.

   3. Nodule.

   4. Wheal.

7. The history and physical of a client indicates past occurrences of lichenification. The nurse practitioner identifies the characteristics of this lesion as:

   1. Dried, crusty exudate, slightly elevated.

   2. Rough thickened epidermis, accentuated skin markings.

   3. Keratinized cells shaped in an irregular pattern with exfoliation.

   4. Loss of epidermis with hollowed-out area and dermis exposed.

8. Clubbing of the nails occurs in clients with chronic respiratory conditions. The nurse practitioner assesses for this condition by:

   1. Evaluating the nail for transverse depressions and ridges.

   2. Placing the client's hands together with palms inward and index fingers aligned.

   3. Placing nail beds of each index finger together to determine angle of nail plate.

   4. Determining if there is diffuse discoloration of the nail bed from decreased oxygenation.

9. A circumscribed, elevated lesion >1 cm in diameter and containing clear serous fluid is best described as a:

   1. Papule.

   2. Vesicle.

   3. Bulla.

   4. Pustule.

10. In performing a skin assessment, the nurse practitioner understands that the following characteristic of a mole would necessitate immediate intervention:

    1. A 5-mm, symmetric, uniformly brown mole on the thigh that has not changed in appearance for more than 5 years.

    2. Multiple small (1–3 mm) flat moles across the upper back that are dark brown in color, round, and have smooth edges.

    3. A 3-cm, waxy papule with a "stuck-on" appearance, noted on the face.

    4. A new, 2-mm brown mole with an irregular red border that is occasionally pruritic.

11. Dermatophyte skin infections can be diagnosed from skin scrapings and prepared with which solution for microscopic examination?

    1. Hydrochloric acid.

    2. 20% potassium hydroxide (KOH) solution.

    3. Gram's stain.

    4. Distilled water.

12. When administering skin tests to an immunocompromised client, the nurse practitioner must consider:

    1. The importance of not applying more than one skin test at a time.

    2. That the skin test may react more aggressively than expected.

    3. Identifying a known allergen for the client and using it as a control.

    4. That an immunocompromised client should not have skin testing.

13. The nurse is examining a 6-week-old infant of Latin American descent. There are irregular areas of deep-blue pigmentation across the infant's buttocks. The nurse would identify this as characteristic of:

    1. Child abuse.

    2. Telangiectatic nevi.

    3. Cutis marmorata.

    4. Mongolian spots.

Skin Disorders

14. A client complains of intolerable itching in the pubic hair. On examination the nurse practitioner notes erythematous papules and tiny white specks in the pubic hair. The differential diagnosis includes all **except**:

    1. Pediculosis pubis.
    2. Scabies.
    3. Impetigo.
    4. Atopic dermatitis.

15. An elderly woman has an area of vesicles in clusters with an erythematous base that extend from her spine, around and under her arm and breast, to the sternum on her left side. She states that the area was very tender last week and that the vesicles started erupting yesterday. She is complaining of severe pain in the area. What is the probable diagnosis for this condition?

    1. Psoriasis.
    2. Herpes zoster.
    3. Contact dermatitis.
    4. Cellulitis.

16. What is a chronic skin condition that is sometimes associated with arthritis?

    1. Eczema.
    2. Psoriasis.
    3. Neurodermatitis.
    4. Pityriasis rosea.

17. Which is a **true** statement about psoriasis?

    1. It is usually worse in the summer.
    2. It is highly contagious.
    3. It can be aggravated by stress.
    4. All clients have accompanying pruritus.

18. A mother brings her school-age child in for examination. She reports that the child frequently scratches and that the itching seems to be worse at night. On examination the family nurse practitioner notes lesions on the sides of the fingers and inner aspect of the elbows. These lesions are short, irregular runs approx-

imately 2–3 mm long and the width of a hair. The nurse practitioner tells the mother she suspects:

    1. Scabies.
    2. Hives.
    3. Fleas.
    4. Ticks.

19. What information should be provided to a client with actinic keratosis?

    1. The affected areas are a normal part of aging and are benign.
    2. These lesions can develop into squamous cell carcinomas.
    3. This is part of an allergic reaction, and the offending allergen needs to be identified.
    4. This skin condition responds well to sunlight, which will help alleviate the symptoms.

20. The following are all true statements regarding urticaria **except**:

    1. Most cases of acute urticaria involve IgE-mediated mast cell degranulation.
    2. Chronic urticaria may be related to occult infections.
    3. Urticaria is characterized by red itchy swellings a few millimeters to a few centimeters in size.
    4. Laboratory studies are necessary to identify the causative agent.

21. A client known to be positive for human immunodeficiency virus (HIV) presents with several painless, persistent, raised purple lesions on the face. What is the most likely diagnosis of the lesions?

    1. Seborrheic dermatitis.
    2. Molluscum contagiosum.
    3. Kaposi's sarcoma.
    4. Fungal infection.

22. In making a differential diagnosis between nummular eczema (dermatitis) and dyshidrotic eczematous dermatitis, the nurse practitioner knows:

    1. Nummular eczema is characterized by flushing and clusters of papulopustules on the cheek and forehead.

    2. Dyshidrotic eczematous dermatitis is a chronic vesicular type of hand-and-foot eczema characterized by vesicles (tapioca-like), scaling, lichenification, and pruritus.

    3. Nummular eczema is a hereditary disorder characterized by chronic, usually bilateral scaly plaques on exposed areas (knees, elbows).

    4. Dyshidrotic eczematous dermatitis affects primarily young adults, is contagious, and is characterized by firm papules with a cleft surface and multiple conical vegetations.

23. A middle-aged male client presents to the clinic with a complaint of being bitten last night by another individual during a fight. He has a bite mark on his forearm, and the skin has been broken. He reports he has had a tetanus shot about 8 years ago. Recommended treatment by the family nurse practitioner should include all the following **except**:

    1. Administer tetanus toxoid 0.5 ml IM.

    2. Instruct client to watch for signs of infection.

    3. Initiate treatment with penicillin plus a penicillinase-resistant penicillin.

    4. Close the wound with sutures or Steri-Strips.

24. Nail involvement secondary to primary foot-and-hand tinea, characterized by accumulation of subungual keratin that produces thickened, distorted, crumbling nails, is termed:

    1. Hippocratic nails.

    2. Onychomycosis.

    3. Koilonychia.

    4. Anonychia.

25. A middle-aged client presents for an office visit with a complaint of a measles-like rash on his trunk and spreading to his extremities. He was seen several days ago for bronchitis and started on trimethoprim-sulfamethoxazole (TMP-SMX; Septra) DS 1 tab PO bid. What is the recommended action for the family nurse practitioner?

    1. Instruct client to continue medication and see if any change occurs in the rash.

    2. Discontinue TMP-SMX.

    3. Take the client off medication for 3 days, then restart the drug.

    4. Decrease TMP-SMX to half-dose.

26. When treating atopic dermatitis in children, all the following instructions are applicable **except**:

    1. Eliminate foods thought to induce flares, one food at a time.

    2. Avoid bubble baths.

    3. Avoid overheating.

    4. Encourage bathing two or three times a day.

27. A client complaining of hyperhidrosis should be counseled that:

    1. This is a normal occurrence.

    2. There are no therapies for this complaint.

    3. Bathing in 20% alcohol solution of aluminum chloride hexahydrate (Drysol) may be beneficial.

    4. A history and physical examination need to be completed to rule out any medical etiologies.

28. During the physical examination the nurse practitioner assesses a maculopapular skin lesion on a client's back that is warty, scaly, greasy in appearance, and light tan in color. What would be the probable diagnosis?

    1. Actinic keratosis.

    2. Basal cell carcinoma.

    3. Seborrheic keratosis.

    4. Senile lentigines.

29. The nurse practitioner is assessing an older client diagnosed with herpes zoster (shingles) in the prodromal stage. What would the practitioner expect to find on the assessment of this client?

    1. Erythematous lesions present over four different parts of the body.

    2. Red, pinpoint, painless rash.

3. Burning pain in a line on only half the client's chest that does not cross the midline.

4. Painless purulent lesions for 2 days followed by complaints of itching, burning, and nausea.

30. What would be the appropriate management for a client with herpes zoster (shingles)?

1. Acyclovir (Zovirax).

2. Miconazole (Monistat-Derm).

3. Clotrimazole (Lotrimin).

4. Corticosteroid (prednisone).

31. An elderly retired farmer presents with a dome-shaped, pearly, firm nodule with telangiectasia on his nose. In making a diagnosis, the nurse practitioner recognizes this to be:

1. Compound nevus.

2. Melanoma.

3. Bullous pemphigoid.

4. Basal cell carcinoma.

32. An adult female presents with an irregular, variegated nevus on her lower left back that has doubled in size in the past 3 months. What would be an appropriate action for the nurse practitioner?

1. Do a punch biopsy to confirm the diagnosis.

2. Take a photograph of the lesion and recheck it in 1 month.

3. Refer immediately to a dermatologist.

4. Reassure the client that these are normal changes related to hormone variations.

33. An elderly client presents with pain in his right chest wall for the past 48 hours. On examination the nurse practitioner notices a vesicular eruption along the dermatome and identifies this as herpes zoster. The nurse practitioner informs the client that:

1. All symptoms will disappear in 3 days.

2. Oral medication can dramatically reduce the duration and intensity of symptoms.

3. He has chickenpox and may be contagious to his grandchildren.

4. The eruptions will recur at regular intervals.

34. A young adult female presents to the nurse practitioner's office stating that she has had an itchy red rash over her trunk for 2 weeks. She has tried over-the-counter lotions and creams, with no relief of symptoms. The rash started as a small, round red patch on her chest and has since spread across her chest, back, arms, and legs. Physical examination reveals a generalized distribution of erythematous, scaly macular lesions that run parallel to each other, creating a "Christmas tree" pattern. The nurse practitioner should:

1. Do a thorough medication history, investigate any potential allergens, and send the client to an allergy specialist.

2. Have physician prescribe triamcinolone 0.025% cream (Aristocort A) bid for 2 weeks.

3. Teach the client this viral disease is self-limiting and to avoid prolonged or excessive exposure to sunlight.

4. Refer the client to a dermatologist for a biopsy.

35. An adult male client presents to the nurse practitioner's office complaining of flulike symptoms, a large red spot in the right groin, headaches, and generalized muscle pain. These symptoms have persisted for about 4–5 weeks. In taking the history, it would be most important to determine whether the client:

1. Was using new skin care products, detergents, etc.

2. Was taking any new medications, vitamins, herbal therapies, etc.

3. Has had a recent insect bite, or was potentially exposed to insects such as ticks.

4. Has been exposed to a person with tuberculosis.

36. A nurse practitioner is teaching the mother of a child how to use permethrin 1% cream rinse (Nix) for treatment of pediculosis capitis. What is the most important information the nurse practitioner should give to the mother?

1. Shampoo the child's hair daily for 1 week with permethrin.

2. After hair is shampooed and towel-dried, apply permethrin to scalp and hair and wait 10 minutes before rinsing.

3. The shampoo should not be used again because it is toxic and may absorb systemically and cause acute respiratory problems.

4. It is not necessary to treat other children in the family or to launder bedding or clothing.

37. The nurse practitioner understands that accidental scalding in young children usually occurs:

    1. On the back of the body.
    2. On the front of the body.
    3. In a circular or glove pattern.
    4. With no specific pattern.

38. An infant has pruritus caused by eczema. The nurse practitioner teaches the mother the following regarding the infant's care:

    1. Dress the infant in cotton shorts and short-sleeved shirts.
    2. Dress the infant in wool blend long-sleeved jump suits.
    3. Give the infant cornstarch or Aveeno baths.
    4. Give the infant salt baths three times a day.

39. A new mother is concerned about the hemangioma on her infant's neck. What is the treatment of choice for the majority of infants with hemangioma?

    1. Cryosurgery.
    2. Intralesional injection of steroids.
    3. Observation.
    4. Injection of a sclerosing agent.

40. The nurse practitioner is examining an infant with atopic dermatitis. What would the physical examination reveal?

    1. Dry, scaly rash with pruritus.
    2. Distribution of rash on face and extensor surfaces.
    3. Erythematous raised areas on flexor surfaces.
    4. Moist, crusting rash with no pruritus.

41. The nurse practitioner is examining a 6-year-old child and identifies 8 to 10 patches of coffee-colored areas on the trunk. The areas are nontender, the border is irregular, and most of the areas are larger than 1.5 cm and nonpalpable. What is the best recommendation to this child's parents?

    1. The child should be evaluated further by a pediatrician for possible referral to a neurologist.
    2. These areas are normal pigmentation and will disappear.

3. A dermatologist should be consulted for removal of lesions.

4. Emollients should be applied to keep skin moist, and sunlight on the areas should be avoided.

42. An infant is noted at his well-child visit to have a yellowish, greasy scaly rash on his scalp, forehead, and ears. What is the most likely diagnosis?

    1. Seborrheic dermatitis.
    2. Atopic dermatitis.
    3. Erythema toxicum.
    4. Eczema.

43. A 1-month-old infant is being seen by the nurse practitioner for a diaper rash. On examination the practitioner notes moderate erythema and poorly marginated, dry patches of skin localized to the buttocks. The deep folds are not affected. There are no satellite lesions. What is the most likely diagnosis?

    1. Infantile seborrheic dermatitis.
    2. Allergy to disposable diapers.
    3. Contact dermatitis.
    4. Candidal diaper rash.

44. A mother brings her preschool child to see the nurse practitioner because of sores on his arms and legs. On examination the nurse practitioner notes several honey-colored crusted lesions with an erythematous base on the arms and legs. There is a history of exposure to mosquitoes. The rest of the exam is essentially negative. What is the most likely diagnosis?

    1. Scabies.
    2. Impetigo.
    3. Pityriasis rosea.
    4. Varicella.

45. A mother returns to the clinic with her 6-month-old infant to have his ears rechecked after a 10-day course of antibiotics for an ear infection. During the visit the mother states that the child is now eating better and appears to be recovering, but he now has a bad diaper rash. What is the most likely cause of this rash?

    1. Poor hygiene.
    2. Cellulitis

3. Seborrheic diaper dermatitis.

4. *Candida albicans.*

46. A school-age child presents with erythematous papular lesions and scaly plaques in the antecubital and popliteal fossae and on the neck, wrists, and ankles. The mother states that the child has been scratching the areas, especially at night. History reveals that the child also has been treated for asthma. The nurse practitioner would make the diagnosis of:

    1. Scabies.

    2. Atopic dermatitis.

    3. Tinea corporis.

    4. Contact dermatitis.

47. While attending a rural public school, a 7-year-old child was bitten on the hand by a raccoon. At the rural clinic the nurse practitioner cleansed the wound. What would be the next action?

    1. Administer tetanus antitoxin.

    2. Contact local animal control authorities.

    3. Administer rabies immune globulin (RIG) and human diploid cell vaccine (HDCV).

    4. Teach the family how to do hourly soaks to the hand using normal saline and peroxide.

48. A toddler is brought to the clinic with a history of an insect bite last evening. What presenting symptom would be associated with the bite of a brown recluse spider?

    1. Paresthesias in all extremities.

    2. Edematous, erythematous area with coalescing macules.

    3. Tissue sloughing in the bite area within 8–10 hours.

    4. Development of a central black eschar of "sinking infarct" within 6–12 hours.

49. The nurse practitioner understands that cat bites become infected more often than dog bites because:

    1. Dogs have a "cleaner mouth" than cats.

    2. Cat bites are often deep puncture wounds.

3. Dog bites are usually on the face, which makes them less susceptible to infection.

4. Cat bites are usually associated with clawing and spreading of microorganisms.

50. When do bites from insects, spiders, snakes, and bees most often occur?

    1. Fall.

    2. Spring to fall.

    3. Winter.

    4. Any time of the year.

51. An adolescent was bitten by a neighbor's dog 3 days ago. He has developed an infection in a large wound on his lower leg. What would be appropriate management of this client?

    1. Prescribe amoxicillin-clavulanate (Augmentin) 250 mg PO tid × 14 days.

    2. Approximate the edges of the wound together with suture.

    3. Prescribe cephalexin (Keflex) 500 mg PO tid × 7 days.

    4. Have the adolescent return to the clinic for follow-up in 2 weeks.

52. Medical management for a brown recluse spider bite includes:

    1. Warm moist soaks to the affected area.

    2. Ice pack and elevation of the area.

    3. Active and passive range of motion (ROM) to area.

    4. Avoidance of antihistamines.

53. A young adolescent has been bitten by a black widow spider while doing yard work. He is having a severe reaction; the nurse practitioner expects:

    1. Hypotension and shock.

    2. Localized pain, erythema, and edema in the area.

    3. Black eschar of sloughing tissue within 4 hours of the bite.

    4. Abdominal rigidity, nausea, and headache.

54. A scout leader is explaining about snakes and snake bites and says to his group about the coral snake, "Red on yellow, kill a fellow; red on black, venom lack." Later, one of the boys is bitten by a snake described a having broad rings of red and black separated by narrow rings of yellow. The nurse practitioner understands that this client will probably experience all the following **except**:

    1. Numbness and change in sensation.

    2. Local swelling at the fang mark site.

    3. Dizziness and diplopia.

    4. No symptoms, as the snake was not poisonous.

Childhood Diseases

55. Phone consultation with a mother reveals that her child has been taking TMP-SMX (Septra) for 3 days for a urinary tract infection. She has been treated with the drug previously with no problems. Currently, the child is experiencing blisterlike sores in the skinfold areas (axilla, groin), oral ulceration, and a few genital sores. Her temperature is 40°C (104°C), and she is very weak. Differential diagnosis includes:

    1. Kawasaki disease.

    2. Erythema multiforme (major).

    3. Viral exanthem.

    4. Early scalded-skin syndrome.

56. A day care center director calls to confirm when a child can return to the center after having fifth disease (erythema infectiosum). The nurse practitioner's response is based on the knowledge that the period of communicability lasts until:

    1. The rash is gone.

    2. The rash appears.

    3. Upper respiratory symptoms are gone.

    4. The transient joint pain disappears.

57. Examination of a nontoxic but ill-appearing 6-year-old reveals vesicular and ulcerative oral lesions and a maculopapular rash on the hands and feet; temperature is 38°C (100.4°F) and the child has feelings of malaise. Differential diagnosis includes:

    1. Hand-foot-and-mouth disease.

    2. Coxsackievirus group B.

    3. Echovirus 11.

    4. Varicella.

58. The nurse practitioner understands that the rash of roseola differs from that of rubella. Which statement is correct?

    1. Rash of roseola starts on the trunk.

    2. Rash of rubella is pruritic.

    3. Rash of roseola fades in 3–5 days.

    4. Rash of rubella clears on the extremities, when facial rash erupts.

59. What is appropriate treatment for a child with roseola?

    1. Antiviral medications, fluids, rest.

    2. NSAIDs, rest, and hydration.

    3. Antibiotics, hydration, and rest.

    4. Hospitalization, antipyretics, and IV fluid replacement.

Pharmacology

60. An obese woman presents to the clinic with complaints of tenderness and irritation under both of her breasts. The examination reveals a very irritated, moist, inflamed area with macules and papules present. What is the best treatment for this woman?

    1. Nystatin cream bid/tid × 10 days, with thorough drying of area and exposure to light and air.

    2. Systemic antistaphylococcal antibiotics (dicloxacillin) and soaking with moist pads of normal saline three times daily.

    3. Gentle washing of the area and removal of crusts, then application of antibiotic ointment.

    4. Antiviral treatment (acyclovir) and topical ointment to prevent secondary infection.

61. Which classification of drugs has the potential to aggravate psoriasis?

    1. Beta-blockers.

    2. Thiazide diuretics.

    3. Vasodilators.

    4. Tricyclic antidepressants.

62. In treatment of severe inflammatory acne for a female adolescent, the nurse practitioner understands that:

    1. Isotretinoin (Accutane) provides an effective first-line therapy.

    2. The benefits of treatment will be noted in 5–7 days.

    3. Counseling on stringent dietary changes is important.

    4. Systemic antibiotics are effective treatment.

63. A young mother brings her infant to the family nurse practitioner with a complaint of diaper rash present for about 1 week. The diaper area appears beefy red with sharply marginated dermatitis. Satellite lesions are also noted. The family nurse practitioner recommends:

    1. Changing from disposable diapers to cloth diapers with plastic pants.

    2. Nystatin cream (Mycostatin) after each diaper change.

    3. Wet soaks three times daily.

    4. Liberally applying oil after bathing.

64. All the following are true of postherpetic neuralgia **except**:

    1. Capsaicin cream (Zostrix) may alleviate some of the discomfort.

    2. In most clients the postherpetic pain gradually subsides over several weeks.

    3. Acyclovir (Zovirax) 200 mg 5 caps qd PO in divided doses is an effective therapy.

    4. It is more common in clients over age 60.

65. When treating genital warts with topical podophyllin, it is important for the family nurse practitioner to:

    1. Apply preparation directly to the wart and approximately 5 mm around the base.

    2. Cover with a dressing so that solution remains moist, and caution client not to remove for 24 hours.

    3. Instruct client to wash off medication in 4–6 hours.

    4. Treat with liquid nitrogen before applying podophyllin.

66. What is the recommended treatment of rosacea?

    1. Oral hydrocortisone.

    2. Oral ketoconazole.

    3. Low-dose tetracycline.

    4. Topical 5-fluorouracil.

67. When using lidocaine with epinephrine 1%–2% as a local anesthetic in the repair of an injury, it is essential to remember that the maximum allowable dose is:

    1. 7 mg/kg.

    2. 2 mg/kg.

    3. 10 mg/kg.

    4. 5 mg/kg.

68. An elderly client presents to the nurse practitioner complaining of a painful, tingling rash across the right side of his abdomen. Examination reveals vesicles with erythematous bases; some of the vesicles are draining cloudy fluid, whereas others are crusted. The nurse practitioner makes the diagnosis of herpes zoster infection, and the client is prescribed antiviral therapy. The patient states that the painful rash has kept him from sleeping for the past 4 nights. What would be appropriate therapy for this client's pain?

    1. Amitriptyline (Elavil) 10 mg PO hs and NSAIDs prn as directed.

    2. High-dose corticosteroid therapy.

    3. Application of heat directly to the area involved.

    4. No appropriate therapy is currently available to treat neuropathic pain.

69. On a return visit to the clinic, a client receiving sulfonamide therapy exhibits generalized rash, mucous membrane lesions, skin sloughing on the palms and feet, high fever, and generalized malaise. These findings would alert the nurse practitioner to consider:

    1. Hepatitis B.

    2. Stevens-Johnson syndrome.

    3. HIV infection/acquired immunodeficiency syndrome (AIDS).

    4. *Pneumocystis carinii* pneumonia.

70. The nurse practitioner is examining lesions around a child's nose and mouth. His mother states that the lesions appeared several days ago and now seem worse. Some of the vesicular, edematous, red, and tender lesions have yellow crusts and an erythematous base. What is the recommended treatment for this child?

    1. Mupirocin ointment (Bactroban) qid × 10 days.

    2. Gently soaking the lesions with antibacterial soap and removing the crusts.

    3. Dicloxacillin (Dynapen) 15 mg/kg/day in four divided doses × 10 days.

    4. Diphenhydramine (Benadryl) 5 mg PO q6h to decrease itching and spreading.

71. A mother brings her 1-year-old child to the clinic for problems with a "rash." She states the child has not been feeling well since the rash started 2 days ago. The nurse practitioner observes numerous macules and vesicles in clusters over the child's trunk and mucous membranes; some are clear, some are crusting. The child is irritable but does not have a fever. What would be the diagnosis and treatment for this child?

    1. Varicella; immunize with varicella-zoster vaccine to decrease symptoms, and begin acyclovir (Zovirax) therapy to prevent/decrease complications.

    2. Impetigo; treat with amoxicillin-clavulanate (Augmentin) for 10 days, and return to clinic in 2 weeks.

    3. Contact dermatitis; apply diphenhydramine (Benadryl) spray over rash, cut child's fingernails to decrease scratching, and thoroughly review any changes in care with the mother.

    4. Varicella; treat first with diphenhydramine (Benadryl) in age-appropriate dose, apply hydroxyzine (Atarax) for itching, and give daily baths with colloidal oatmeal (Aveeno).

72. A 6-month-old infant is brought to the clinic for a rash on the face and diaper area that consists of linear erythematous burrows. An older sibling has a similar rash on his wrists and between his fingers. An appropriate intervention would be:

    1. Neosporin ointment.

    2. Mycitracin ointment.

    3. Acitretin (Soriatane).

    4. Permethrin 5% cream (Elimite).

73. A mother brings her school-age child to the nurse practitioner's office. She states that the child developed a blistering rash on his face 2 days ago that has since spread to his hands and forearms. Examination reveals multiple small vesicular lesions across the child's face, arms, and hands. Some of the lesions are covered with a honey-colored crust. The nurse practitioner diagnoses impetigo and recommends:

    1. Frequent scrubbing of the lesions with a washrag and antibacterial soap.

    2. Isolation of the child from other children for 7 days and discarding the clothing the child has been wearing since the lesions appeared.

    3. Dicloxacillin (Dynapen) suspension 25 mg/kg/ day in four divided doses for 10 days and gentle washing of the lesions to remove any loose crusts.

    4. Referral to a dermatologist and that the mother practice better personal hygiene.

74. An adolescent female presents to the office with a long history of facial acne. She has been seen by several dermatologists and has been treated over the past 3 years with multiple therapies, including topical antibiotics, drying agents, intralesional injections of corticosteroids, and multiple systemic antibiotics, without success. After consulting with the collaborating physician, the nurse practitioner prescribes isotretinoin (Accutane). Teaching/counseling related to the use of this medication includes:

    1. No dietary/alcohol restrictions are necessary.

    2. Exposure to sunlight without burning can be helpful in hastening the healing process.

3. Eliminate all fat from the client's diet.

4. Emphasize the importance of effective contraception if the client is sexually active.

75. A father brings in his 4-year-old son to the emergency department after the boy ingested a small bottle of aspirin. What is the nurse practitioner's priority?

   1. Insert a nasogastric tube and attach to low suction.

   2. Give 16 oz of orange juice.

3. Give 8 oz of milk.

4. Give 30 ml of syrup of ipecac followed by a glass of water.

76. The nurse practitioner is aware that the toxic symptoms of salicylate poisoning are:

   1. Tinnitus and nausea.

   2. Itching and blurred vision.

   3. Fruity odor to the breath.

   4. Fever and chills.

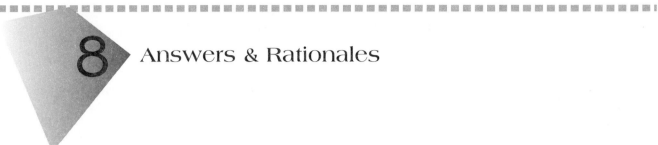

Answers & Rationales

Physical Examination & Diagnostic Tests

1. **(4)** Annular skin lesions may be arranged in a circular manner or in an arciform (arc-shaped) pattern (e.g., tinea corporis). Multiple groups of vesicles erupting unilaterally following the course of cutaneous nerves are described as herpetiform or zosteriform (herpes zoster). Linear lesions are arranged in a line (allergic contact dermatitis to poison ivy). Confluent lesions merge and are not discrete (scarlet fever rash).

2. **(1)** Psoriasis, peripheral vascular disease, diabetes, tuberculosis, and other infectious diseases such as syphilis are associated with pitting deformities of the nail that may vary from pinpoint to pinhead size and may be linear or irregular in distribution. Iron deficiency anemia, eczema, malnutrition, and pellagra are associated with koilonychia (spoon nails). Hyperthyroidism and hypothyroidism are associated with onycholysis, which is a separation of the nail from the nail bed starting at the free edge and progressing proximally.

3. **(1)** The place to inspect is in that portion of the sclera that is observed when the eye is open. If jaundice is suspected, the posterior portion of the hard palate should be examined for a yellowish cast. Pallor and cyanosis can be noted in the nail beds, palms, and soles.

4. **(1)** On an adult the best place is just below the clavicle or on the abdomen. The best place to evaluate skin turgor for hydration status in children is the fleshy part of arms or legs since a child with a distended abdomen may have a tight abdomen, which appears to have adequate turgor, even though the child may actually be dehydrated.

5. **(1)** Fungal lesions will be visualized as a green-yellow fluorescence when viewed with the Wood's lamp in a dimly lit room.

6. **(1)** A macule is less than 1 cm in diameter, nonpalpable, and brown, red, purple, or tan (freckles, flat moles, rubella). A papule is elevated and palpable (warts, pigmented nevi). A nodule is 1–2 cm in diameter, elevated, and deeper (lipoma). A wheal is elevated and irregular and has a variable diameter (insect bites, urticaria).

7. **(2)** Lichenification occurs with chronic irritation, often of an exposed extremity (chronic dermatitis). Crusts are dried exudate; scales are heaps of keratinized cells from exfoliation (psoriasis); and loss of epidermis is excoriation, as seen in an abrasion.

8. **(3)** The angle of the nail beds should form a diamond when the nail beds are approximated. Transverse ridges and grooves may occur from trauma. Placing the palms together provides no assessment data. Diffuse discoloration may be from a fungal infection or an injury.

9. **(3)** Bulla is the correct term. A papule is solid, a vesicle is less than 1 cm in diameter, and a pustule contains a purulent exudate.

10. **(4)** The appearance of a new mole with high-risk features, including irregular border, color changes, and changes in sensation (e.g., pruritus), would necessitate immediate biopsy to rule out melanoma and/or referral to a dermatologist. Uniform moles, those that are symmetric and have smooth borders, and those

not showing signs of change can be followed with annual skin assessments. Seborrheic keratosis is a benign skin growth, usually on sun-exposed areas and appearing waxy or "stuck-on," that requires no treatment.

11. **(2)** Under microscope examination, fungal scrapings in KOH solution will appear as threadlike hyphae crossing cell walls. The other solutions are not indicated to identify dermatophytes.

12. **(3)** It is important to remember to apply controls when skin testing the immunocompromised client. Ask clients what diseases they believe they have immunity to, such as measles. Apply the "known" allergen and appropriate skin test. If the client is unable to mount an immune response at all, the known allergen will not react. By not applying the controls, the nurse practitioner may assume a skin test is negative, when in fact the client's immune system is unable to respond.

13. **(4)** This best describes mongolian spots that are characteristic in newborns of African, Asian, or Latin descent. When closely evaluated, these spots do not resemble the ecchymoses that occur with trauma. Telangiectatic nevi are commonly known as "stork bites" and are deep-pink lesions most often found on the back of the neck. Cutis marmorata is the transient mottling that occurs when an infant is cold.

Skin Disorders

14. **(3)** Intense itching is characteristic of pediculosis pubis, scabies, and atopic dermatitis. Impetigo starts out as a tender erythematous papule and progresses through a vesicular to a honey-crusted stage with no itching.

15. **(2)** Herpes zoster typically presents with a history of tenderness followed by eruptions and vesicles that follow a dermatome on one side of the body. This condition is very painful. Other symptoms may include fever, headaches, and malaise.

16. **(2)** Approximately 10%–30% of people with psoriasis develop an accompanying form of arthritis called psoriatic arthritis. The other

options are dermatologic conditions but are not directly associated with arthritis.

17. **(3)** Stress can aggravate psoriasis. Sunlight helps psoriasis, so it is usually better in the summer. It is not contagious, and only about 30% of clients with psoriasis itch.

18. **(1)** The location and appearance of the lesions is typical of scabies: short, irregular runs approximately 2–3 mm long and the width of a hair.

19. **(2)** Actinic keratoses are potentially precancerous lesions and are found in areas of skin exposed to sunlight. Due to the increasing popularity of sunbathing, the lesions may be seen even in persons 30 to 50 year old.

20. **(4)** Laboratory studies are not likely to be helpful in evaluation of urticaria. Identification of causes is usually based on history and physical findings. The other statements are true of urticaria.

21. **(3)** Although any of these conditions can affect the skin, particularly of an HIV-positive client, the description relates most closely to Kaposi's sarcoma and warrants a biopsy.

22. **(2)** Despite the name "dyshidrotic" eczematous dermatitis (bullous form called pompholyx), there is no evidence of sweating. Most clients have an atopic history, and emotional stress is often a precipitating factor in the appearance of the vesicles. Nummular (discoid) eczema is a chronic, pruritic, inflammatory dermatitis that occurs as coin-shaped plaques composed of papules and vesicles on an erythematous base. Option #1 describes rosacea. Option #3 describes psoriasis. Option #4 describes a verruca or common wart.

23. **(4)** Delay wound closure until determination of no infection in approximately 24–48 hours. Mouth flora of humans is abundant, and a bite carries the risk of heavy bacterial inoculum and severe infection. Tetanus toxoid is indicated because the client has had no booster in last 5 years.

24. **(2)** Onychomycosis is the correct term. Hippocratic nails are clubbed nails and fingers associated with chronic heart and lung disorders. Koilonychia is a concavity of the nail plate often associated with iron deficiency anemia. Anonychia is a total congenital absence of the nail.

25. **(2)** In case of suspected drug reactions, it is recommended that the drug be eliminated and documented in the client's record so it is not reintroduced.

26. **(4)** Excessive bathing dries the skin, which irritates the atopic dermatitis. Food allergies and other causative triggers should be identified and avoided. Bubble baths can irritate skin, as can sweating.

27. **(4)** Excessive sweating may be normal, but history and physical exam are needed to rule out underlying causes. Therapies can be offered. Drysol is for use only on the feet and axilla. Full bathing is not recommended with this solution.

28. **(3)** The assessment describes a seborrheic keratosis. The actinic keratosis is an irregular, rough, scaly, white to erythematous macular lesion found most often on the dorsal surface of the hands, arms, neck, and face. It has malignant potential. The basal cell carcinoma is a smooth, round nodule with a pearly gray border and central induration. Senile lentigines are gray-brown, irregular, macular lesions on sun-exposed areas of the face, arms, and hands.

29. **(3)** Herpes zoster (shingles) is a vesicular dermatomal eruption related to a reactivation of latent varicella virus. It increases with advanced age and is characterized by burning pain and paresthesia along one or two dermatomes and not crossing the midline and may be accompanied by fever, malaise, or headache. The vesicular stage lasts 2–3 weeks. The vesicles are initially clear or blood filled and become purulent. The area along the dermatome is erythematous, and the vesicles crust and then scab, which may leave hypopigmented scars. The other options discuss painless lesions and are not specific to this prodromal stage.

30. **(1)** Antiviral therapy with acyclovir 800 mg five times daily for 7 days may speed healing if started within 2–3 days of onset, especially in immunocompromised individuals. Miconazole and clotrimazole are antifungal creams. Prednisone would only be used to decrease the incidence of postherpetic neuralgia and may increase the incidence of disseminated infection.

31. **(4)** These are classic signs of a basal cell carcinoma, also supported by the client's employment history. Melanoma would be pigmented; compound nevus would not be firm or have telangiectasia; and bullous pemphigoid results in bullous lesions.

32. **(3)** Refer immediately to a dermatologist because these findings are highly suspicious for a melanoma. Biopsy should never be done on a melanoma, and any delay could be detrimental to the outcome.

33. **(2)** Oral acyclovir is very effective in reducing intensity and duration of symptoms if started early in the course of the disease. Herpes zoster does not usually recur at regular intervals but frequently lasts for several weeks.

34. **(3)** This client presents with a classic case of pityriasis rosea, a benign self-limiting skin eruption of unknown etiology. Although a medication/allergen history would be warranted, referral to an allergy specialist or dermatologist would not be necessary. Triamcinolone would not be indicated because the treatment is mainly symptomatic. Sunlight in moderate amounts has been shown to hasten healing in some clients.

35. **(3)** The signs and symptoms presented are classic for Lyme disease, which is transmitted by ticks. Therefore it would be important to inquire about potential exposure to ticks before the signs and symptoms developed. Exposure to new skin care products would be important if the practitioner suspected an allergic reaction, which is not consistent with the signs and symptoms. Although always important, a thorough medication history probably will not reveal the cause of the signs and symptoms in this case. Tuberculosis does not present in this manner.

36. **(2)** This is the correct procedure for the permethrin cream rinse. After rinsing, remove nits with a nit comb. Repeat shampoo treatment after 7 days if living lice are still observed. Clothing and bedding should be washed or dry-cleaned. Family members should also be treated.

37. **(2)** Accidental scalding is usually splash-related and occurs on the front of the body. The nurse practitioner should be suspicious of any burns on the back of the body or any well-defined, uniform burn areas on the buttocks or extremities, which they may indicate physical

abuse. Immersion burns on the buttocks may be seen as punishment for toileting or wetting "accidents."

38. **(3)** The cornstarch or Aveeno baths will temporally help relieve the itching. The shorts and short-sleeved shirt would expose too much skin, which would be scratched by the infant. Wool irritates the skin. Salt would also be an irritant.

39. **(3)** The most common treatment is observation because most hemangiomas resolve over time, usually beginning about 18 months of age. The other treatments may be performed, especially for hemangiomas proliferating rapidly.

40. **(2)** Infantile atopic dermatitis, as contrasted to atopic dermatitis in older children and adolescents, is a moist, oozing, crusting pruritic rash found mainly on the extensor surfaces of the body and the face. It usually begins about 2 months of age, often with a family history of atopy.

41. **(1)** In prepubertal children, café au lait spots larger than 1 cm and present in more than five areas are a concern and may be associated with neurofibromatosis. The child should be referred to a pediatrician for further evaluation.

42. **(1)** Seborrheic dermatitis is usually salmon in color and has a yellowish, greasy appearance. It occurs in infants under 6 months of age. It does not itch. The distribution is mainly to the face, postauricular scalp, axillae, and groin. Rashes in atopic dermatitis and eczema are pink, or red if inflamed, and have a whiter, nongreasy appearance. Rash may begin at 2–12 months and continues through childhood and is associated with a family history of allergy. Itching may be severe. The distribution is to the cheeks, trunk, and extensors of extremities. Erythema toxicum consists of yellow or white papules on the face. It occurs in 30%–50% of term infants and disappears in 2 weeks.

43. **(3)** Given the distribution of the rash, the most likely cause is a contact dermatitis, such as that caused by the use of baby wipes. Allergy to disposable diapers would involve the entire diaper area. Seborrheic dermatitis presents as large confluent sharply marginated bright plaque on the anterior surface of the groin. Candidal rashes are bright red with satellite lesions that involve the deep folds and may spread to the entire diaper area.

44. **(2)** Impetigo presents with honey-colored crusted lesions with an erythematous base. Staphylococci and group A streptococci are important pathogens in this disease. Scabies presents with linear burrows about the wrists, ankles, finger webs, areolars, anterior axillary folds, genitalis, or face (in infants). Pityriasis rosea presents as erythematous papules that coalesce to form oval plaques preceded by a large oval plaque with central clearing and a scaly border (the herald patch). Varicella (chickenpox) presents as crops of red macules that rapidly become tiny vesicles with surrounding erythema that form pustules. The pustules become crusted, then scabs form. The rash appears predominantly on the trunk and face.

45. **(4)** After a course of antibiotics the normal flora is destroyed, making the child a prime target for *Candida albicans*. The classic signs of a yeast infection include a beefy red, sharply marginated, maculopapular rash with satellite lesions. Poor hygiene and a contact dermatitis would present as erythema and thickening of the skin in the perianal area. Seborrheic dermatitis consists of an erythematous scaly dermatitis accompanied by overproduction of sebum in areas rich in sebaceous glands (face, scalp, perineum).

46. **(2)** Atopic dermatitis typically presents in the flexural areas of children. The lesions are characteristically erythematous and papular, with scales and pruritus often noted. A personal or family history of atopy is noted in about 70% of clients with atopic dermatitis. Scabies lesions appear as gray or skin-colored ridges, vesicles, and papules. Tinea corporis lesions are generally distributed over the entire body and face, with an area of clearing in the center of the lesion. Contact dermatitis usually produces vesicular lesions in the shape of the object causing the reaction.

47. **(3)** Any bite potentially associated with an animal that may harbor rabies (skunks, bats, raccoons, foxes, coyotes, rats) should be treated with both active and passive rabies immunization. Tetanus antitoxin would be indicated if the client was not current on the immunization. Animal authorities would be called after the initial treatment to locate the animal and sacrifice it so that the brain could be examined for rabies.

48. **(4)** Brown recluse spiders produce sharp pain at the instant of the bite, with subsequent minor swelling and erythema. Tissue necrosis may occur within 4 hours. A blue-gray to black macular halo may surround the bite, with eventual widening and sinking of the center of the lesion, leading to a "sinking infarct." This leaves a deep ulcer requiring weeks or months to heal.

49. **(2)** Deep puncture wounds are more likely to become infected with anaerobic organisms. The narrow, sharp feline incisors deeply puncture tissue and may easily penetrate a bone or joint. Bites on the hand have the highest infection rate, whereas bites on the face have the lowest rate.

50. **(2)** Insects are more active, reproduce, and are present in greater numbers in the warm months of spring to early fall.

51. **(1)** Amoxicillin-clavulanate an excellent choice for the empiric treatment of animal bites. Cephalexin is not indicated due to resistant strains of *Pasteurella multocida*, an organism present in 25% of dog bites and 50% of cat bites. An infected bite should be followed up daily until the infection clears. Open wound management is indicated, not suturing.

52. **(2)** Heat application is contraindicated; ice packs are preferred, as is elevation, to decrease the edema. The area should be immobilized. Tetanus toxoid may be given along with antihistamines to reduce swelling and relieve itching.

53. **(4)** In addition to these symptoms, bronchospasm, hypertension, seizures, and altered mental status may occur. Black eschar is associated with a brown recluse bite.

54. **(4)** This was a poisonous coral snake bite. The typical symptoms are those listed, as well as nausea, vomiting, and muscle fasciculations.

Childhood Diseases

55. **(2)** Erythema multiforme is a major side effect of sulfa drug use that presents with a sudden onset of high fever, weakness, blisters, bulla, and ulcerations of the mucous membranes. Kawasaki disease presents with a more diffuse erythematous rash. Viral exanthems are centrally located and do not resemble blisters. Scalded skin syndrome is staphylococcal in origin and causes the skin to peel off and turn bright red.

56. **(2)** The incubation period for erythema infectiosum is 4–14 days, with communicability until the rash appears.

57. **(1)** The symptoms are indicative of coxsackievirus 5 or 16 group A (usually A16), called hand-foot-and-mouth disease. The lesions may appear in one or all three areas. Children are usually uncomfortable, but not seriously ill, and may refuse fluids with severe oral lesions. Varicella lesions begin on the trunk with classic "teardrop" vesicles.

58. **(1)** In roseola an erythematous maculopapular rash appears on the trunk after abrupt onset of fever and spreads to the extremities, neck, and face. It fades within 24 hours. The pink maculopapular rash of rubella begins on the face and spreads down the trunk. Often the facial rash will disappear as the rash erupts on the extremities, clearing in 3–5 days.

59. **(2)** The primary treatment for roseola is supportive, including control of fever, adequate rest, and hydration. No preventive measure or immunization is available.

Pharmacology

60. **(1)** The description is consistent with intertriginous candidiasis, which is treated with an antifungal ointment or oral medication. It is not a staphylococcal infection; the area needs to be kept dry, not moist. An antibiotic ointment will not relieve the problem. Herpes zoster is treated with antiviral medications; this case is not described as particularly painful, and it is bilateral.

61. **(1)** Beta-blockers can exacerbate psoriasis. They are believed to decrease cAMP-dependent protein kinase, an inhibitor of cell proliferation. Drugs in the other classifications have no known effect on psoriasis.

62. **(4)** Systemic antibiotics (e.g., tetracycline) offer the most effective treatment in inflammatory acne. Isotretinoin is also very effective but,

because of serious teratogenic side effects, it is not first-line treatment. Improvement in acne will not be noted for 4–8 weeks and dietary changes have not been demonstrated to have any beneficial effect.

63. **(2)** The appearance is indicative of *Candida albicans*, which is best treated with nystatin. The other choices would aggravate the diaper rash by promoting overhydration.

64. **(3)** Acyclovir treats the acute phase during initial eruption of vesicular lesions and offers no benefit for postherpetic pain.

65. **(3)** Clients need to be instructed to wash off podophyllin. It should be applied sparingly, only to the wart and avoiding normal skin, and allowed to dry thoroughly before the client dresses. No rationale exists to treat with both liquid nitrogen and podophyllin.

66. **(3)** Systemic treatment with low-dose tetracycline is very effective for rosacea; topical treatment with metronidazole or low-dose hydrocortisone may also be useful. Oral cortisone and antifungal agents are not known to be effective. Topical 5-fluorouracil is used in the treatment of actinic keratosis, a precancerous skin condition.

67. **(1)** The maximum allowable dose for adults is 7 mg/kg of lidocaine with epinephrine and 5 mg/kg of lidocaine without epinephrine. Although local anesthetics are often used, the maximum allowable doses are rarely emphasized, and overdose can result in anaphylactic shock.

68. **(1)** Amitriptyline in low doses is effective in treating neuropathic pain. NSAIDs may also be effective in treating the inflammatory component of herpes zoster pain. The most effective nonpharmacologic method of treating pain from shingles is the application of cool compresses. Heat may exacerbate neuropathic pain in some clients. Antidepressants and anticonvulsants are effective adjuvant therapy in the treatment of neuropathic pain.

69. **(2)** Stevens-Johnson syndrome is a severe form of erythema multiforme that can be fatal. The clinical picture is mucous membrane lesions, conjunctival and corneal lesions, fever, malaise, arthralgia, and sloughing of the skin of the hands and feet. Distinguishing characteristics of the syndrome are eruption of vesicles, mucosal ulcerations, and sloughing skin.

70. **(3)** The child's lesions are characteristic of impetigo and should be treated with an antibiotic if present on the face; dicloxacillin is acceptable therapy. However, compliance may improve with twice-daily (bid) dosing (amoxicillin-clavulanate). The ointment, soaking, and Benadryl will not stop the spread of the infection, which could lead to poststreptococcal glomerulonephritis.

71. **(4)** Varicella (chickenpox) should be treated symptomatically unless the child is at high risk secondary to other medical problems. Acyclovir is not recommended for routine treatment of uncomplicated varicella. The current bathing therapy is with colloidal oatmeal products, taking preference over the traditional baking soda baths. Impetigo usually occurs on the face and neck with no diffuse lesions over the trunk. Contact dermatitis is characterized by erythema and scaling, possibly with weeping vesicles. The area of distribution of rash offers clues to diagnosis.

72. **(4)** Permethrin 5% cream is used in infants but is not recommended in those under 2 months of age. Neosporin could be used to treat secondary infections but would not help eradicate the scabies. Mycitracin is also not effective for the treatment of scabies. Acitretin is used for the treatment of psoriasis.

73. **(3)** Impetigo is communicable until the client has been on antibiotic therapy for 48 hours. Washing clothing and linens separately with hot water is recommended, along with surveillance of close contacts for the appearance of lesions. Isolation is not necessary, except to keep the child home from school until 48 hours of antibiotic therapy has been completed. Dicloxacillin is effective treatment, although for those children in day care whose parents request bid dosing, amoxicillin-clavulanate 25–45 mg/kg/day is an alternative. Gentle washing is recommended to keep the lesions clean and to prevent scarring (potentially caused by vigorous scrubbing).

74. **(4)** Because isotretinoin is extremely teratogenic, sexual assessment and pregnancy testing (as appropriate) and contraceptive counseling should be done for all clients. The combination of alcohol and isotretinoin can

cause a disulfuram-like reaction, so alcohol should be avoided. Isotretinoin can cause photosensitivity, so the nurse practitioner should counsel the client to avoid sunlight, wear protective clothing and sunglasses, and apply sunscreen to all sun-exposed areas without acne. No conclusive relationship between diet and acne has been established.

75. **(4)** An age-appropriate dose of syrup of ipecac followed by a glass of water would be indicated. The nurse practitioner would lavage the child, not insert a nasogastric tube and attach to suction.

76. **(1)** Tinnitus and nausea are toxic symptoms of salicylate poisoning. Fruity odor to the breath is usually associated with diabetic ketoacidosis.

Endocrine

Physical Examination & Diagnostic Tests

1. What is the correct procedure for palpation of a client's thyroid gland?

   1. Stand behind the client, hyperextend the head, and palpate both sides simultaneously.

   2. Have the client lower the chin and lean head slightly toward the side being evaluated.

   3. Hyperextend the head and have the client lean away from the side being evaluated.

   4. Have the client lean away from the side being examined and take a swallow of water.

2. When a client sips water and swallows, the thyroid gland:

   1. Moves downward and slightly posterior and feels smooth on palpation.

   2. Elongates and enlarges during the swallow and immediately returns to a resting position.

   3. Moves slightly out during the sipping and backward during the swallowing.

   4. Moves upward during the swallow and feels symmetric and smooth to palpation.

3. Which question is **not** part of the Carville Diabetic Foot Screen?

   1. Has there been a change in the foot since the last evaluation?

   2. Does the foot hurt when walking?

   3. Does the foot have an abnormal shape?

   4. Are the nails thick, too long, or overgrown?

4. While conducting the interview for a physical examination, the nurse practitioner identifies which finding in the client's history as being commonly associated with thyroid carcinoma?

   1. Family history of thyroid cancer.

   2. History of hyperthyroidism.

   3. Irradiation of the neck.

   4. Smoking for 15 years.

5. When doing a physical examination on a client with hyperthyroidism, a common neurologic finding is:

    1. Memory, attention, and problem-solving deficits.

    2. Diminished deep tendon reflexes.

    3. Severe cognitive impairment.

    4. Delusions and psychosis.

6. The treatment goal for glycemic control in a person with type 2 diabetes is to achieve and maintain hemoglobin A level ($HgbA_{1c}$) of:

    1. <10%.

    2. 6%–9%.

    3. <7%.

    4. >8%.

7. Which finding would alert the nurse practitioner that a client might be experiencing a problem with the endocrine system?

    1. Coagulation abnormalities and fatigue.

    2. Growth abnormalities and glucose intolerance.

    3. Hypoxia and jaundice.

    4. Steatorrhea and abdominal distention.

8. The nurse practitioner notes a solitary thyroid nodule on a client during a routine physical examination. The preferred diagnostic test of choice is:

    1. Thyroid scan and antibody level.

    2. Thyroid-stimulating hormone (TSH) level and ultrasound.

    3. X-ray film of the thyroid.

    4. Fine-needle aspiration (FNA) biopsy.

9. An adult female client presents to the nurse practitioner's office complaining of fatigue, weakness, and weight gain over the past 4 months. Physical examination reveals elevated blood pressure (BP), facial and supraclavicular fullness, hirsutism noted on the face, proximal muscle weakness, and facial and truncal distribution of acne. Appropriate laboratory tests the nurse practitioner should order include:

    1. Antinuclear antibody (ANA) and rheumatoid factor (RF).

    2. Three-hour glucose tolerance test and lipid profile.

    3. Red blood cell (RBC) count and a calcium level.

    4. Dexamethasone suppression test, urinary free cortisol level, and TSH/thyroxine (T_4).

10. The nurse practitioner would anticipate which laboratory values in the client with Graves' disease?

    1. TSH levels to be increased.

    2. TSH levels to be decreased.

    3. TSH levels to be within normal limits (WNL).

    4. T_4 levels to be decreased.

11. Which information is correct regarding foot screening using a nylon filament (5.07 Semmes-Weinstein)?

    1. Use a 25-gm filament and apply along perimeter of any scar or ulcer tissue.

    2. Apply the filament at a 45-degree angle to the skin surface.

    3. Apply sufficient force for approximately 1.5 seconds to cause the filament to bend.

    4. Slide the filament across the skin and make repetitive contact to each of the 10 sites.

12. To make the diagnosis of diabetes, the client must have two fasting plasma glucose levels documented on two occasions greater than or equal to ($\geq$):

    1. 200 mg/dl

    2. 140 mg/dl

    3. 126 mg/dl

    4. 110 mg/dl

Disorders

13. The etiology of type 1 diabetes can be best described as:

    1. An autosomal dominant genetic disorder.

    2. Autoimmune destruction of the beta cells.

3. Overnutrition and resulting obesity as the major risk factor.

4. Prevented by exercise, which increases the concentration of insulin receptors.

14. A client has been diagnosed with diabetes for more than 5 years. To whom should the nurse practitioner maintain an annual referral for this client?

1. Cardiologist.

2. Dietitian.

3. Vascular surgeon.

4. Ophthalmologist.

15. Hirsutism presenting in a female with normal menstruation and normal plasma androgens is most likely:

1. An ovarian tumor.

2. Cushing's syndrome.

3. Idiopathic.

4. Polycystic ovary disease.

16. Pathophysiologic causes of decreased testosterone levels develop in the:

1. Hypothalamus.

2. Anterior pituitary.

3. Testes.

4. All the above.

17. A common cause of poor control of type 1 diabetes during the adolescent period is:

1. Too frequent evoluation of blood sugar.

2. Increased intake of protein.

3. Too much exercise.

4. Denial of the severity of the condition.

18. When counseling a diabetic client on foot care, it is important to emphasize:

1. Daily foot soaks in warm, soapy water.

2. Careful daily foot inspections.

3. Trimming corns and calluses regularly.

4. Trimming toenails close to the nail bed.

19. An adult client presents to the nurse practitioner for evaluation of polyuria, polydipsia, and weight loss. Which laboratory result would require immediate intervention by the practitioner?

1. HgbA$_{1c}$ of 14%.

2. Serum glucose of 150 mg/dl.

3. HgbA$_{1c}$ of 6.0%.

4. Serum glucose of 65 mg/dl.

20. An adult client is being evaluated for hypoglycemia due to a blood sugar of 58 mg/dl. The nurse practitioner would begin the differential diagnosis by:

1. Deciding if the hypoglycemia is fasting or postprandial.

2. Ascertaining if it is related to alcohol use.

3. Deciding if the client has other medical problems.

4. Reassuring the client that it is a benign problem.

21. An elderly male client complains of lethargy, cold intolerance, weight gain, and yellowing of the palms. The most important laboratory study ordered by the nurse practitioner in diagnosing this condition is:

1. Complete blood count.

2. Liver enzymes.

3. Thyroid panel.

4. Cardiac enzymes.

22. A middle-aged, normally healthy female presents for evaluation of intermittent palpitations. She also reports mood variability, tremulousness, difficulty falling asleep, and a 10-lb weight loss despite a normal appetite. She feels warm most of the time and wonders if she is perimenopausal. She has no history of heart disease. The objective data that would yield the most useful information would be:

1. Electrocardiogram (ECG).

2. TSH, free T$_4$.

3. Electrolytes.

4. Holter monitor.

23. An adult woman presents to the clinic complaining of fatigue, weakness, weight gain despite lack of appetite, and feelings of depression. Physical examination reveals an obese, alert client with thinning hair, bilateral chest puffiness, increased facial hair, supraclavicular fat pad, thin arms and legs, purple striae on the abdomen, and multiple ecchymotic areas on extremities. Her vital signs are BP 158/96, pulse 88, and respirations 22. Laboratory results show fasting blood sugar (FBS) of 200 mg/dl, electrolyte panel WNL except for potassium 3.0 mEq/L, hemoglobin 11.8 gm, and hematocrit 34%. This assessment information would support the nurse practitioner's diagnosis of:

    1. Addison's disease.
    2. Pheochromocytoma.
    3. Cushing's syndrome.
    4. Hypoaldosteronism.

24. Which of the following is the best alternative for treating hyperthyroidism diagnosed during the first trimester of pregnancy?

    1. Radioactive iodine in smaller than usual dose during first trimester.
    2. Propylthiouracil (PTU) during first trimester, subtotal thyroidectomy during second trimester, no thyroid replacement.
    3. PTU during first trimester, subtotal thyroidectomy during second trimester, thyroid replacement.
    4. No treatment until after delivery.

25. Clinical findings in a client with hypothyroidism include:

    1. Hyperactive bowel sounds.
    2. Oily skin and acne.
    3. Postural tremors of the hands.
    4. Edema of the face and eyelids.

26. A young adult male reports anxiety, tremulousness, headaches, palpitations, and sweating 2–4 hours after eating. Physical exam is normal. No lab results are currently available. No medical conditions are noted in the history. What is the most likely diagnosis?

    1. Dumping syndrome.
    2. Hypoglycemia.
    3. Alcohol abuse.
    4. Hyperthyroidism.

27. Which of the following is the most likely etiology for hypercalcemia in the medically well asymptomatic adult?

    1. Hyperthyroidism.
    2. Hyperparathyroidism.
    3. Hyperpituitarism.
    4. Hypothyroidism.

28. A middle-aged male with no previous medical history presents with a 30-lb weight gain in 2.5 months. He denies any medication use or allergies. He was recently laid off of a very active job and has been sedentary. Physical exam reveals BP 172/111, central obesity, FBS 200 mg/dl. What is the most likely cause of client's weight gain?

    1. Cushing's disease.
    2. Hypothyroidism.
    3. Depression.
    4. Diabetes.

29. A middle-aged woman presents with agitation, confusion, fever, tachycardia, and diaphoresis. Her daughter states that nausea, vomiting, and abdominal pain preceded these symptoms. The client has no history of cardiac disease, diabetes, or substance abuse. She was started on some "anti-drug" 2 weeks ago and is scheduled for some form of throat surgery next week (per daughter). Based on this history, the nurse practitioner immediately orders:

    1. TSH, T_4.
    2. Urinalysis.
    3. Spinal tap.
    4. Computed tomography of head.

30. A 45-year-old female client presents to the office complaining of a 6-month history of fatigue, 15-lb weight gain, lethargy, an inability to tolerate cold temperatures, forgetfulness, hair loss, and constipation. Physical findings include dry coarse skin, periorbital edema and puffy facies, bradycardia, hyporeflexia and muscle weakness, and a smooth goitrous thyroid. The nurse practitioner would make the diagnosis of:

    1. Congestive heart failure (CHF).
    2. Diabetes mellitus (DM).
    3. Hypothyroidism.
    4. Thyroid cancer.

31. A diabetic client has been taking 6 U of regular insulin and 12 U of Lente insulin in the morning. In the evening she has been taking 3 U of regular insulin and 8 U of Lente insulin. The client has been monitoring her blood glucose levels (mg/dl) and shows the nurse practitioner the following chart:

	7 am	Noon	5 pm	Bedtime
Monday	100	76	98	109
Tuesday	119	75	88	110
Wednesday	119	66	86	100
Thursday	123	70	111	122
Friday	128	60	99	110

    The nurse practitioner adjusts the client's insulin by:

    1. Increasing the regular insulin.
    2. Decreasing the regular insulin.
    3. Decreasing the Lente insulin.
    4. Increasing both insulins.

32. The role of the nurse practitioner in the initial management of a client with a thyroid nodule involves:

    1. Referring the client to an endocrinologist for further evaluation.
    2. Obtaining fine-needle aspiration (FNA) biopsy of the nodule and sending to cytology.
    3. Ordering an ultrasound and a thyroid scan.
    4. Ordering levothyroxine (Synthroid) to reduce the size of the nodule.

33. When teaching a client with diabetes about "sick day" guidelines, the nurse practitioner explains that the client should:

    1. Stop measuring blood glucose and only check urine for ketones.
    2. Not take the usual dose of insulin at the usual time.
    3. Be sure to take metformin (Glucophage) and acarbose (Precose), even if nausea and vomiting are present.
    4. Administer extra doses of regular insulin according to instructions for blood glucose levels above 240 mg/dl.

34. A young adult female client presents to the clinic with complaints of nervousness, tremulousness, palpitations, heat intolerance, fatigue, weight loss, and polyphagia. After a complete history and physical examination, along with thyroid function tests, the nurse practitioner makes the diagnosis of hyperthyroidism, recognizing that the most common cause of this condition is:

    1. Thyroid cancer.
    2. Graves' disease.
    3. Pituitary adenoma.
    4. Postpartum thyroiditis.

35. A young adult male client presents to office stating that he found a lump in his neck while shaving. Physical examination reveals a firm, 2-cm nodule that is fixed and nontender located on the right lobe of the thyroid gland. Right posterior cervical lymphadenopathy is also noted. The nurse practitioner should:

    1. Order a TSH level to determine thyroid function, and refer to a surgeon for FNA biopsy of the nodule.
    2. No intervention is necessary at this time; schedule a follow-up visit in 6 months.
    3. Prescribe levothyroxine (Synthroid) 0.1 mg PO daily, and schedule a 6-week follow-up visit.
    4. Immediately ablate the client's thyroid with radioactive iodine, and refer to an endocrinologist.

36. A client with Graves' disease is to have radioactive iodine (I^{131}) therapy. Which information is important for the nurse practitioner to include when teaching about this treatment?

    1. Clients are highly radioactive for approximately 7 days after treatment and need to be isolated.

    2. Clients should not become pregnant during or after receiving this therapy because of the teratogenic effects to the fetus that occur due to chromosomal abnormalities.

    3. Clients may become hypothyroid after this treatment and therefore need to have regular TSH and T_4 levels drawn, with the potential for thyroid hormone replacement therapy.

    4. This therapy is contraindicated in clients with cardiac disease.

37. An infant with congenital hypothyroidism is being discharged home. The nurse would instruct the parents to:

    1. Watch for constipation and slow pulse as signs of toxicity.

    2. Reduce the medication as symptoms decrease.

    3. Give the medication as a single dose in the early morning.

    4. Expect weight loss until the child adjusts to the dose.

38. A goal in the management of a child with diabetes would be to maintain blood sugar level in a target range according to what?

    1. The target blood sugar level must be individualized based on the child's age and ability to recognize the symptoms of hypoglycemia.

    2. The target range for blood sugar level depends on the provider's judgment, the health care team, and the goals set with the child and parents.

    3. The overall goal is to maintain the child's blood sugar level in the range that allows the lowest $HgbA_{1c}$ without significant hypoglycemia.

    4. All the above.

39. A mother presents her school-age child to the nurse practitioner and expresses her concern that her son is the shortest child in his class and asks if something is wrong with him.

Initial differentiation of cause by the nurse practitioner of the child's short stature would include:

    1. History with familial height patterns, physical exam with Tanner stage, and radiography to assess skeletal maturation, if indicated.

    2. History with familial height patterns, physical exam, and trial treatment with growth hormone.

    3. Immediate referral to an endocrinologist.

    4. Physical exam and complete blood count (CBC), thyroid function panel, urinalysis, karyotyping, chemistry profile, and insulin sensitivity tests.

40. Which of the following findings would the nurse practitioner expect to find in a child with pubertal gynecomastia?

    1. Tanner stage II with testes ≤4 cm in length.

    2. Breasts and nipples nontender and equal in size.

    3. Breast tissue enlargement mainly glandular, movable, and nonadherent to skin or underlying tissue.

    4. Lymphadenopathy, goiter, asymmetrical testes, and repaired hypospadias.

41. Which of the following is true regarding hyperthyroidism in children?

    1. Boys have a higher incidence of Graves' disease.

    2. Autoimmune response is most often triggered by the body's reaction to a bacterial or viral infection.

    3. Decreased production and secretion of thyroid hormone and presence of goiter.

    4. Common, endemic congenital disorder caused by iodine deficiency.

42. On physical examination of a 14-year-old girl complaining of amenorrhea, the nurse practitioner notes BP 138/90, pulse 98, broad chest with widely spaced nipples, Tanner stage I, webbing of neck, low hairline, and prominent, anomalous ears. The nurse practitioner suspects:

    1. Klinefelter's syndrome.

    2. Marfan's syndrome.

3. Fragile X syndrome.

4. Turner's syndrome.

43. The nurse practitioner understands that growth retardation that appears after age 12 in boys is usually caused by:

    1. Chromosomal abnormalities.

    2. Hyperthyroidism.

    3. Hyperpituitarism.

    4. Hypogonadism.

44. Which of the following conditions is associated with growth failure?

    1. Fanconi's syndrome.

    2. Tourette's syndrome.

    3. Klinefelter's syndrome.

    4. Angelman's syndrome.

45. The nurse practitioner understands that blood glucose level in diabetic children 7–12 years of age who can recognize the symptoms of hypoglycemia need to be maintained in which range?

    1. 60–75 mg/dl.

    2. 100–175 mg/dl.

    3. 80–140 mg/dl.

    4. >180 mg/dl.

46. An adolescent male client presenting with recent-onset nocturia, polydipsia, polyphagia, weight loss, and blurred vision is most likely experiencing the symptoms of:

    1. Type 1 diabetes.

    2. Type 2 diabetes.

    3. Urinary tract infection (UTI).

    4. Mononucleosis.

47. In which of the following groups of clients is tight glycemic control contraindicated?

    1. Adolescent males.

    2. Middle-aged females.

    3. Middle-aged males.

    4. Children under age 6.

48. An infant with an abnormally pitched cry may demonstrate a genetic disorder or other problems such as:

    1. Hypothyroidism.

    2. Hypertelorism.

    3. Cleft palate.

    4. Pyloric stenosis.

49. During an evaluation of a client with pre-onset diabetes, the nurse practitioner identifies what finding in the client's objective data as being associated with the dysmetabolic syndrome (insulin resistance syndrome)?

    1. Triglycerides >150 mg/dl.

    2. High-density lipoprotein >40 mg/dl in men and >50 mg/dl in women.

    3. Blood pressure <130/85.

    4. Fasting blood sugar <110 mg/dl.

50. While taking a history on a client, the nurse practitioner identifies what finding that may be associated with osteopenia/osteoporosis?

    1. High calcium intake.

    2. Minimal alcohol intake.

    3. Smoking 1 pack/day for 20 years.

    4. Walking 30 minutes 4 days a week.

51. Of the following risk factors for osteoporosis, which would the nurse practitioner see primarily with men?

    1. Smoking 2 packs of cigarettes a day.

    2. Excessive use of alcohol.

    3. Low testosterone level.

    4. Minimal exercise.

52. When prescribing a meal plan for a client with type 2 diabetes, the nurse practitioner tells the client that the macronutrient with the most influence on postprandial glucose levels is:

    1. Fiber.

    2. Fat.

    3. Protein.

    4. Carbohydrate.

Pharmacology

53. When prescribing oral medications for an overweight client with type 2 diabetes who also has a voracious appetite, the nurse practitioner is likely to prescribe which medication to encourage weight loss and reduce appetite?

    1. Nateglinide (Starlix).

    2. Pioglitazone (Actos).

    3. Metformin (Glucophage).

    4. Glyburide (Micronase).

54. Glargine (Lantus) is an insulin analog that essentially has no peak and is usually administered:

    1. Before meals.

    2. With lispro insulin (Humalog).

    3. Before breakfast and dinner.

    4. Once a day.

55. An adult male client with type 2 diabetes has a creatinine level of 1.8 mg/dl. Which of the following drugs is **contraindicated**?

    1. Pioglitazone (Actos).

    2. Metformin (Glucophage).

    3. Rapaglinide (Prandin).

    4. Acarbose (Precose).

56. Clients started on metformin (Glucophage) need to be monitored closely for what potential side effect?

    1. Significant increase in weight.

    2. Elevation of low-density lipoprotein (LDL) cholesterol level.

    3. Lactic acidosis.

    4. Increase in insulin requirements.

57. A client with type 2 diabetes is taking glipizide (Glucotrol) 10 mg PO bid. In evaluating the medication's effectiveness, the nurse practitioner knows that glipizide reduces blood glucose by:

    1. Delaying the cellular uptake of potassium and insulin.

    2. Stimulating insulin release from the pancreas.

    3. Decreasing the body's need for and utilization of insulin at the cellular level.

    4. Interfering with the absorption and metabolism of fats and carbohydrates.

58. The nurse practitioner would expect which symptom to be a side effect of metformin (Glucophage)?

    1. Gastrointestinal (GI) upset.

    2. Photophobia.

    3. Hyperglycemia.

    4. Skin eruptions.

59. A client is receiving antithyroid medication. The nurse practitioner understands that:

    1. Lifelong daily treatment is necessary to keep TSH levels within the normal range.

    2. Antithyroid medications do not cross the placenta.

    3. The drugs are somewhat expensive and have serious cardiac and hematologic side effects.

    4. Clients remain on drug therapy for 1–2 years and then the medication is gradually withdrawn.

60. When prescribing an antihypertensive medication for a type 2 diabetic client, the drug classifications that would tend to reduce insulin sensitivity are:

    1. Diuretics and calcium channel blockers.

    2. Diuretics and beta-blockers.

    3. Calcium channel blockers and angiotensin-converting enzyme (ACE) inhibitors.

    4. Alpha-blockers and ACE inhibitors.

61. A 35-year-old female sees the nurse practitioner with a complaint of cold intolerance, fatigue, dry skin, weight gain, and heavy menstrual periods. Physical examination shows a pulse of 58, a "waxy" sallow complexion, and a firm goiter. Her TSH level is 176 mU/L. What is the best treatment choice for this client?

    1. Begin levothyroxine (Synthroid) at 0.025 mg PO qd and repeat TSH in 2 weeks.

    2. Administer loading dose of PO levothyroxine and start full replacement dose.

3. Administer loading dose of IV levothyroxine and start on half replacement dose.

4. Begin levothyroxine at 0.1 mg PO qd and recheck TSH in 6 weeks.

62. The nurse practitioner is performing the preoperative evaluation of a man scheduled to undergo coronary artery bypass grafting. Physical examination shows mild facial puffiness, hoarse voice, and dry skin. Thyroid function results show that the client has TSH level of 34 mU/L. What is the recommended treatment for this client?

1. Give loading IV bolus of levothyroxine (Synthroid) 0.5 mg and proceed with surgery.

2. Cancel surgery and send him home to begin levothyroxine PO 0.1 mg, reschedule surgery.

3. Begin PO levothyroxine and monitor in the hospital until he is euthyroid.

4. Proceed with surgery and treat hypothyroidism postoperatively.

63. The nurse practitioner is seeing an obese, middle-aged female client for a follow-up visit. She was diagnosed with type 2 diabetes 3 months ago and started on a regimen of diet and exercise. Today her fasting plasma glucose is 200 mg/dl and $HgbA_{1c}$ is 10%. She has lost 2 lb. She reports her home glucose monitoring has ranged from 180–300 mg/dl. The rest of her chemistry profile is WNL. What is the best treatment choice for this client?

1. Review her diet and exercise plan, increase exercise regimen, and reduce caloric intake. Schedule her for another follow-up in 3 months.

2. Start her on sliding-scale insulin and instruct her on recording glucose and insulin requirements. Schedule her to return in 1 week for reevaluation regarding long-acting insulin.

3. Initiate treatment with metformin (Glucophage).

4. Initiate treatment with an oral sulfonylurea agent (e.g., glyburide).

64. What is associated with chronic overtreatment with levothyroxine (Synthroid)?

1. Tachycardia.

2. Severe osteoporosis.

3. Insomnia.

4. Sweating.

65. A middle-aged male presents for a diabetes follow-up exam. He has been in good health without identified complications of diabetes. His FBS is 100 mg/dl, and his personal records indicate that he is taking insulin in the prescribed amounts and times. Vital signs are BP 142/98, pulse 80, and respirations 20. Today's plan would include:

1. Begin diuretics and a beta-blocker.

2. Begin ACE inhibitor and consider a diuretic.

3. Obtain ECG and chest x-ray.

4. Return for BP check in 5–7 days.

66. An adult male has recently been started on insulin. His regimen is two daily injections with two thirds of the total daily insulin in the morning and one third in the evening. He is using the 70/30 mixture of intermediate- and short-acting insulin in both injections. He presents for a follow-up visit with his FBS log. The nurse practitioner notes that his recorded glucose levels before the evening meal have been 60–70 mg/dl. Other checks during the day are 100–120 mg/dl. What adjustment needs to be made?

1. Intermediate insulin: change 70/30 combination to self-mix and reduce AM dose.

2. Regular insulin: reduce AM dose of 70/30.

3. Intermediate insulin: reduce AM dose of 70/30.

4. Regular insulin: change 70/30 combination to self-mix and reduce AM regular dose.

67. A client on antithyroid drug therapy for hyperthyroidism presents with complaints of palpitations and dry mouth for the past 2 days. He has had a cough and cold symptoms for the past 3 days, which he has been treating with over-the-counter medications. Which medication would the nurse practitioner encourage the client to avoid?

1. Benzocaine (Chloraseptic) lozenges.

2. Guaifenesin (Robitussin).

3. Ibuprofen (Advil).

4. Pseudoephedrine (Sudafed).

68. What is the most frequent complaint of clients who use insulin pumps?

    1. Problems with elevated glucose after changing the catheter-type (nonneedle) infusion set.

    2. Skin and site problems with dressing adhesive not sticking; redness and pain at infusion site.

    3. Mechanical problems with the pump's digital readout.

    4. Understanding "sick day" management modifications.

69. The nurse practitioner understands that pioglitazone (Actos) or rosiglitazone (Avandia) is indicated for:

    1. Prenatal clients with gestational diabetes.

    2. "Brittle" type 1 diabetic clients.

    3. Type 2 diabetic clients requiring insulin who have poor glycemic control and insulin resistance.

    4. Type 2 diabetic clients, to prevent the rapid postprandial blood glucose surges by delaying carbohydrate absorption.

70. An older client with a history of hypertension and coronary bypass surgery has been diagnosed with hypothyroidism. Appropriate medication management is:

    1. Levothyroxine (Synthroid) 0.1 mg qd and return in 6 weeks for follow-up.

    2. Desiccated thyroid extract 2 grains qd and return in 6 weeks for follow-up.

    3. Levothyroxine (Synthroid) 0.025 mg qd for 6 weeks with gradual increase in dosage every 4–6 weeks until therapeutic level obtained.

    4. Methimazole (Tapazole) 15 mg daily in three divided doses, gradually increasing dose every 4 weeks until therapeutic level obtained.

71. A client is newly diagnosed as being hypothyroid and is placed on levothyroxine (Synthroid) 0.1 mg PO qd. What should be the nurse practitioner's approach to follow-up?

    1. No follow-up visits are necessary.

    2. The client should return to the clinic in 4–6 weeks for TSH measurement and determination of any symptomatic improvement.

    3. The client should have weekly levothyroxine levels drawn.

    4. The client should have monthly CBCs while on levothyroxine (Synthroid) because the medication has been found to be myelosuppressive.

72. Classes of medications typically used to treat hyperthyroid conditions include:

    1. Antibiotics and corticosteroids.

    2. ACE inhibitors, anxiolytics, and antithyroid medications.

    3. Beta-blockers, nonsteroidal antiinflammatory drugs (NSAIDs), and antithyroid medications.

    4. Calcium channel blockers and corticosteroids.

73. A client with hypothyroidism receiving daily levothyroxine (Synthroid) for 3 weeks presents to the clinic with complaints of chest pain. What is the appropriate therapeutic response?

    1. Discontinue levothyroxine because chest pain is a contraindication to its continuance.

    2. Schedule the client for a stress test.

    3. Decrease dose of levothyroxine, order an ECG, and consult with a collaborating physician.

    4. Prescribe an anxiolytic agent for the client.

74. A 6-year-old child with hypothyroidism diagnosed shortly after birth is seen by the nurse practitioner for a routine physical exam. Temperature is 96.8°F and pulse 68. The mother states that the child has been constipated and seems to be more tired than usual. Based on this history, what should the nurse practitioner suspect?

    1. The child has been taking too much levothyroxine and is exhibiting symptoms of toxicity.

    2. The child needs to add more fluids to his diet to correct the constipation.

    3. The child needs to have the dose of levothyroxine (Synthroid) increased because he is exhibiting signs of hypothyroidism.

    4. The child has "outgrown" the hypothyroidism and no longer needs levothyroxine.

75. A 6-year-old client has been discharged home on DDAVP (desmopressin acetate) for diabetes insipidus after removal of a pituitary tumor. On examination the nurse practitioner notes that the child is lethargic but has 4+ deep tendon reflexes. The practitioner suspects:

    1. Noncompliance with therapy.

    2. Water intoxication.

    3. Increased vasopressor effect.

    4. Interaction with OTC cough medicine products.

76. When monitoring an adolescent's insulin therapy regimen, the nurse practitioner is aware that the NPH/regular insulin proportions are:

    1. 2:1 in the AM and 1:1 in the PM.

    2. 1:1 in the AM and 1:2 in the PM.

    3. 1:2 in the AM and 2:1 in the PM.

    4. 1:1 in the AM and PM.

77. The nurse practitioner understands that lispro insulin (Humalog):

    1. Can be injected just before eating.

    2. Is less costly than regular insulin.

    3. Increases the likelihood of late postprandial hypoglycemia due to its length of action.

    4. Has a long-term safety profile and does not cause teratogenic effects.

78. When prescribing sulfonylureas, the nurse practitioner educates the client that the most common side effect of therapy is

    1. Upset stomach.

    2. Diarrhea.

    3. Angina.

    4. Hypoglycemia.

79. The primary action of pioglitazone (Actos) and rosiglitazone (Avandia) is to:

    1. Decrease hepatic glucose output.

    2. Increase secretion of insulin from the pancreas.

    3. Increase glucose uptake into the muscle and fat.

    4. Increase postprandial uptake of glucose into the intestine.

Answers & Rationales

Physical Examination & Diagnostic Tests

1. **(2)** When examining the thyroid, it is important that the client relax the sternocleidomastoid muscles, which is done by having the client lean toward the side being evaluated.

2. **(4)** The thyroid gland is fixed to the trachea and thus ascends during swallowing. This assists the nurse practitioner to distinguish thyroid structures from other neck masses. The gland's size, degree of enlargement, consistency, and surface characteristics and the presence of nodules or bruits are noted during the examination.

3. **(2)** The five questions in the Carville Diabetic Foot Screen are as follows:

   - Has there been a change in the foot since the last evaluation?
   - Is there a foot ulcer now or a history of foot ulcer?
   - Does the foot have an abnormal shape?
   - Is there weakness in the ankle or foot?
   - Are the nails thick, too long, or overgrown?

   There is no reference to pain on this screening.

4. **(3)** Papillary carcinoma, the most common form of thyroid cancer, is associated with a history of exposure to radiation. Family history, history of hyperthyroidism, and smoking are not considered significant risk factors for this malignancy.

5. **(1)** The high level of thyroid hormone affects the nervous system, causing sympathomimetic symptoms such as brisk deep tendon reflexes, fine rapid tremor of the hands, restlessness, irritability, insomnia, dreams, nightmares, and rarely severe cognitive impairment and psychosis.

6. **(3)** The American Diabetes Association recommends <7% as an important treatment goal to decrease risk of long-term complications. A lab result of >8% $HgbA_{1c}$ is an indication that action needs to be taken, either by a change of medication or a reinforcement of education.

7. **(2)** Growth abnormalities are associated with anterior pituitary dysfunction and glucose intolerance with diabetes related to pancreas dysfunction. Coagulation abnormalities and fatigue would be associated with hematologic dysfunction. Hypoxia would be associated with oxygenation problems and jaundice with liver or biliary problems. Steatorrhea is associated with malabsorption syndrome and cystic fibrosis.

8. **(4)** Although the primary care provider may obtain TSH and antibody levels, the preferred diagnostic tool for the endocrinologist is the FNA biopsy. Scans, sonography, and x-ray tests can be used in initial screening; they do not assist in the determination of whether the nodule is malignant or not. The aspirate is sent for cytology and interpretation.

9. **(4)** The dexamethasone suppression test is the best screening test and 24-hour urine for free cortisol is the best confirmatory test for Cushing's disease. TSH/T_4 may also be appropriate to rule out a thyroid condition because some of the client's signs and

symptoms are consistent with thyroid dysfunction. ANA and RF are ordered when rheumatoid arthritis or systemic lupus erythematosus (SLE) is suspected; this client's clinical picture is not consistent with these conditions. RBC count would be done to rule out anemia, a potential problem for this client based on the history of fatigue, but the rest of the clinical picture indicates more than anemia. No clinical findings support a calcium level being drawn.

10. **(2)** TSH levels should be decreased in a client with Graves' disease because thyroid-stimulating immunoglobulins bind to TSH receptors, which increase T_4 synthesis and release, subsequently suppressing TSH levels.

11. **(3)** Correct procedure is to use a 10-gm (5.07 Semmes-Weinstein) filament and apply it to 10 sites on the foot (one on the top of the foot, nine on the heel, sole, and toes). The filament is applied perpendicular (90-degree angle) to the skin surface with sufficient force for 1.5 seconds to cause the filament to bend. The filament should not be allowed to slide across the skin or make repetitive contact with each test site. Randomizing the selection of test sites (start with big toe→heel→instep area→little toe) and the time between successive tests to reduce client guessing and having the client close the eyes are also helpful.

12. **(3)** In 1997 the American Diabetes Association revised the classification and diagnostic criteria for diabetes to include any one of the three following methods, which must be confirmed on a subsequent day:

- Random plasma glucose ≥200 mg/dl and acute symptoms (polyuria, polydipsia, polyphagia)
- Fasting plasma glucose ≥126 mg/dl
- Two-hour plasma glucose ≥200 mg/dl

Disorders

13. **(2)** Type 1 diabetes is caused by destruction of the beta cells mediated through the immune system. The other three choices refer to type 2 diabetes.

14. **(4)** An annual eye examination with the pupils dilated should be done by a specialist who can recognize subtle abnormalities. Although the other referrals can offer important contributions to diabetic care, these would be done on an as-needed basis rather than annually.

15. **(3)** Because of the normal menstrual periods and androgen plasma level, this hirsutism would be considered idiopathic. Diseases related to the ovaries would cause changes in the menstrual cycle and with Cushing's syndrome would be associated with adrenal androgen overproduction.

16. **(4)** Testosterone production is regulated by the hypothalamic-pituitary-testicular (HPT) axis, so abnormalities in any of these areas can affect the production of testosterone.

17. **(4)** All these contribute significantly to difficulty controlling diabetes in the teenage years. Hormonal changes and the desire to become independent increase emotional conflicts. Teens have a great desire to be like their peers and do not want to be regimented in following a specific diet and adhering to a treatment plan.

18. **(2)** It is important for clients with diabetes to have their feet inspected daily either by self-examination or by a family member. Feet should be washed daily but never soaked. Corns and calluses should receive a professional's care. Nails should be trimmed straight across to avoid injury to the nail beds.

19. **(1)** The normal serum glucose for adults ranges from 70–120 mg/dl. Diabetic acidosis is not of concern until the glucose is >300 mg/dl. An $HgbA_{1c}$ >8.0% indicates poor glucose control over the past few months.

20. **(1)** True hypoglycemia can be organized around whether it is fasting or postprandial. Postprandial hypoglycemia may be caused by early adult-onset diabetes or postgastrectomy syndrome. Fasting hypoglycemia is most often caused by excessive doses of insulin, sulfonylureas alone or with biguanides, and thiazolidinediones.

21. **(3)** The symptoms suggest hypothyroidism, and thyroid studies (TSH) would be most useful.

22. **(2)** This middle-aged female client presents with many of the classic symptoms of early hyperthyroidism. A suppressed TSH with an elevated free T_4 establishes the diagnosis of hyperthyroidism.

23. **(3)** The client's physical findings and habitus, along with hypertension and hypokalemia, are associated with Cushing's syndrome, which is a state of excessive cortisol production due to a pituitary tumor. A Cushing's-like syndrome is often associated with prolonged glucocorticoid administration. Obesity is the primary finding in Cushing's syndrome, along with the "moon face," "dowager/buffalo" hump, truncal obesity, hirsutism in women, and impotence and loss of body hair in men. Addison's disease is characterized by hyperkalemia, hyponatremia, hypoglycemia, anemia, and hypercalcemia. Clients with hypoaldosteronism (impaired renin secretion) have hyperkalemia. Pheochromocytoma would be in the differential diagnosis of this client because of the hypertension; the other findings are not consistent with this diagnosis.

24. **(3)** Low-dose antithyroid drugs are considered a good alternative to prevent the effects of hyperthyroidism on the mother and developing fetus until surgery can be performed. Another option is using an antithyroid drug until after delivery and then having surgery. Removal of the thyroid during the second trimester can be performed safely and is the usual recommendation. Replacement is essential after removal of the gland.

25. **(4)** Accumulation of hyaluronic acid in interstitial tissues increases capillary permeability to albumin and causes the interstitial edema of the face and eyelids in clients with hypothyroidism.

26. **(2)** Although alcohol abuse may be a cause of hypoglycemia, this client is presenting with classic symptoms of postprandial hypoglycemia. Assessment for alcohol abuse as the etiology of the hypoglycemia would be advisable.

27. **(2)** Hyperparathyroidism accounts for more than 60% of clients and is likely to be the explanation for elevated serum calcium levels.

28. **(1)** Although Option #3 may explain the weight gain, Cushing's disease is correct for the constellation of symptoms of rapid weight gain, hypertension, and elevated blood sugar. These symptoms suggest adrenal dysfunction. Serum cortisol and adrenocorticotropic hormone (ACTH) levels should be checked.

29. **(1)** This woman is likely experiencing the life-threatening syndrome that can occur in decompensated hyperthyroidism. The clues are her symptom presentation and progression, the new "anti-drug," and upcoming throat surgery.

30. **(3)** The symptoms describe the classic presentation of a client with hypothyroidism. A client with CHF would have jugular venous distention, rales, and peripheral edema. The criteria for diagnosing DM are polydipsia, polyphagia, polyuria, and weight loss. Thyroid cancer typically presents without physical symptoms, and often the only physical finding is a hard, fixed nodule on the thyroid gland.

31. **(2)** The client's blood sugar levels are low around lunchtime, which is when the regular insulin is peaking (3–4 hours), so a reduction in the regular insulin would address this problem.

32. **(1)** The nurse practitioner's role in primary care for a client with a thyroid nodule involves initially the early identification of the thyroid nodule on physical examination, referring the client to an endocrinologist for further evaluation, and possibly obtaining some preliminary TSH and antibody testing. The endocrinologist performs the FNA. Levothyroxine may or may not be used to diminish the size of the nodule based on the findings from the FNA and the endocrinologist's chosen treatment plan.

33. **(4)** Clients with diabetes must understand that when they are sick, blood glucose level will probably increase, even when they are not eating. They need to monitor blood glucose levels every 2–4 hours and check urine for ketones if glucose level >240 mg/dl. The medications in Option #3 should **not** be given until the client's nausea and vomiting have subsided and the client has resumed a normal diet (blood glucose monitoring is important during this time).

34. **(2)** Graves' disease, an autoimmune condition also known as diffuse toxic goiter, is the most common cause of hyperthyroidism in this age group. Much less common causes include cancer of the thyroid, adenoma of the pituitary gland, and postpartum (or silent) thyroiditis.

35. **(1)** The TSH should be ordered to determine whether the client is euthyroid, hypothyroid, or hyperthyroid. The client should also be sent to an endocrinologist or surgeon because all nodules of the thyroid should be biopsied to

rule out malignancy. "Watching and waiting" is inappropriate without having a biopsy performed. Thyroid hormone replacement therapy would be indicated only in clients found to be hypothyroid and in whom thyroid cancer has been ruled out. Thyroid ablation may be indicated in clients whose FNA biopsy results are positive for thyroid cancer, but this cannot be determined without a surgeon's intervention.

36. **(3)** Hypothyroidism often follows this treatment, with 50% of clients requiring replacement therapy in the first year and almost 100% requiring therapy in 10 years. For this reason, regular monitoring of TSH/T$_4$ levels should be performed. Clients emit a small amount of radioactivity after receiving the dose used to treat this condition and do not require isolation for 7 days. Radioactive iodine is very safe, without an increased risk of chromosomal abnormalities; therefore no contraindication exists to becoming pregnant after therapy, although clients are counseled to avoid pregnancy while on treatment and to avoid children and pregnant women after receiving the oral ablation dose. This therapy is recommended for clients who have cardiac disease associated with their thyroid condition.

37. **(3)** Thyroid replacement is lifelong maintenance therapy and should be given as one dose in the morning. Weight loss, diarrhea, and tachycardia are signs of overmedication.

38. **(4)** No consensus exists on adapting glycemic goals in the pediatric population. The goals for glucose control must be individualized with each family based on the child's age and ability to recognize symptoms of hypoglycemia and a past history of hypoglycemia or seizures.

39. **(1)** This is the best choice for the initial examination because the history may reveal normal variation in pattern of growth related to race, heredity, size of other family members, and psychosocial status. Skeletal maturation ("bone age") can be assessed through radiography if child is in the fifth growth percentile or lower. Other choices are inappropriate without history and physical exam, and growth hormone would not be administered without lab evaluation.

40. **(3)** Pubertal (physiologic) gynecomastia is a visible or palpable glandular enlargement of the male breast that can occur in healthy adolescents. Typically the breasts are unequal in size and may be tender; nipples are often irritated from rubbing against clothing; and Tanner stages II–IV of pubertal development are noted. The symptoms in Option #4 are associated with pathologic gynecomastia.

41. **(2)** Hyperthyroidism in children most often affects girls and is an autoimmune disorder (Graves' disease) in which the body produces antibodies that stimulate TSH receptors, causing overproduction of thyroid hormones and goiter. Hypothyroidism is associated with iodine deficiency.

42. **(4)** These findings are consistent with Turner's syndrome: short stature, gonadal dysgenesis, lymphedema (usually appearing in infancy), left-sided heart or aortic abnormalities, primary amenorrhea, and delayed onset of puberty. Fragile X syndrome is an inherited condition usually affecting males and characterized by long narrow face and prominent ears, mild to profound mental retardation, hyperactivity and poor attention span, and autistic-type behavior. Marfan's syndrome is a connective tissue disorder of tall and thin adolescent characterized by long limbs, narrow hands, long slender fingers, and nearsightedness. Klinefelter's syndrome is characterized by small testes, sterility, gynecomastia, and long legs.

43. **(4)** Hypogonadism, associated with delayed sexual development, sexual infantilism, and small testes, is most often the contributing factor to growth retardation after age 10 years for girls and 12 years for boys. Other causes of decelerated growth or short stature include hypothyroidism, diabetes, and hypopituitarism. Chromosomal abnormalities would be noted at an earlier age.

44. **(1)** Fanconi's syndrome is most often a hereditary problem caused by an inborn error of metabolism, such as galactosemia or Wilson's disease, and usually presents as growth failure in children. Tourette's syndrome is a disorder characterized by multiple vocal or motor tics. Klinefelter's syndrome is characterized by small testes, sterility, gynecomastia, and long legs. Angelman's syndrome is associated with mental retardation, seizures, wide-based ataxic gait, pleasant happy disposition, and limited vocabulary or absent speech.

45. **(3)** Most children have a target goal to maintain blood sugar at 80–140 mg/dl if they can recognize the symptoms of hypoglycemia. Option #1 is too low and may predispose the child to hypoglycemia. Options #2 and #4 are too high.

46. **(1)** Type 1 diabetes usually (but not always) appears before age 30 and is heralded by the three "Ps": polydipsia, polyuria, and polyphagia.

47. **(4)** Tight glycemic control is contraindicated in infants <2 years of age and should be instituted with extreme caution in children <7 years of age to avoid injuring the developing brain.

48. **(1)** Infants with hypothyroidism often have an abnormally pitched cry due to lethargy and delayed mental responsiveness. Hypertelorism does not produce an abnormal cry unless accompanied by microcephaly.

49. **(1)** The National Cholesterol Education Program Adult Treatment Panel III states that the metabolic syndrome exists when a client has met three of the following criteria:

    - Triglycerides >150 mg/dl
    - HDL <40 mg/dl in men and <50 mg/dl in women
    - Waist circumference >102 cm (>40 inches) in men and >88 cm (>35 inches) in women
    - BP >130/85 mm/Hg
    - FBS >110 mg/dl

50. **(3)** Smoking causes thinning of the bones and can lead to osteopenia/osteoporosis. Options #1, #2, and #4 are all self-care practices that may prevent or delay onset of osteopenia/osteoporosis.

51. **(3)** Low testosterone levels may result from prostate cancer treatment and longstanding liver disease. Options #1, #2, and #4 are risk factors of osteoporosis that can occur with men and women alike.

52. **(4)** Carbohydrate is the macronutrient with the greatest impact on the postprandial glucose levels. Ingested protein has minimal effect on the blood glucose levels. A diet high in fat may be associated with cardiovascular disease. Fiber has little effect on the plasma glucose response but may result in decreased low-density lipoprotein (LDL) cholesterol.

Pharmacology

53. **(3)** Metformin is associated with weight loss and appetite suppression, although the actual cause of weight loss is unknown. Nateglinide and glyburide are considered insulin secretagogues, which tend to stimulate insulin secretion from the pancreas, thus causing a slight weight gain. Pioglitazone is an insulin sensitizer and increases glucose uptake in the muscle and fat. Common side effects include fluid retention and increase in central adiposity.

54. **(4)** Glargine, introduced in 2001 and considered a long-acting (background) insulin, is usually given once daily and may last 24 hours without a peak. This clear insulin must be given alone and not mixed with other insulin. Lispro insulin is usually given three times daily with meals.

55. **(2)** Metformin should not be given to men with a serum creatinine ≥1.5 mg/dl and women with a serum creatinine ≥1.4 mg/dl because it can predispose the client to lactic acidosis. Pioglitazone and rapaglinide are metabolized primarily in the liver and require monitoring of liver function tests. Acarbose is metabolized mainly in the gastrointestinal tract.

56. **(3)** Lactic acidosis is a potentially severe and fatal reaction to metformin. Metformin does not contribute to weight gain; it often helps with weight loss and decreases LDL/triglyceride levels and insulin requirements.

57. **(2)** The sulfonylureas reduce blood glucose by stimulating insulin release from the pancreas. Over time these drugs also may actually increase insulin effects at the cellular level and decrease glucose production by the liver, which is why sulfonylureas are used in clients with type 2 diabetes who still have a functioning pancreas.

58. **(1)** Anorexia, nausea, and a metallic taste in the mouth are common side effects. Over time the GI symptoms subside and can be relieved by taking the medication with food or by starting at a lower dose.

59. **(4)** Antithyroid medications (propylthiouracil, methimazole) are relatively inexpensive and do cross the placenta. The client remains on the medications for 1–2 years with the hope of a

permanent remission of symptoms when they are withdrawn.

60. **(2)** Both these drug classifications tend to reduce insulin sensitivity and can cause hyperglycemia. ACE inhibitors, calcium channel blockers, and selective alpha-blockers are metabolically neutral; some may actually have a beneficial effect.

61. **(4)** The client's symptoms indicate hypothyroidism, as does the elevated TSH (normal 0.5–4.7 mU/L). Full replacement dose of levothyroxine should be started based on the client's age, and TSH level should be checked in 6 weeks, the time it may take for a given dose to become effective. Loading doses should never be given except for coma, which is treated by IV medication in the hospital.

62. **(4)** Coronary disease clients found to be mildly to moderately hypothyroid can safely undergo urgent surgery (including bypass procedures) without prior replacement. The rate of complications is no greater than for nonhypothyroid clients, and the cardiac risks are less compared with initiating replacement therapy preoperatively.

63. **(3)** Metformin is a better option in an obese client because it is frequently associated with weight loss, whereas sulfonylureas may actually cause a weight gain. Insulin is an overaggressive approach to mildly elevated glucose; clients also tend to be less receptive to treatment requiring injections. Diet and exercise were unsuccessful, and the longer her blood sugar remains elevated, the greater the risk for end-organ damage.

64. **(2)** Chronic overtreatment is associated with osteoporosis; the other options are related to *acute overdosage* of levothyroxine and can be relieved by omitting the dose for 3 days and then starting on a lower dose.

65. **(4)** To initiate treatment for elevated BP, it is recommended that three elevated readings be recorded on three separate occasions. No evidence suggests that this client had increased BP on prior visits.

66. **(1)** This is the best answer because the AM intermediate dose affects the glucose level before dinner. Altering the regular insulin will affect levels before lunch and before bedtime; however, these levels are acceptable. To reduce

the intermediate dose while maintaining the level of regular insulin, the client will need to self-mix the intermediate and regular insulin, using less of the intermediate.

67. **(4)** Pseudoephedrine and other decongestant medications that contain sympathomimetics lead to adverse reactions of central nervous system (CNS) overstimulation, palpitations, headache, hypertension, and nervousness. Guaifenesin in combination with dextromethorphan and phenylpropanolamine (Robitussin-CF) or pseudoephedrine (Robitussin-PE) can also cause palpitations and CNS overstimulation. Guaifenesin with dextromethorphan (Robitussin-DM) may cause GI upset, drowsiness, headache, and rash.

68. **(2)** Infusion site problems and skin irritation are by far the most frequent complaints of clients who use an insulin pump and often why the pump is discontinued. Clients also find it is more time consuming and costly. However, the Diabetes Control and Complications Trial (DCCT, 1993) reported a reduced risk of microvascular complications when insulin pumps and multiple daily injections were used.

69. **(3)** Prenatal clients are managed with insulin, not an insulin sensitizer. Pioglitazone and rosiglitzone act by decreasing peripheral insulin resistance in skeletal muscle and adipose tissue without enhancing insulin secretion and improving glucose tolerance in clients with type 2 diabetes. Option #4 refers to the action of α-glucosidase inhibitors, such as acarbose (Precose) and miglitol (Glyset).

70. **(3)** Older clients, especially with heart disease, need to be started on the smallest amount of thyroid medication replacement (0.025 mg, not 0.1 mg) and gradually increased until a therapeutic level is achieved. If thyroid replacement occurs too quickly, the heart may decompensate; 2 grains of thyroid extract is too much. Methimazole is an antithyroid medication used to treat hyperthyroidism.

71. **(2)** The response to therapy is based on clinical symptomatology and a TSH assay approximately 4–6 weeks after initiation of therapy. This is continued until a stable dose is obtained. TSH and a free T_4 level are the two standard tests that can be used to monitor the status of the thyroid; a levothyroxine level cannot be drawn. Levothyroxine is not a myelosuppressive.

72. **(3)** Beta-blockers are initially prescribed to reduce the signs and symptoms of the condition and to reduce the peripheral conversion of T_4 to triiodothyronine (T_3); NSAIDs are indicated for reducing inflammation associated with thyroiditis; and antithyroid medications (PTU, methimazole) are used to treat severe hyperthyroidism. Corticosteroids are sometimes used in the treatment of thyroiditis, but the remaining classes (antibiotics, ACE inhibitors, calcium channel blockers, anxiolytics), are not routinely used in the management of hyperthyroidism.

73. **(3)** Decreasing the dose of levothyroxine and evaluating the client's cardiac status are the appropriate interventions in this situation, in addition to involving the collaborating physician regarding further work-up. Discontinuing the thyroid replacement would be inappropriate because the client remains hypothyroid and requires therapy for life. An anxiolytic may be a helpful adjunct but is not appropriate as the sole intervention, as it ignores the cardiac symptoms.

74. **(3)** A low temperature and pulse, constipation, and fatigue are all signs of hypothyroidism, and therefore the dose of levothyroxine needs to be increased. Levothyroxine toxicity would manifest with signs of hyperthyroidism. Constipation is a symptom of hypothyroidism and is not related to the child's fluid intake. Congenital hypothyroidism requires lifelong drug therapy.

75. **(2)** DDAVP promotes reabsorption of water in the renal tubules, which can lead to water intoxication. The signs of water intoxication are lethargy, behavioral changes, disorientation, and neuromuscular excitability.

76. **(1)** Insulin injections for the child/adolescent are 2:1 proportion NPH/regular in the AM and 1:1 in the PM. Changes are made based on blood sugar level done four times daily. The proportion is based on the periods of insulin activity.

77. **(1)** Lispro (Humalog), introduced in 1996, is the first analog of human insulin and has several advantages over regular insulin, including more rapid onset and shorter duration of action. It reaches peak activity in 1–2 hours and has a 4-hour duration, versus 6–8 hours for regular insulin. It is convenient because it can be injected immediately before eating (10–15 minutes). No long-term safety profile has yet been established, and its teratogenicity is unknown. It is also more expensive than insulin, and some third-party payers may not reimburse clients.

78. **(4)** Hypoglycemia and weight gain are the most common side effects of sulfonylurea therapy.

79. **(3)** Pioglitazone and rosiglitazone are insulin sensitizers, which increase the glucose uptake in the muscle and fat. Metformin decreases hepatic glucose output. Oral sulfonylureas increase insulin secretion in the pancreas. The α-glucosidase inhibitors increase postprandial glucose uptake in the intestine.

10

Musculoskeletal

Physical Examination & Diagnostic Tests

1. A goniometer is a measurement device in the musculoskeletal examination of a client. The nurse practitioner uses this tool to determine:

   1. Strength of the muscles in the extremities.

   2. Degree of joint flexion and extension.

   3. Range of motion of the extremities.

   4. Point of joint flexion that is painful.

2. The nurse practitioner places a client in the prone position with the knee flexed 90 degrees. The tibia is firmly opposed to the femur by exerting downward pressure on the foot. The leg is rotated externally and internally. If locking of the knee occurs, this is accurately called a positive:

   1. Drawer sign.

   2. McMurray's test.

   3. Apley's sign.

   4. Bulge sign.

3. A client has numbness and tingling in the thumb and first two fingers when pressing the backs of the hands together (flexes wrists at 90 degrees) for 60 seconds. This is a positive:

   1. Tinel's sign.

   2. Drawer sign.

   3. McMurray's test.

   4. Phalen's maneuver.

4. What is the sign that occurs when compressing the suprapatellar pouch back against the femur and feeling for fluid entering the spaces?

   1. Drawer sign.

   2. Kernig's sign.

   3. Balloon sign.

   4. Bulge sign.

5. De Quervain's disease can be diagnosed in part by a positive:

    1. Finkelstein's sign.

    2. Tinel's sign.

    3. Phalen's maneuver.

    4. Lachman's sign.

6. The primary examination techniques to use to assess the musculoskeletal system are:

    1. Inspection and percussion.

    2. Auscultation and palpation.

    3. Inspection and palpation.

    4. Palpation and percussion.

7. What can the nurse practitioner use to confirm a diagnosis of polymyalgia rheumatica (PMR)?

    1. Chest radiograph.

    2. Serum protein electrophoresis.

    3. Corticosteroid challenge.

    4. Erythrocyte sedimentation rate (ESR).

8. When performing an assessment, the nurse practitioner understands that the metacarpophalangeal (MCP) joints are frequently involved with:

    1. Gout.

    2. Rheumatic fever.

    3. Rheumatoid arthritis (RA).

    4. Osteoarthritis (OA).

9. In the evaluation of polyneuropathy, which study would **not** be recommended?

    1. Sedimentation rate.

    2. Complete blood count (CBC).

    3. Hemoglobin A (HgbA$_{1c}$).

    4. Electromyography (EMG).

10. In accurately assessing a client who reports back injury, it is critical to question:

    1. Family history of back problems.

    2. Previous injury.

    3. Personal history of chronic illness.

    4. Mechanism of injury.

11. Tinel's sign and Phalen's maneuver are used in identifying a common workplace illness that the nurse practitioner recognizes as:

    1. Lateral epicondylitis.

    2. Carpel tunnel syndrome.

    3. Dupuytren's disease.

    4. Thoracic outlet syndrome.

12. An elderly client complains of fatigue, weakness, lightheadedness, and anorexia. He also complains of hot, swollen proximal interphalangeal (PIP) and metacarpophalangeal (MCP) joints. These symptoms occurred 5 months ago and recurred a few days ago. Which laboratory findings would be most conclusive of these assessments?

    1. Mean corpuscular volume (MCV) 104, low serum ferritin.

    2. Mean corpuscular volume (MCV) 92, high serum ferritin.

    3. Elevation in uric acid level.

    4. Elevation in white blood cell (WBC) count.

13. How is the talar tilt test conducted?

    1. The tibia is grasped with one hand, and backward pressure is applied to the heel.

    2. The ankle is gently inverted, and laxity of the ligament is graded.

    3. The examiner passively inverts, everts, dorsiflexes, and plantar-flexes the ankle.

    4. The client actively inverts, everts, dorsiflexes, and plantar-flexes the ankle.

14. Varus pressure on a knee that is slightly flexed (30 degrees) tests:

    1. Medial collateral ligament stability.

    2. Lateral collateral ligament stability.

    3. Medial cruciate ligament stability.

    4. Lateral meniscus tear.

15. The nurse practitioner is assessing a preadolescent girl for scoliosis. How is this test conducted?

    1. Have the girl bend at the waist, and look for asymmetry in the back and hip area.

2. Examine the child fully clothed, paying particular attention to the hips and back.

3. Have the child walk heel-to-toe, and observe the gait and pelvis.

4. Place the child on her back, and flex the knees and observe for misalignment.

16. In doing a physical assessment on a newborn, the nurse practitioner notes a "hip click." What other findings are associated with this condition?

1. Shortened quadriceps.

2. Lateral deviation of patella.

3. Limited abduction.

4. Lax hamstrings.

Disorders

17. An adolescent complains of right knee pain immediately after running in track practice. On examination the knee is warm to touch, and a tender, swollen tibial tuberosity is noted. The nurse practitioner suspects:

1. Osgood-Schlatter disease.

2. Rheumatoid arthritis.

3. Acute tendinitis.

4. Posttraumatic knee effusion.

18. The nurse practitioner realizes that the most common cause of shoulder pain is:

1. Frozen shoulder.

2. Thoracic outlet syndrome.

3. Impingement syndrome.

4. Osteoarthritis.

19. A 45-year-old female complains of knee pain when kneeling and a "clicking" noise when walking up steps. The nurse practitioner notes slight knee effusion and tenderness when palpating the patella against the condyles. The diagnosis for this client is:

1. Anterior cruciate tear.

2. Dislocated patella.

3. Chondromalacia patella.

4. Tendinitis.

20. A client has been diagnosed with a complete rotator cuff tear of the left shoulder. The nurse would expect the client to have difficulty in:

1. Abducting the left arm.

2. Supinating the left forearm.

3. Shrugging the shoulders.

4. Touching the left hand to the right shoulder.

21. Nighttime extremity pain in school-age children that is deep but not present in the joints and that may be caused by inflammation of the muscle bodies in tight fascial sheaths and by periods of high activity is:

1. Osgood-Schlatter disease.

2. Patellofemoral stress syndrome.

3. Growing pains.

4. Shin splints.

22. A client has been diagnosed with polymyalgia rheumatica (PMR). The nurse practitioner understands that this disorder is:

1. An autoimmune, multisystem problem in which the body makes antibodies to its own proteins.

2. A degenerative disorder with no inflammatory changes in which joint cartilage wears away with age and eventually causes bone spurs.

3. An inflammatory disorder involving the axial skeleton and large peripheral joints.

4. An inflammatory connective tissue disorder that primarily affects older women and is associated with giant cell (temporal) arteritis.

23. In teaching a client about fibromyalgia, the nurse practitioner includes what information?

1. Diagnostic studies such as ESR and CBC are important tools to confirm disease progression.

2. Avoid stretching exercises and daily low-impact aerobics.

3. Take ibuprofen (Motrin) 200 mg q4–6h prn for pain and amitriptyline (Elavil) 10 mg 1–2 hours before bedtime.

4. Apply heat or massage "trigger points" to reduce pain.

24. The nurse practitioner understands that chronic synovitis with pannus formation is the basic pathophysiologic finding in clients with:

    1. Systemic lupus erythematosus (SLE).

    2. Ankylosing spondylitis (AS).

    3. Rheumatoid arthritis (RA).

    4. Osteoarthritis (OA).

25. The nurse practitioner is examining a client who is complaining of pain in her hips and knees. She has a history of osteoarthritis. On examination the joints are painful to movement and are warm to touch. The best immediate therapy for this client is:

    1. Physical therapy for range of motion of affected areas.

    2. Decreased physical activity and immobilizing splints for affected joints.

    3. Moist heat and/or cold therapy on painful joints.

    4. ESR to determine level of activity.

26. The history of a client who may have contracted Lyme disease may include what characteristic?

    1. Erythematous rash on bridge of nose and cheeks with discoid patches on the trunk.

    2. Immediate development of arthritis symptoms, especially in the knees.

    3. Expanding rash with central clearing within a month of being bitten.

    4. Early symptoms of meningitis and myocarditis.

27. The nurse practitioner understands that finding Heberden's nodes on physical examination of a client is a cardinal sign of:

    1. Septic arthritis.

    2. Rheumatoid arthritis.

    3. Gouty arthritis.

    4. Osteoarthritis.

28. The nurse practitioner is teaching crutch walking to an adolescent with a lower leg cast for a fractured tibia. Instructions for assisting the adolescent to walk up the stairs would include:

    1. Place both crutches on the upper step and step up with unaffected leg while balancing on crutches.

    2. Position the affected leg on the upper step and use the crutches to move up.

    3. Place the unaffected leg on the upper step and move affected leg and crutches up together.

    4. Position the affected leg and the crutch on the upper step and bring the unaffected leg up with the crutch.

29. Competing diagnoses for an adult male client who presents with acute onset of unilateral inflammation, pain, and erythema of the first metatarsophalangeal (MTP) joint could be:

    1. Gout, cellulitis, and osteoporosis.

    2. Cellulitis, rheumatoid arthritis, and gout.

    3. Osteoporosis, fibromyalgia, and cellulitis.

    4. Septic arthritis, rheumatoid arthritis, osteoarthritis.

30. Diseases that often present as polyarthritic disorders include:

    1. Lyme arthritis, rheumatic heart disease, ankylosing spondylitis, and psoriatic arthritis.

    2. Rheumatoid arthritis, gout, Reiter's syndrome, and osteoarthritis.

    3. Gonococcal arthritis, systemic lupus erythematosus, and septic arthritis.

    4. Polymyalgia rheumatica, Lyme arthritis, pseudogout, and psoriatic arthritis.

31. A common injury can most often cause a meniscus tear under which circumstances?

    1. The knee is almost completely extended, and the tibia is externally rotated.

    2. An applied external force is sufficiently strong to cause external rotation or hyperextension of the knee.

    3. Valgus or varus pressure on the knee occurs at full extension and at 30 degrees of flexion.

    4. The knee is simultaneously twisted and flexed during an injury.

32. Pain in lumbosacral strain typically begins:

    1. Immediately with the injury.

    2. 1–2 hours after injury.

    3. 6–8 hours after injury.

    4. 12–36 hours after injury.

33. An acute onset of pain descends down to the lower leg and foot of a 25-year-old obese adult is likely to be a symptom of:

    1. Lumbosacral strain.

    2. Herniated intervertebral disk injury.

    3. Osteomyelitis.

    4. Osteoporosis.

34. The nurse practitioner sees a client with trauma to the knee that caused it to "give out," followed by severe pain and effusion. Later, he had "locking" of the knee with pivoting or turning. This client has probably suffered:

    1. Patellofemoral stress syndrome.

    2. Growing pains.

    3. Shin splints.

    4. Patellar subluxation.

35. A client with patellofemoral syndrome has quadriceps setting as a recommended exercise. The nurse practitioner would teach the client to:

    1. Lie supine on the floor with legs extended, dorsiflex the foot, and push the thigh into the floor.

    2. Sit on the floor leaning back on the elbows, flex one knee to 90 degrees, and extend the other completely and hold for 5 seconds.

    3. Lie on the floor and flex both knees to about 20 degrees with a rolled towel underneath them, and extend one leg and hold for 5 seconds.

    4. Use resistive exercises with an elastic band.

36. Which risk factor is associated with gout?

    1. Female gender.

    2. Age 20 years.

    3. Ingestion of salicylate medications.

    4. Overuse of extremity.

37. A third-degree ankle sprain is associated with:

    1. Minimal ecchymosis, moderate edema, and a stable joint.

    2. Moderate ecchymosis, moderate edema, and an unstable joint.

    3. Marked ecchymosis, marked edema, and a stable joint.

    4. Marked ecchymosis, marked edema, and an unstable joint.

38. A client with rheumatoid arthritis presents for follow-up. What is the best evaluative question the nurse practitioner can ask that will help determine the severity of disease?

    1. "Were you able to drive the car to your appointment today?"

    2. "Were you able to fix your dinner last night?"

    3. "How long does it take for your joints to loosen up after you get up in the morning?"

    4. "How many pounds can you carry?"

39. A 35-year-old woman is seen with a complaint of diffuse musculoskeletal pain, stiffness, and fatigue for the past 3 months. The pain is worse in the morning and also with changes in weather. She states she wakes up in the morning feeling tired. Physical examination is normal except for pain on digital palpation in 12 tender points. Laboratory results are unremarkable. The most likely diagnosis is:

    1. Fibromyalgia.

    2. Myofascial syndrome.

    3. Rheumatoid arthritis.

    4. Depression.

40. When counseling a postmenopausal female client on prevention of osteoporosis, all the following are therapeutic recommendations **except**:

    1. Cessation of smoking.

    2. Daily intake of 200 mg of calcium and 40 IU of vitamin D.

    3. Continue hormone therapy.

    4. Monitor bone loss by dual-energy x-ray absorptiometry (DEXA) every 1–2 years.

41. A client tells the nurse practitioner that she has a "whiplash." The nurse practitioner understands that this is:

    1. Cervical facet joint dysfunction.
    2. Cervical flexion injury.
    3. Cervicothoracic injury.
    4. Cervical strain.

42. A client presents with a complaint of sudden pain and swelling in the knee. He also has chills and fever. On examination the knee is warm, tender, and swollen with evidence of effusion. What action would the nurse practitioner take?

    1. Splint the affected joint.
    2. Obtain aspiration of synovial fluid from the affected joint.
    3. Initiate treatment with nonsteroidal antiinflammatory drugs (NSAIDs).
    4. Recommend rest, ice, compression, and elevation of affected joint.

43. When determining the specific etiology of polyarticular complaints, which clinical clues are most helpful for diagnosis?

    1. Laboratory identification of antinuclear antibodies (ANA) and sedimentation rate.
    2. Radiograph of affected joints.
    3. Affected joint pattern and presence or lack of inflammation.
    4. Sexual history of client.

44. A client with ankylosing spondylitis is receiving education on managing her disease. The nurse practitioner would teach the client all the following **except**:

    1. Regular exercise program.
    2. Maintenance systemic corticosteroid therapy.
    3. Use of indomethacin (Indocin) for discomfort.
    4. Observation for signs and symptoms of iritis.

45. An adolescent client is being evaluated by the nurse practitioner for knee pain. The client is active in sports in his school but can recall no specific injury to the knee. On examination the nurse practitioner finds unilateral swelling of the anterior aspect of the tibial tubercle that is tender. The most likely diagnosis is:

    1. Stress fracture.
    2. Patellar dislocation.
    3. Osgood-Schlatter disease.
    4. Neuman's syndrome.

46. An adult client comes to the office complaining of foot pain. He can recall no specific injury but gives a history of being an occasional runner who drinks 6 to 10 beers on weekends. What physical findings would the nurse practitioner expect to find?

    1. Redness, swelling, and warmth of first metatarsophalangeal joint.
    2. Swelling, ecchymosis, and decreased range of motion.
    3. Swelling and decreased circulation.
    4. Decreased range of motion and obvious bone deformity.

47. Which of the diet selections indicate that the older client understands the health education regarding the prevention of osteoporosis?

    1. Chicken and baked potato.
    2. Glass of skim milk and toasted cheese sandwich.
    3. Hamburger and salad.
    4. Ice cream sundae with whipped cream.

48. During the history, which of the following questions would best assist the nurse practitioner in diagnosing osteoarthritis (OA) versus rheumatoid arthritis (RA)?

    1. "Is your joint pain symmetric and localized?"
    2. "Does your morning stiffness usually last several hours?"
    3. "Have you experienced fatigue, weakness, and weight loss?"
    4. "Is your joint pain asymmetric and worse with movement and relieved by rest?"

49. The number-one cause of disability in adults under age 45 is:

    1. Cancer.
    2. Fracture.

3. Low back pain.

4. Migraines.

50. Which of the following is the most accurate statement about juvenile rheumatoid arthritis (JRA)?

    1. Symptoms present in much greater severity than in adult RA.

    2. Complete remission occurs in three fourths of clients.

    3. More than 90% of cases progress to severe joint destruction.

    4. Cytotoxic drugs should be initiated as early as possible in the treatment regimen.

51. Primary treatment of joint injury involves:

    1. Rest, ice, compression, and elevation.

    2. Narcotic pain control and radiograph.

    3. Specialist referral and magnetic resonance imaging.

    4. NSAIDs and exercise.

52. The most common complaint in a client with back injury who had cauda equina syndrome, a surgical emergency, is:

    1. Urinary retention.

    2. Numbness below the level of injury.

    3. Weakness in the lower extremities.

    4. Pain.

53. Recognition of annular tears is important in the diagnosis of back pain because:

    1. They require immediate surgery.

    2. They are often misdiagnosed as strain or sprain, leading to herniation.

    3. They result in rapid paralysis.

    4. Radiograph would reveal them, but x-rays are usually not ordered initially.

54. What chronic musculoskeletal problem may occur after an injury and is characterized by a 3-month history of pain on both sides of body (above and below waist) and tenderness in at least 11 of 18 specified points?

    1. Chronic osteoarthritis.

    2. Reflex sympathetic dystrophy.

3. Tendinitis.

4. Fibromyalgia.

55. Which client is at highest risk for osteoporosis?

    1. 55-year-old male smoker and retired athlete.

    2. 60-year-old, 105-lb postmenopausal white female switchboard operator.

    3. 42-year-old black female intensive care nurse who is lactose intolerant.

    4. 50-year-old obese white woman with three children living on a farm.

56. A 38-year-old secretary complains of pain in her hands at night. On examination the nurse practitioner notes wasting of the thenar eminence of both hands and dry skin on the thumb, index, and middle fingers. The nurse practitioner suspects:

    1. Carpal tunnel syndrome.

    2. Transient ischemic attack.

    3. Osteoarthritis.

    4. Raynaud's phenomenon.

57. A 53-year-old woman presents with complaints of morning stiffness in the neck and back. She has pelvic and shoulder pain, and fatigue. Her laboratory studies reveal elevated ESR, normal rheumatoid factor, normal creatine phosphokinase, and normochromic normocytic anemia. Physical examination reveals an elevated temperature, bilateral pain, and stiffness of the pectoral and pelvic muscles. Based on this information, the most appropriate diagnosis is:

    1. Polyarteritis nodosa.

    2. Wegener's granulomatosis.

    3. Polymyalgia rheumatica.

    4. Rheumatoid arthritis.

58. A 55-year-old woman with a prior diagnosis of PMR presents with headache, low-grade fever, aching, stiffness, fatigue, malaise, and anorexia. Based on this information, the nurse practitioner would make a preliminary diagnosis of:

    1. Influenza.

    2. Pneumonia.

    3. Temporal arteritis.

    4. Rheumatoid arthritis.

59. Children with JRA must be screened regularly for:

    1. Ulcerative colitis.

    2. Iridocyclitis.

    3. Diabetes mellitus.

    4. Adrenal insufficiency.

60. An adolescent who twisted his knee while skateboarding comes to the clinic complaining of knee pain. He also states that in the past few weeks his knee has "locked up a couple of times." On examination a positive McMurray's test is elicited. This is consistent with a diagnosis of:

    1. Anterior cruciate ligament tear.

    2. Dislocated patella.

    3. Medial meniscus tear.

    4. Chondromalacia patella.

61. In young children a complaint of hip pain without a history of trauma suggests several differential diagnoses. Which diagnosis is considered a true orthopedic emergency?

    1. Toxic synovitis of the hip.

    2. Legg-Calvé-Perthes disease.

    3. Increased femoral anteversion.

    4. Avascular necrosis of the femoral head.

62. Differentiation between structural and functional scoliosis can be done by placing the child in Adam's position. Which of the following occurs in this position?

    1. Structural scoliosis disappears, and functional scoliosis is enhanced.

    2. Persistent functional scoliosis is indicated.

    3. Functional scoliosis disappears, and structural scoliosis is enhanced.

    4. Curves greater than 10 degrees are indicated.

63. A man comes into the clinic complaining of low back pain that radiates down the lateral thigh. The pain began suddenly on the job after lifting a heavy object. The nurse practitioner would further evaluate the client for:

    1. Compression fracture of lower lumbar vertebrae.

    2. Spinal cord injury.

    3. Compression of a lumbar disk.

    4. History of spinal cord injury.

64. A male child with pectis excavatum and associated scoliosis should be evaluated for:

    1. Pulmonary dysfunction.

    2. Cardiac compromise.

    3. Marfan's syndrome.

    4. Joint deformities.

65. An 80 year-old resident of a long-term care facility with a history of multi-infarct dementia (MID) is alert but is disoriented to person, place, and situation. His only health problems are MID and osteoarthritis. Over the past 2 weeks he has become agitated and exit seeking and is constantly rubbing his knees. The nurse practitioner suspects that this client is experiencing:

    1. Worsening dementia.

    2. Pain.

    3. Urinary tract infection (UTI).

    4. Acute infarct.

Pharmacology

66. The nurse practitioner is seeing a middle-aged severely arthritic woman receiving maintenance therapy of prednisone 10 mg/day for the past 6 weeks. She now presents as acutely ill with signs and symptoms of acute pneumonia. She is fatigued and weak with loss of appetite, and BP is lower than on previous visits. Which action should be taken in regard to prednisone?

    1. Immediately discontinue the medication.

    2. Increase dosage to 60 mg/day, then taper back to 10 mg/day.

    3. Gradually taper from 10 to 1 mg/day.

    4. Maintain dose at 10 mg/day.

67. What is the drug of choice for a client with rheumatoid arthritis (RA)?

    1. NSAIDs.

    2. Aspirin.

3. Methotrexate.

4. Hydrocortisone.

68. A client with RA is placed on prednisone 5 mg PO qd. In teaching the client about her medication, it would be important for the nurse practitioner to include what information?

1. When the symptoms of arthritis subside, she will be able to quit taking her medication.

2. It is important to take the medication as prescribed, even after the redness and swelling decrease.

3. Increased fluid intake is important to prevent renal damage by the steroids.

4. The medication should be taken about 30 minutes before eating.

69. What is the correct drug therapy for an adult with an acute episode of gout?

1. Indomethacin (Indocin) 25 mg PO prn.

2. Naproxen (Naprosyn) 100 mg PO bid.

3. Colchicine 0.6 mg qid.

4. Indomethacin (Indocin) 50 mg q8h × 6–8 doses, then 25 mg q8h until resolution.

70. If a 24-hour urine test indicates that a client is secreting too much uric acid (>900 mg/day), the nurse practitioner would prescribe:

1. Aspirin 325 mg PO qd.

2. Tylenol 325 mg PO q4–6h prn.

3. Indomethacin (Indocin) 25 mg PO q8h, then increase at weekly intervals by 25 mg daily.

4. Allopurinol (Zyloprim) 100 mg PO qd × 1 week, then increase daily dose by 100 mg to a maximum of 300 mg/day.

71. Disease-modifying drugs for rheumatoid arthritis in adults include:

1. Ibuprofen (Motrin, Advil), sulindac (Clinoril), and salicylates (aspirin, Disalcid).

2. Corticosteroids (prednisone, methylprednisolone).

3. Misoprostol (Cytotec).

4. Hydroxychloroquine (Plaquenil), sulfasalazine (Azulfidine), methotrexate, and gold sodium thiomalate (Myochrysine).

72. Gold compounds are contraindicated in clients with all the following conditions **except**:

1. Renal disease.

2. Hepatic disease.

3. Rheumatoid arthritis.

4. Blood dyscrasia.

73. The most appropriate medication used to control pain for a client with osteoarthritis would be:

1. Acetaminophen.

2. Systemic corticosteroids.

3. Gold salts.

4. Misoprostol.

74. What is a serious side effect of ibuprofen in the elderly client?

1. Rebound headaches.

2. Impairment of renal function.

3. Neuropathy.

4. Liver failure.

75. A client has been on methotrexate (Rheumatrex) for 6 weeks. This was the medication of choice for her severe refractory RA. What parameters should the nurse practitioner monitor?

1. Monthly platelet count, complete blood count (CBC), and differential.

2. Urinalysis, blood sugar, and electrocardiogram (ECG) every 2 weeks.

3. Monthly CBC, urinalysis, and electrolytes.

4. Coagulation studies, electrolytes, and CBC every week.

76. A middle-age male client presents with a complaint of waking up yesterday morning with his big toe swollen and painful. The client reports he has "never had anything like this before" and has not had previous health problems. On examination the big toe is red, hot, and tender in the joint with inflammation extending into the surrounding tissue. His temperature is 99.8°F and WBC count is mildly elevated. Needle aspiration of joint fluid reveals urate crystals. What is the best treatment choice that

the nurse practitioner could recommend for this client?

1. Bed rest, very-low-calorie diet, and increased fluid intake.

2. Allopurinol (Zyloprim) 200 mg PO qd, continuing dose for maintenance therapy once symptoms resolve.

3. Naproxen (Naprosyn) 500 mg PO tid, continuing full-dose until symptoms resolve, then tapering and discontinuing over 72 hours.

4. Injection of intraarticular corticosteroid to the affected joint.

77. An elderly woman comes into the clinic complaining of "sores" in her mouth. The nurse practitioner observes several inflamed ulcers on her gums and lips. Which medication would the nurse identify as most likely to cause this problem?

1. Propranolol (Inderal)

2. Spironolactone (Aldactone)

3. Fexofenadine (Allegra)

4. Alendronate (Fosamax).

Answers & Rationales

Physical Examination & Diagnostic Tests

1. **(2)** The goniometer is used to determine the degree of joint flexion and extension. It provides a means of measuring the degree of angle flexion and extension.

2. **(3)** Apley's sign, locking of the knee or the sound of clicks and pain, may indicate a loose body, such as torn cartilage. It is performed to detect a torn meniscus. The drawer sign tests the cruciate ligaments with the client in a sitting and lying position, not prone. In McMurray's test for medial meniscus injury the knee is fully flexed and the tibia externally rotated, with varus pressure applied to the knee while extended. For medial meniscus tear the test is performed while applying valgus pressure to the knee.

3. **(4)** Phalen's maneuver, when present, suggests carpal tunnel syndrome. Tinel's sign also tests for carpal tunnel syndrome but is performed by lightly percussing over the median nerve on the volar (palmar) side of the wrist, with characteristic tingling or shocklike sensations across the palm, thumb, and first two fingers. Drawer sign and McMurray's test are used to assess the knee.

4. **(3)** The balloon sign occurs when considerable fluid is in the suprapatellar pouch, with possible ballottement of the patella. The bulge sign is for testing fluid in the knee joint and is elicited with the knee extended by applying pressure to the medial aspect and watching for a bulge or fluid wave. A patellar tap suggests fluid in the knee as the patella clicks against the femur. The drawer sign tests the cruciate ligaments with the client in a sitting and lying

position. Kernig's sign for meningeal irritation is the inability to extend the lower leg when that leg is flexed at the hip, or there may be resistance or pain during elicitation of the sign.

5. **(1)** Pain with gentle deviation of a fist (thumb tucked under other four fingers) to the ulnar side is a positive Finkelstein's sign and an indication of De Quervain's disease, which is swelling and tenderness over the volar portion of the "snuffbox" resulting from chronic tenosynovitis. Treatment is usually a thumb splint, NSAIDs, and possible steroid injection into the area. A positive Tinel's sign (tapping gently over carpal tunnel causing tingling in thumb, index finger, and middle and radial half of ring finger) and positive Phalen's maneuver (holding dorsum of hands flexed 90 degrees back to back with the same distribution of tingling) are indicative of carpel tunnel syndrome. Lachman's sign indicates stability of the cruciate ligament of the knee.

6. **(3)** The musculoskeletal system is examined by a visual inspection and palpation of bones, joints, and surrounding musculoskeletal soft tissue. Percussion is generally not done, and auscultation is not appropriate to the system being examined.

7. **(3)** Clients with PMR have a rapid, dramatic clinical response to corticosteroid therapy. The serum protein electrophoresis is used to rule out myeloma. The ESR is elevated in a number of diseases and is not specific to PMR. The chest radiograph is used to diagnose diseases affecting the lungs and thorax.

8. **(3)** The wrist, MCP, and proximal interphalangeal (PIP) joints and other small joint of the hands and feet are involved with RA. The great toe is most often involved with gout. The large joints of the hip, knee, and shoulder along with the distal interphalangeal (DIP) joint and base of the thumb are involved with degenerative joint disease (osteoarthritis).

9. **(2)** It would not be necessary to obtain a CBC. The $HgbA_{1c}$ would be ordered to evaluate the relative control of diabetes. The EMG is most often performed to evaluate both nerve conduction and needle electrode examination. Many toxins and inflammatory processes are involved with polyneuropathy, so sedimentation rate would be a helpful diagnostic tool.

10. **(4)** A thorough history is very important in assessing any client with injury, but with a back injury the mechanism will provide the best indication as to extent of injury and proper diagnostic and treatment approach.

11. **(2)** Carpel tunnel syndrome, a compression neuropathy of the median nerve at the wrist, is commonly caused by repetitive finger and wrist motion and results in positive Tinel's sign and Phalen's maneuver. Tinel's sign is considered positive when tapping over the nerve with a reflex hammer causes tingling in the distribution of the nerve. Phalen's maneuver is performed by fully flexing the wrist passively and noting tingling in the thumb or fingers.

12. **(2)** The clinical assessments point to a chronic inflammatory process such as RA. The dizziness, fatigue, lightheadedness, and weakness may be a problem with anemia. The anemia of chronic disease is either a microcytic or normocytic anemia. The value that differentiates the anemia of chronic disease from other anemias is the serum ferritin (iron stores). The value will be either normal or high. The MCV of 104 indicates a macrocytic anemia, which would not include the anemia of chronic disease. The low serum ferritin would not be considered a possibility with this disorder. The uric acid level would be elevated in gout. The WBC count does not address the signs of anemia.

13. **(2)** Gentle inversion of the affected ankle in an ankle injury is compared with the unaffected ankle in the talar tilt test. Anterior ankle stability is tested in the anterior drawer test, in which the tibia is grasped by the examiner's one hand while the heel is firmly grasped and backward pressure is applied to the tibia with the examiner's other hand. In passive range of motion the examiner inverts, everts, dorsiflexes, and plantar-flexes the foot and ankle. The client puts the foot and ankle through the complete range in active range of motion.

14. **(2)** Varus pressure on a slightly flexed knee tests for lateral collateral ligament stability. Valgus pressure tests for medial collateral ligament stability. Cruciate ligaments are tested with the anterior drawer test. McMurray's test is for medial meniscus injury (see rationale for Answer 2).

15. **(1)** The child should remove her shirt (leave on bra or swimsuit top) and bend at the waist. The nurse practitioner should examine for uneven hips and shoulders.

16. **(3)** Typical findings include Ortolani's (hip click) sign, limited abduction, shortening of the extremity on the affected side, and asymmetric gluteal folds. The lax hamstrings allow for full extension of the hip when the knee is fully flexed.

Disorders

17. **(1)** Osgood-Schlatter disease (tibial tubercle apophysitis) is characterized by a painful, self-limiting tibial tubercle swelling that leads to knee pain, especially during periods of rapid growth. Extension of the knee against resistance or application of pressure over the tibial tubercle aggravates the pain. Pain worsens with activity and subsides with rest.

18. **(3)** Impingement syndrome is usually caused by rotator cuff tendinitis, which occurs when internal/external rotation is impaired. Frozen shoulder can occur after a rotator cuff injury, especially if a sling is used for a prolonged period. With Adson's or Wright's maneuver, thoracic outlet syndrome would indicate a decrease or loss of the radial pulse when the client abducts the arm and holds a deep breath, while simultaneously hyperextending the neck and turning the chin toward the raised arm.

19. **(3)** These are common symptoms of chondromalacia patella. With anterior cruciate tears the client generally cannot bear weight on the extremity without it buckling or giving way. With a dislocated patella the client would have severe pain associated with considerable effusion (loss of normal knee hollow on sides of patella) and possible patellofemoral compartment.

20. **(1)** With a complete rotator cuff tear (rupture of supraspinatus tendon) the client would have difficulty abducting the arm and impaired internal/external rotation. Touching the hand to the opposite shoulder is adduction.

21. **(3)** Growing pains usually occur at night and resolve by morning. The pain is deep and does not involve the joints. Osgood-Schlatter disease results from degeneration of the tibial tubercle due to overuse and a rapid growth spurt. Pain and swelling occur over the tibial tubercle. Symptoms are exacerbated by activities that involve the quadriceps muscle. Another form of overuse syndrome is patellofemoral stress syndrome. Pain of a dull, aching quality is present in the knee, sometimes with clicking. Long periods of sitting or activities that involve knee flexion as well as compression of the patella in the groove cause increased pain. In shin splints, inflammation of muscles along the medial shaft of the tibia results from overuse and causes aching pain. Rest improves the pain. Improper warm-up exercises or extended exercise by an unconditioned person, especially in unsuitable shoes, can lead to this pain.

22. **(4)** Anemia is common in PMR, along with an elevated ESR. There is a common complaint of morning stiffness; rheumatoid factor is negative. Option #1 is characteristic of SLE. Option #2 is characteristic of osteoarthritis. Option #3 is characteristic of ankylosing spondylitis.

23. **(3)** Diagnostic studies are of little value and benefit, except to rule out other causes, such as PMR or hypothyroidism. Treatment is symptomatic; the usual drugs are amitriptyline (Elavil), NSAIDs, cyclobenzaprine (Flexeril), temazepam (Restoril), and triazolam (Halcion). Daily, slow, low-impact aerobics, preferably in the late afternoon or early evening, is encouraged. Heat and massage are helpful, but not on the "trigger points."

24. **(3)** The chronic inflammatory disorder of RA has synovial hypertrophy from chronic synovitis and pannus formation that results in progressive destruction of the cartilage, ligament, tendons, and bone. AS usually involves the large peripheral joints (e.g., sacroiliac) and is characterized by extreme kyphosis. There is no inflammation with OA. SLE has a distribution of symptoms similar to that of RA, but no pannus formation.

25. **(3)** Moist heat or cold, whichever relieves the pain more effectively, is appropriate to use on acutely affected joints. Physical therapy is recommended after the acute involvement of the joint; care must be taken to decrease repetitive movements. Immobilization is avoided because it tends to increase the stiffness of the joint. The ESR is not an appropriate indicator of activity of osteoarthritis.

26. **(3)** Expanding rash with central clearing may also be described as the "bull's-eye rash" associated with Lyme disease. Option #1 describes the malar or "butterfly" rash of SLE. The arthritis symptoms and other complications (meningitis and myocarditis) occur later in the disease process, especially if the client is not treated with antibiotics, usually tetracycline, doxycycline, or amoxicillin.

27. **(4)** Deformities (bony protuberances) of the DIP are called Heberden's nodes and are cardinal signs of osteoarthritis. The DIP joints are seldom involved with RA. Gouty arthritis most often affects the great toe. Joints are warm, red, tender, and swollen with septic arthritis.

28. **(3)** The unaffected leg goes up the step first, then the crutches and affected leg follow. This allows for stability and weight bearing on the unaffected leg, with the crutches supporting the affected leg.

29. **(2)** Cellulitis usually presents with warm, erythematous, painful areas of the skin. Symptoms of erythema, edema, and pain of the first MTP joint are a common presentation for gout. Symptoms present in RA are similar: red, swollen, painful joint(s). The inflammation of RA is usually symmetric but can present as erythematous, swollen joints. Systemic symptoms may also be present. Osteoporosis most often occurs in postmenopausal women

due to bone loss that occurs with the decline of the estrogen in the blood. Bone thinning leads to fractures, not inflammation of joints or skin. Osteoarthritis presents as pain and stiffness with decreased range of motion, stiffness in the morning for a few minutes, and occasionally joint effusions. Point tenderness in 11 of 18 sites with digital palpation is present in fibromyalgia. Joint swelling and erythema are not present. In septic arthritis, joint pain, inflammation, and erythema would be accompanied by systemic symptoms of fever and chills. It would be considered in the differential for this client.

30. **(1)** Lyme arthritis, rheumatic heart disease, ankylosing spondylitis, psoriatic arthritis, RA, Reiter's syndrome, osteoarthritis, gonococcal arthritis, SLE, and PMR typically occur as polyarthritic disease. Gout, septic arthritis, and pseudogout most often occur as monoarthritis.

31. **(4)** A client who sustained a meniscal tear can usually recall a twisting injury of the knee followed by pain and effusion over the joint line. A strong force or injury that causes external rotation or hyperextension of the knee is a common mechanism of injury for collateral or cruciate ligament injuries. A test for stability of the knee joint involves applying medial and lateral pressure to the knee during full extension and flexion of 30 degrees.

32. **(4)** As the soft tissue swells, pain onset is usually about 12–36 hours after injury.

33. **(2)** Herniated intervertebral disk pain typically descends to the lower leg and foot. Lumbosacral strain causes pain in the back, buttock, and sometimes thigh. Osteomyelitis must be preceded by an event that permits an infectious agent to enter the bone. Osteoporosis occurs most often in postmenopausal women.

34. **(4)** At the time a patellar subluxation occurs, a traumatic event causes the knee to "give out," and the patella is usually laterally displaced. Severe pain and an effusion result. Subsequent to the injury, the client will notice a locking sensation in the knee with pivoting or turning. Patellofemoral stress syndrome is a form of overuse syndrome. Pain of a dull, aching quality is present in the knee, sometimes with clicking. Long periods of sitting or activities that involve knee flexion as well as compression of the patella in the groove cause increased pain. Growing pains usually occur at night and resolve by morning. The pain is deep and does not involve the joints. In shin splints, inflammation of muscles along the medial shaft of the tibia due to overuse causes aching pain. Rest improves the pain. Improper warm-up exercises or a sudden increase in exercise by an unconditioned person, especially while wearing worn or improper athletic shoes, can lead to this pain.

35. **(1)** In quadriceps setting, with the foot dorsiflexed, the thigh is pressed down against the floor and held for 5 seconds. The straight leg raise involves lifting an extended leg while sitting on the floor and leaning back on the elbows with the opposite leg flexed to 90 degrees. A terminal arc extension requires that the client lie on the floor supine with extended legs flexed to 20 degrees over a rolled towel. The client then extends one leg and holds for 5 seconds. The exercise is repeated with the opposite leg. All these exercises can be used to stretch and strengthen the quadriceps muscles in those with patellofemoral stress syndrome. Resistive exercises with an elastic band are general exercises that can be done with the extremities.

36. **(3)** Gout generally affects men over age 30 and is associated with obesity, lead intoxication, starvation, and use of some medications, including salicylates, diuretics, pyrazinamide, and alcohol.

37. **(4)** A third-degree sprain is a complete tear of the ligament resulting in marked edema, ecchymosis, pain, and an unstable joint.

38. **(3)** Morning stiffness or activity and the length of time required for maximal improvement are American Rheumatism Association Classification criteria for RA and useful, measurable tools for effects of treatment. The other questions are good indicators of quality of activities of daily living but do not give a full, overall, measurable picture of the client's joint discomfort.

39. **(1)** This client meets the classification criteria for fibromyalgia based on history of widespread pain and pain in 11 of 18 tender points. Myofascial syndrome symptoms are more focal, with no associated fatigue or sleep disorder. RA would have abnormal serologic studies. Depression may cause musculoskeletal pain and fatigue but would not have reproducible tender points.

40. **(2)** This is a subtherapeutic amount of calcium and vitamin D. The other choices are recommendations for prevention of osteoporosis.

41. **(4)** Most whiplash injuries are associated with a cervical neck strain due to a motor vehicle accident. These injuries take considerable time to heal, usually five times longer than a strain involving another part of the body.

42. **(2)** This client's symptoms are indicative of septic arthritis, which is a medical emergency; if not treated promptly, the joint may be severely damaged or destroyed. Examination of the joint fluid is the most important diagnostic test. The other choices may provide some symptomatic relief, but the first goal of treatment is to determine if the joint is septic.

43. **(3)** When developing a differential diagnosis, the history and physical exam will help narrow the differentiation. Other procedures are important in completing the evaluation, but the most important information is the pattern of joints affected and whether it is inflammatory or noninflammatory disease.

44. **(2)** Corticosteroids have limited value in treating AS, and long-term use is associated with many serious side effects. Important treatment includes regular exercise to strengthen supporting muscles and use of NSAIDs for pain. Approximately one third of clients have recurrent attacks of acute iritis.

45. **(3)** Osgood-Schlatter disease is common in late childhood and adolescence. The risk for disease increases in clients who are involved in strenuous activity, especially involving the quadriceps muscle. The usual treatment is NSAIDs and rest.

46. **(1)** Trauma, increased alcohol intake on weekends, and physical stress have all been implicated in acute gout. Gout occurs primarily in adult men. Decreased circulation, ecchymosis, and bone deformity are not likely with acute gout.

47. **(2)** The calcium intake is important in minimizing the development of osteoporosis. Both these foods contain calcium. The other distracters are not focused on the calcium intake.

48. **(4)** Signs and symptoms of osteoarthritis include asymmetric joint pain exacerbated by movement and relieved by rest. Stiffness is of short duration (<15 minutes) after inactivity, or in the morning. Pain may be described as aching and poorly localized. Options #1, #2, and #3 are indicative of RA.

49. **(3)** Low back pain is the number-one cause of disability and accounts for 25% of disabling work-related injuries.

50. **(2)** Most do not have disease persistent into adulthood. JRA symptoms present very similar to adult arthritis. Most disease activity diminishes with age; although some do have some residual joint damage, the percentage is not this high. Aspirin is the treatment of choice, and cytotoxic drugs are reserved for clients in whom other therapies have failed.

51. **(1)** The RICE principle is used for initial treatment: **R**est, **I**ce, **C**ompression, and **E**levation. All other treatments mentioned may be appropriate, but not as the primary treatment.

52. **(1)** Although all these symptoms may be associated with cauda equina syndrome, urinary retention is the most important clue to the immediate need for surgery.

53. **(2)** Annular tears are the first step toward herniation, and early recognition can help to avoid the need for surgical repair of a subsequent herniation.

54. **(4)** Fibromyalgia is a poorly understood condition that can prolong the normal treatment course of an injury considerably and is very difficult to treat. Osteoarthritis may follow an injury, as can reflex sympathetic dystrophy and tendinitis, but they do not have specified tender points.

55. **(2)** This example demonstrates five of the risk factors for osteoporosis, which include female gender, Caucasian or Asian, over age 45, low body weight, postmenopausal, sedentary lifestyle, low calcium intake, and smoker.

56. **(1)** The client's occupation and symptoms both suggest carpal tunnel syndrome. Initial treatment would involve night splinting, ice, and antiinflammatory medication.

57. **(3)** PMR is an inflammatory disorder of the proximal muscles presenting as described. Polyarteritis nodosa, an inflammatory disorder affecting the small arteries, presents with muscle weakness, myalgias, headache, and subcutaneous nodules along leg and arm arteries. Wegener's disease presents with mild anemia, dyspnea, cough, chest pain, hemoptysis, and abnormal urinalysis.

58. **(3)** Up to 40% of clients with temporal arteritis have a previous history of PMR. Presenting complaints include headache, low-grade fever, aching and stiffness of PMR, fatigue, malaise, and anorexia.

59. **(2)** Development of iridocyclitis may be insidious and asymptomatic and if untreated may cause blindness. Although children may develop any of the other listed diseases, there is no correlation with JRA.

60. **(3)** A positive McMurray's test (palpable click and pain when rotating the foot laterally and extending the leg) along with the symptoms is indicative of a medial meniscus tear. The drawer test evaluates for anterior cruciate ligament tears (knee flexed with foot on table; sit on foot and grasp both sides of tibia at knee; pull tibia forward; abnormal if movement of tibia away from the joint).

61. **(4)** Avascular necrosis results in death of the femoral head with revascularization. Toxic synovitis and increased femoral anteversion, while causing pain, are not bone threatening. Legg-Calvé-Perthes disease results in necrosis of the proximal femoral epiphysis; however, there is later revascularization.

62. **(3)** In Adam's position (forward bending, arms loose at side, thumbs hooked together), true scoliosis (structural) is demonstrated (by an elevated rib hump), whereas the functional type related to other conditions is not apparent. Persistent functional scoliosis can eventually become structural.

63. **(3)** The client is presenting with the classic symptoms of nerve root compression secondary to pressure from a protruding lumbar disk. The sciatic stretch test (straight leg raise) maneuver will increase the radiation of pain down the hip.

64. **(3)** Pectus excavatum can affect cardiopulmonary function, but when associated with scoliosis, the child should be evaluated for Marfan's syndrome.

65. **(2)** This client is likely experiencing an acute exacerbation of his osteoarthritis, since his is constantly rubbing his knees. Because 85% of the residents of long-term care facilities have uncontrolled pain, he probably has uncontrolled pain. Starting him on routine acetaminophen (Tylenol) would be an excellent start to pain management in this client. It is unlikely that the client's dementia is worsening because this is an acute problem. Although UTI is a good choice, the cues of rubbing the major joints would likely rule out a UTI as the problem. The client is not exhibiting any neurologic symptoms, which would rule out an acute infarct.

Pharmacology

66. **(2)** Clients on chronic steroid therapy should be evaluated for adrenal insufficiency during an acute illness, which increases stress. Signs and symptoms indicate subtle clinical manifestations of adrenal insufficiency. Recommended treatment is to treat empirically with stress-dose corticosteroid during acute illness. Stopping the medication or maintaining the same dose may precipitate acute adrenal insufficiency.

67. **(2)** Aspirin is the first choice. NSAIDs can be used, but the antiinflammatory and antipyretic effects of aspirin, plus low cost, make it the drug of choice. Methotrexate is used for severe cases that do not respond to aspirin or NSAIDs. Steroids may be given but are not the drug of choice.

68. **(2)** The client needs to understand the importance of maintaining her dose of the steroids. When symptoms decrease, the medication is effective. It is not influenced by fluids and should be taken with food.

69. **(3)** This is the only effective dose listed for the treatment of an acute episode of gout. The other doses are incorrect and insufficient as dosed.

70. **(4)** Allopurinol works to keep the serum uric acid level lower. The goal of therapy is a serum uric acid level of <6.5 mg/dl. The other

medications listed do not help to lower serum uric acid levels, and aspirin can precipitate a gout attack.

71. **(4)** These drugs modify the disease when NSAIDs (ibuprofen, sulindac, salicylates) have not worked. Corticosteroids can be used until the disease-modifying agents begin to work. Misoprostol is used to prevent ulcer development related to long-term medication use.

72. **(3)** Gold is indicated for treatment of RA and is contraindicated in the presence of the other listed diseases.

73. **(1)** Acetaminophen or a NSAID is generally used for pain relief for clients with osteoarthritis. Systemic corticosteroids are not indicated in osteoarthritis. Gold salts may be one of several pharmacologic approaches to the treatment of RA. Misoprostol is used to minimize the development of NSAID-induced gastric ulcers.

74. **(2)** Renal function may already be reduced in elderly persons, and ibuprofen can further impair renal function, which in turn can result in nephrosis, cirrhosis, and congestive heart failure.

75. **(1)** This client should be monitored for blood dyscrasias on a monthly basis. Women of childbearing age should avoid pregnancy.

76. **(3)** NSAIDs (naproxen) are recommended treatment for an acute gout attack in clients able to tolerate NSAID therapy. Allopurinol is contraindicated in an acute attack and can even precipitate an attack in the early stages of treatment. Low-calorie diets increase risks of gouty attacks. Joint injection would not be first-line treatment choice, but for refractory cases in clients unable to take oral medication, it may be an option.

77. **(4)** Gastritis and oral ulcers are common complications of Fosamax. Alendronate is used to increase calcium absorption in patients with osteoporosis. If these effects occur, the medication should be discontinued. The medications in the other options do not cause this problem.

Neurology

Physical Examination & Diagnostic Tests

1. To evaluate the neurologic system for appropriate sensory system functioning in the geriatric client, it is appropriate to determine the presence of stereognosis. This is done by having the client: *ability to distinguish familiar objects*

   1. Rapidly touch the index finger and then the nose.

   2. Distinguish between a coin and a key by touch.

   3. Stand with heels together and eyes closed.

   4. Close eyes and identify familiar odors.

2. To determine cerebellar functioning in the geriatric client, the nurse practitioner evaluates:

   1. Ability to balance on one foot, then the other.

   2. Ability to discriminate between two familiar objects by sensation.

   3. Ability to recall names of three U.S. presidents.

   4. Range of motion and ability to move extremities.

3. What is considered a "soft" (or equivocal) neurologic sign?

   1. Positive Babinski's reflex in an adult.

   2. Mirroring hand movements of the extremities.

   3. Brudzinski's sign.

   4. Kernig's sign.

4. A client is having problems controlling her seizures and is referred to have an electroencephalogram (EEG). The nurse practitioner explains to the client that:

   1. This test will cause some discomfort and she will be given a sedative before the test.

   2. It will be important for her to take her regular dose of paroxetine (Paxil) and phenytoin (Dilantin) before the test.

   3. The procedure is painless and she will not experience discomfort or electrical shock.

   4. After the test she will be on bed rest for 8 hours and will be given full liquids for 12 hours.

5. Which cranial nerve is being tested when the nurse practitioner asks the client to raise the eyebrows, smile, frown, or puff out the cheeks?

   1. Hypoglossal nerve.

   2. Acoustic nerve

   3. Glossopharyngeal nerve.

   4. Facial nerve.

6. The nurse practitioner notes an absent patellar reflex in a healthy client. What might the practitioner ask the client to do?

   1. Lift both arms above the head and count to 5 slowly as the reflex is tested.

   2. Raise both legs slowly and then lower and immediately test for the reflex.

   3. Clench both hands together and pull while the reflex is tested.

   4. Close eyes and hold breath while examiner tests for the reflex.

7. With the client in the supine position, the nurse practitioner gently flexes the client's neck in the direction of the chin touching the chest. If there is pain and resistance to the flexion, and if the hips and knees flex at the same time, the nurse accurately describes this finding as:

   1. Phalen's sign.

   2. Romberg's sign.

   3. Kernig's sign.

   4. Brudzinski's sign.

8. The nurse practitioner understands that dysdiadochokinesia refers to:

   1. Trouble with speech.

   2. Memory impairment.

   3. Trouble with attempts at rapidly alternating movements.

   4. Neurologic triad of symptoms with gait, memory, and speech.

Disorders

9. The nurse practitioner understands that the most common form of facial paralysis in the adult client is:

   1. Facial nerve fasciitis.

   2. Trigeminal neuralgia.

   3. Bell's palsy.

   4. Herpes zoster.

10. A client has a history of injury at the fifth thoracic vertebra (T5), and his condition has stabilized. The nurse practitioner understands that, with this level of injury, the client most likely will not be able to:

    1. Perform coordinated movements with his hands, such as writing.

    2. Achieve lower body strength and coordination for walking.

    3. Have adequate upper body strength to drive a car.

    4. Maintain the upper body coordination required for eating.

11. An older client, who as a young child recovered quickly after extensive initial impairment due to poliomyelitis, is diagnosed with post-polio syndrome. The most common symptom is:

    1. Gastrointestinal upset, headache, and malaise.

    2. New onset of weakness, fatigue, and pain.

    3. Sudden onset of lower limb paralysis after an acute infection.

    4. Headache, fever, and elevated blood pressure and pulse.

12. The nurse practitioner is discussing safety measures for the home environment of a client with Parkinson's disease. It would be important for the nurse practitioner to include what information for this client?

    1. Sleep on a firm mattress that is high off the floor to facilitate getting into and out of bed.

    2. Pour hot liquids with the cup or container placed on the table to avoid spilling.

3. Place a sheepskin pad on the bed to decrease the development of decubiti.

4. Perform passive and active range of motion twice daily to prevent contracture.

13. A client is admitted to a rural clinic after a diving accident. The nurse practitioner suspects a spinal cord injury at the fifth cervical vertebra (C5). While awaiting emergency transport services, the practitioner assesses for the development of complications by:

1. Checking for voluntary movement of extremities and sensation below the level of injury.

2. Assessing breath sounds and evaluating movement of diaphragm with respiration.

3. Maintaining cervical flexion to facilitate airway until cervical traction is initiated.

4. Beginning neurologic checks with careful documentation of location of pain sensations.

14. Many clients who suffer from recurrent headaches have similar symptoms with each episode. Which is a sign that a headache may be from a more serious cause?

1. It occurs on the right side.

2. Rhinorrhea occurs with the headache.

3. It becomes more and more painful.

4. It increases when the client bends over.

15. Epidemic meningococcal meningitis occurs rarely. This control is a result of:

1. Use of active immunization.

2. Lower community carrier rates.

3. Improved socioeconomic conditions.

4. Earlier detection and recognition of outbreaks.

16. The nurse practitioner understands that benign paroxysmal positional vertigo:

1. Is described as vertigo and nystagmus with positional change and occurs most often in elderly persons.

2. Is more common in young persons and occurs suddenly and in episodes that include vertigo, tinnitus, hearing loss, feeling of fullness in the ears, and nausea and vomiting.

3. Follows a viral syndrome (upper respiratory or gastrointestinal), with exacerbation of the

vertigo with position change without hearing loss or tinnitus.

4. Involves gradual hearing loss and tinnitus along with vertigo, eventually with facial numbness and weakness.

17. All the following conditions are included in the differential diagnosis of a client with facial paralysis **except**:

1. Herpes zoster.

2. Bell's palsy.

3. Trigeminal neuralgia. *pain not paralysis*

4. Otitis media.

18. What would be appropriate to include in the health promotion plan for a client with a diagnosis of multiple sclerosis?

1. Avoid aerobic exercise, due to muscle weakness.

2. Keep warm (especially extremities) to improve neurologic function.

3. Avoid antioxidants (vitamins C/E, beta-carotene); they contribute to loss of myelin sheath.

4. Consume a low-fat, high-fiber diet, with daily cranberry juice and calcium supplement.

19. A client who has had a cerebrovascular accident (CVA) is incontinent of urine. The family should be taught to:

1. Restrict fluid intake.

2. Insert a Foley catheter.

3. Establish a scheduled voiding pattern.

4. Reposition the client often to reduce the discomfort of urgency.

20. What is the best approach to test the hearing of a client with Bell's palsy?

1. Stand out of sight of the client and ask the client to move or do something.

2. Use a tuning fork to test for lateralization of sound.

3. Stand in front of the client and whisper, "Raise your hand."

4. Snap your fingers next to the client's ear and ask if the sound was heard.

21. Physical findings in a 50-year-old female client who wears a left lower leg brace are weight 100 lb, height 65 inches, and vital signs within normal limits. She has developed post-polio symptoms. The nurse practitioner suggests that the client:

    1. Gain weight to prevent further disability.

    2. Exercise all muscle groups vigorously to prevent disuse syndrome.

    3. Avoid exposure to cold or chilling, which may cause a loss of strength in the affected muscle.

    4. Reduce the amount of time using the brace for joint support to prevent further loss of strength.

22. In infants, especially preterm infants, seizures can present as:

    1. Coughing spells.

    2. Poor feeding.

    3. Awake apnea.

    4. Regurgitation.

23. Inflammation and swelling of the seventh cranial nerve with resultant unilateral facial muscle paralysis is called:

    1. Bell's palsy.

    2. Transient ischemic attack.

    3. Facial droop.

    4. Trigeminal neuralgia.

24. The nurse practitioner understands that the following is a trigger that helps to differentiate a migraine from a tension headache:

    1. Alcohol.

    2. Bright lighting and noxious stimuli.

    3. Stressful situations.

    4. Sleep pattern disturbances.

25. All the following statements are true of migraine headache **except**:

    1. Migraine is likely related to sensitization of trigeminal nerve fibers within the meninges.

    2. Migraine and related headaches are disorders of the inflammatory response.

    3. Genetic and environmental factors are influential in migraine.

4. During migraine, serotonin levels decrease in the central nervous system.

26. Which symptom(s) can occur in a client who has experienced a transient ischemic attack (TIA) in the anterior cerebral circulation?

    1. Bilateral vision disturbance and diplopia.

    2. Dysarthria (speech disturbance).

    3. Disorders of behavior and cognition.

    4. Motor and sensory problems on both sides of body at once.

27. Many visits to emergency departments by adults are prompted by headaches. Which symptom may help the nurse practitioner differentiate a migraine headache from a headache that may indicate severe problems?

    1. It is preceded by an "aura."

    2. It occurs mainly behind one eye and tends to be grouped.

    3. Onset is sudden and accompanied by nuchal rigidity.

    4. It occurs mainly on awakening.

28. An adult client presents with a complaint of facial paralysis that started suddenly. In making a diagnosis, the nurse practitioner considers which of the following symptoms of Bell's palsy?

    1. Concurrent paralysis of the opposite arm and leg.

    2. Pain in the (ipsilateral) ear that accompanied or preceded the paralysis.

    3. Loss of bowel control.

    4. Loss of hearing on the opposite side.

29. An elderly lady is present when her husband is admitted for a myocardial infarction. She complains to the nurse practitioner that she is having numbness and tingling in her hands and face. Here heart rate is 98 and respiratory rate 32. What is the best action for the nurse practitioner to take?

    1. Administer oxygen per nasal cannula at 3 L/min.

    2. Schedule magnetic resonance imaging (MRI) appointment.

    3. Have her breathe into a paper bag.

    4. Administer amitriptyline (Elavil) 25 mg PO.

30. The nurse practitioner is evaluating an elderly client's tremor. Which assessment finding would be characteristic of an essential tremor rather than parkinsonian tremor?

   1. The handwriting is not affected.

   2. The tremor occurs with purposeful movements.

   3. The tremor occurs at rest.

   4. The tremor worsens with beta-blockers or alcohol.

31. Which assessment may be evaluated in a client with Parkinson's disease?

   1. Macrographia.

   2. Micrographia.

   3. Exaggeration of rapid successive movements.

   4. Increased swinging of arms while walking.

32. A 3-week-old infant has been diagnosed with bacterial meningitis. The nurse practitioner is aware that the most common causative organism is:

   1. *Streptococcus pyogenes.*

   2. *Escherichia coli.*

   3. *Neisseria meningitidis.*

   4. Group B *Streptococcus.*

33. A client recently diagnosed with multiple sclerosis asks the nurse practitioner about the disease process. The nurse practitioner knows that:

   1. 90% of clients have a quickly progressive form of the disease.

   2. 90% of clients, after the first onset of symptoms, have relapses and remissions.

   3. 10% of clients will respond to corticosteroids.

   4. 10% of clients have problems with optic neuritis and sensory loss.

34. The nurse practitioner is caring for a 10-year-old child with meningitis. To assess for the presence of nuchal rigidity, the nurse practitioner would:

   1. Have the child bend forward at the waist, and observe the line of the spine.

   2. Place hand on child's forehead and ask child to press nurse's hand with his head.

   3. With the child relaxed, attempt to move his head side to side.

   4. Place hand on back of child's head and assist him to put his chin on his chest.

35. An adolescent girl is accompanied to the clinic by her mother, who states the school reports that she "stares off into space a lot" and does not seem to pay attention during these brief periods, which typically last 1–3 minutes. The neurologic examination is within normal limits. What should the nurse practitioner suspect in this client?

   1. Grand mal seizure.

   2. Complex partial seizure.

   3. Absence seizure.

   4. Simple partial seizure.

36. A child is admitted to the rural clinic after a car accident in which she sustained a closed head injury and fractured femur. The child is lethargic and follows commands slowly, and her pupils are equal and reactive. The child is to be transferred to a hospital by air ambulance. In assessing the child, what would the nurse practitioner consider as a significant change in her condition?

   1. Urine output is less than 500 ml in 24 hours.

   2. She complains of a headache in the frontal area.

   3. She is able to move her lower extremities to command.

   4. Vital signs are blood pressure (BP) 130/50 and pulse 70.

37. A parent whose son was recently diagnosed with Tourette's syndrome asks the nurse practitioner about the condition. The nurse practitioner understands that:

   1. Tourette's syndrome is usually treated with antianxiety agents, such as diazepam (Valium).

   2. The tics may occur often throughout the day and may change over time.

   3. Children rarely have attention deficit hyperactivity disorder (ADHD) in conjunction with Tourette's syndrome.

   4. Tics are typically neuromuscular (e.g., facial grimacing, tongue protruding, neck twitching) and rarely vocal.

38. A 30-year-old female client has had several episodes of incontinence, weakness, visual loss, and some ataxia. Physical examination reveals slight swelling of the optic disc on funduscopy, difficulty with heel-to-toe walking, lower extremity weakness, and 2+ deep tendon reflexes. Which condition does the nurse practitioner suspect?

    1. Multiple sclerosis.

    2. Parkinson's disease.

    3. Amyotrophic lateral sclerosis.

    4. Post-polio syndrome.

39. The nurse practitioner is seeing a 3-year-old child with a history of hospitalization at 18 months for bacterial meningitis and treatment with ampicillin and gentamicin. Which test should the nurse practitioner make sure to include in the examination?

    1. Vision testing.

    2. Hearing testing.

    3. Lumbar puncture.

    4. Electrocardiogram (ECG).

40. Which is considered a likely cause of seizures in adolescents and young adults?

    1. Congenital abnormalities and metabolic disturbances.

    2. Metabolic disorders, central nervous system (CNS) infection, and fever.

    3. Idiopathic disease, trauma, and substance abuse.

    4. Trauma, malignant tumor, and cerebrovascular accident.

41. A client has a 3-year history of recurrent headaches once or twice a month lasting 12–18 hours. When the client presents at the clinic, she has taken 6 gm of acetaminophen in the past 12 hours with no relief. The nurse practitioner would:

    1. Refer the client to a neurologist for headache workup.

    2. Consider an analgesic rebound relative to the dose of acetaminophen taken.

    3. Order naproxen (Anaprox) for prophylactic treatment of the headaches.

    4. Order an EEG and MRI to rule out pathology.

42. A child presents with a history of a purpuric rash with a centrifugal distribution and a fever. After the nurse practitioner examines this child, what would be the most important condition to rule out at this time?

    1. Rubella.

    2. Lyme disease.

    3. Meningococcemia.

    4. Roseola.

43. A client presents to the emergency department with the "worst headache of my life." The client reports that the headaches have not responded to the usual over-the-counter headache remedies. What is most important for the nurse practitioner to rule out?

    1. Brain tumor.

    2. Migraine.

    3. Onset of newly diagnosed seizure disorder.

    4. Subarachnoid hemorrhage.

44. A client with a recent history of a left hemisphere stroke returns to the clinic for a checkup. What symptoms would the nurse practitioner anticipate the client to exhibit?

    1. Left-sided weakness.

    2. Bilateral weakness of lower extremities.

    3. Difficulty with speech.

    4. Left visual field deficit.

45. The nurse practitioner is evaluating a group of geriatric clients for risk factors of an embolic stroke. Which condition would be **least** likely to precipitate this type of stroke?

    1. Mitral valve disease.

    2. Atrial fibrillation.

    3. Endocarditis.

    4. Diabetes mellitus.

46. A client returns to the clinic for a follow-up visit. She has a history of simple partial seizures. When questioning the client, the nurse practitioner would identify recurrence of this seizure activity if the client reported:

    1. Short episodes when she loses consciousness but does not fall.

2. No loss of consciousness but jerking and tingling of her right leg, then right hand.

3. Auditory hallucinations, unconsciousness, and urinary incontinence.

4. Short period of unconsciousness, followed by period of confusion.

47. An elderly woman comes to the clinic complaining of having difficulty when she tries to do her needlework. She walks straight, although somewhat slowly, and no rigidity is noted on movement. She states the shaking in her hands stops when she holds her hands in her lap. What tentative diagnosis would the nurse practitioner make?

1. Parkinson's disease.

2. Transient ischemic attack.

3. Benign essential tremor.

4. Simple partial seizure activity.

48. A mother brings her 5-year-old son to the clinic with complaints that he is "acting funny." She states there are brief periods when he does not respond to her, then he suddenly responds and acts as if nothing has happened. The nurse would initially evaluate the child further for the presence of:

1. Petit mal or absence seizures.

2. Attention deficit disorder.

3. Horner's syndrome.

4. Avoidance disorder of childhood.

49. A client with a history of myasthenia gravis presents with ptosis, facial weakness, dysphagia, and generalized weakness. What is important for the nurse practitioner to ask and establish initially?

1. When did the symptoms first begin, and have they increased in severity?

2. What medications is the client taking, and when did he last take them?

3. What activity was the client participating in when the symptoms began?

4. Has the client experienced any seizure activity with the increase in symptoms?

50. A client presents with miosis and ptosis with anhidrosis of the ipsilateral face and neck. The initial diagnosis would be:

1. Horner's syndrome.

2. Damage to cranial nerves III and IV.

3. Meniere's syndrome.

4. Mycotic aneurysm.

51. The nurse practitioner is reviewing the records of a client who is recovering from a stroke (CVA). The records indicate the client is experiencing homonymous hemianopia. This is interpreted as:

1. Partial loss of visual acuity in the peripheral area of the visual field.

2. Diplopia in the eye contralateral to the cerebral lesion.

3. Nystagmus in both eyes, but movements are dissimilar.

4. Loss of vision in both eyes in either the right or the left half of the visual field.

Pharmacology

52. An elderly patient is diagnosed with postherpetic neuralgia. All the following drugs are used initially to treat the associated pain **except**:

1. Anticonvulsants.

2. Tricyclic antidepressants.

3. NSAIDs.

4. Opioids.

53. A client is taking an antiepileptic medication. The nurse practitioner understands that antiepileptic medication:

1. Must be taken indefinitely.

2. Is usually discontinued after 4 years of no seizure activity, and EEG confirms lack of seizure activity.

3. Is usually given in combination with other antiepileptics or sedatives to reduce the seizure threshold.

4. Must be given to all clients who experience a seizure.

54. Pharmacologic management of clients with peripheral vestibulopathy includes:

    1. Meclizine (Antivert) 100 mg PO qid.

    2. Dimenhydrinate (Dramamine) 5 mg PO tid to qid.

    3. Scopolamine transdermal patch, 1 disc applied behind ear and left in place for 3 days.

    4. Prochlorperazine (Compazine) 25–50 mg PO q4h prn.

55. What medication and dose can be used for abortive therapy in an adult client with symptoms of migraine headache?

    1. Sumatriptan (Imitrex) 6 mg IM.

    2. Ergotamine (Ergostat) 2 mg SL.

    3. Ketorolac (Toradol) 100 mg IM.

    4. Amitriptyline (Elavil) 100 mg PO.

56. During physical examination of a child diagnosed with chronic recurrent seizures who is currently receiving antiepileptic medication, the nurse practitioner notes hyperplasia of the gums. The nurse understand that hyperplasia of the gums is:

    1. An unusual side effect of phenobarbital.

    2. A common side effect of phenytoin.

    3. Common with chronic recurrent seizures.

    4. Caused by poor oral hygiene.

57. The family of a Parkinson's client brings him to the clinic because he is experiencing increasing difficulty with ambulation. The nurse practitioner increases the client's carbidopa (25 mg)/levodopa (100 mg) (Sinemet 25-100) from three to four times daily. What is important for the nurse practitioner to teach the family regarding the increase in the dose of this medication?

    1. Sleep disorders and hallucinations are common side effects of carbidopa/levodopa, and the last dose should not be given near bedtime.

    2. Carbidopa/levodopa has shown efficacy in slowing disease progression.

    3. Orthostatic hypotension can be problematic at higher dosing ranges.

    4. The medication should be given on an empty stomach due to its altered absorption with meals, especially in conjunction with protein foods.

58. What information is important for the nurse practitioner to teach the client regarding the use of medications to treat trigeminal neuralgia?

    1. Medications may cause seizure-like activity.

    2. Therapeutic levels of the drug may take up to a month to be reached.

    3. Relief of the symptoms should occur within 24 hours of starting the medication.

    4. It is not necessary to monitor laboratory levels.

11   Answers & Rationales

Physical Examination & Diagnostic Tests

1. **(2)** Stereognosis is the ability to determine familiar objects by shape rather than visual identification. Option #1 determines fine motor and coordination, Option #3 determines proprioception (balance, posture), and Option #4 determines the functioning of the first cranial (olfactory) nerve.

2. **(1)** The cerebellar area controls gross motor movements and balance, as well as fine motor movements of the upper and lower extremities. Discriminatory sensation tests the sensory system, and a remote memory test is a mental status examination involving the cerebral cortex.

3. **(2)** Soft neurologic signs involve slight deviations of the central nervous system (CNS) that are present occasionally or inconsistently. Examples are short attention span, clumsiness, frequent falling (disturbances of gait), hyperkinesis, left-handed but right-footed, language disturbances, anisocoria, and mirroring movements of the extremities (when one hand performs a movement, the other is also in motion). The other three options indicate a CNS problem that occurs consistently; Brudzinski's and Kernig's signs indicate meningeal irritation, and positive Babinski's reflex in an adult may indicate an upper motor lesion in the corticospinal tract.

4. **(3)** The procedure is painless with no danger of electrical shock. All anticonvulsants, antidepressants, stimulants (caffeine, tobacco), and alcohol should be stopped. There is no restriction on movement or diet after the procedure.

5. **(4)** The facial nerve is tested by facial movement, taste, sensation, and corneal reflex. The hypoglossal nerve is tested by the client sticking out the tongue. The acoustic nerve is tested by a hearing test. The glossopharyngeal nerve is tested by taste, gag reflex, and having the client drink and swallow.

6. **(3)** Augmentation of the patellar reflex can be obtained by having the client isometrically tense muscles not directly involved with the reflex arc being tested, called Jendrassik's maneuver.

7. **(4)** This describes Brudzinski's sign. Phalen's sign (maneuver) is elicited in carpal tunnel syndrome. Romberg's test is done to assess gross swaying by asking the client to stand with feet together and eyes closed for 5 seconds. Kernig's sign (inability to extend lower leg when leg is flexed at hip or when there is resistance or pain) along with Brudzinski's sign indicate meningeal irritation and should be evaluated further.

8. **(3)** Dysdiadochokinesia is difficulty with attempts at rapidly alternating movements (e.g., finger to nose).

Disorders

9. **(3)** The most common form of facial paralysis is Bell's palsy, a disorder affecting the facial nerve characterized by muscle flaccidity of the affected side of the face. Trigeminal neuralgia

is a disorder of cranial nerve V characterized by an abrupt onset of pain in the lower and upper jaw, cheek, and lips. Herpes zoster affects the dermatomes and does not cause a paralysis, but rather pain and possible postherpetic neuralgia.

10. **(2)** T5 injuries do not affect the coordination or capacity of the upper body, arms, and hands; the lower body is paralyzed. The client should be able to do all the activities listed except walk.

11. **(2)** The cardinal signs of post-polio syndrome include onset of new weakness, fatigue, and pain along with hot or cold intolerance, and swallowing, speech, breathing, and sleep disturbances.

12. **(2)** Pouring liquids is frequently a complicated task for this client due to his tremors. If the cup or container to be filled is placed on the table, there is less chance of spilling the contents.

13. **(2)** At this level of injury (C5) the intercostal muscles and diaphragm can be affected, and the client may have respiratory compromise. Airway maintenance and avoiding flexion of the neck are critical.

14. **(3)** If a headache becomes more and more severe, if there is new onset of severe headache in a client over 35 years old, if the headache's character or progression is different from other headaches, or if there is vomiting but no nausea, there could be a new and serious cause for the headache. The side on which the headache occurs and accompanying rhinorrhea may or may not be significant. Increasing pain when bending over is characteristic of sinus pressure or infection.

15. **(3)** Improved sanitary and socioeconomic conditions have led to the marked reduction in the number of cases of epidemic meningitis. There is no research to support increased cases in communities with higher carrier numbers.

16. **(1)** Benign paroxysmal positional vertigo usually occurs in older clients. Younger persons who experience a sudden episode of vertigo, tinnitus, hearing loss, sensation of fullness, and nausea and vomiting typically have Meniere's disease. Peripheral vestibulopathy usually follows upper respiratory or gastrointestinal viral illness and involves nearly incapacitating vertigo that increases with positional changes, but not hearing loss or tinnitus. The nurse

practitioner should suspect acoustic neuroma if gradual hearing loss, tinnitus, and vertigo occur before the development of facial numbness and weakness.

17. **(3)** The differential diagnosis for facial paralysis includes bacterial ear infections, Lyme disease, herpes zoster, mumps, temporal bone fracture, acoustic neuroma, other tumors, and demyelinating diseases. Trigeminal neuralgia is associated with intense facial pain, not paralysis.

18. **(4)** In addition to the factors listed, keeping cool, not warm, is associated with improvement of neurologic function. A regular exercise program is encouraged, along with daily intake of a multivitamin, antioxidants, and low-dose aspirin (81 mg). Maintaining ideal body weight, having rest periods or naps daily, and becoming informed about the disease process are important aspects of promoting health.

19. **(3)** Reestablishing regularity will assist in maintaining bladder control. A catheter exposes the client to infection. Fluids should not be restricted.

20. **(1)** Bell's palsy involves a sensorineural hearing loss. In contrast to being able to read lips, this client must be able to hear the direction of sound without any visual prompting. The tuning fork assists in differentiating between air and bone conduction of sound.

21. **(3)** In addition to regular health maintenance visits, the client should be advised to avoid gaining weight and exercising to the point of muscle pain. Cold temperatures can cause a loss of muscle strength in the affected muscle groups and should be avoided. Assistive or orthotic devices (canes, walkers, braces) should be used, along with periodic evaluation of muscle strength and function.

22. **(3)** Although it is important to investigate all episodes of apnea in infants, premature infants may not exhibit the typical tonic-clonic type seizures but may have awake apnea.

23. **(1)** The symptoms describe Bell's palsy, which is thought to be caused by a virus. This sudden onset of unilateral facial paralysis usually resolves within 2 weeks but can endure for months. A few clients may have residual problems. Transient ischemic attacks last less

than 24 hours. Facial droop occurs with Bell's palsy due to paralysis of the muscles innervated by the facial (seventh cranial) nerve. Trigeminal neuralgia is sudden pain along the fifth cranial nerve.

24. **(4)** Sleep pattern disturbances, either too little or too much, may trigger a migraine headache. Lighting and noxious stimuli, along with alcohol use and stress, may trigger both types.

25. **(2)** Headache disorders, including migraine, are disorders of neurovascular regulation. All other responses are part of the current theory of migraine.

26. **(3)** A wide variety of changes can occur in behavior and cognition after TIA. Bilateral vision disturbance, diplopia, dysarthria (speech disturbance), and motor/sensory problems on both sides of the body are problems associated with TIA in the posterior cerebral circulation.

27. **(3)** Classic migraine headaches are accompanied by auras. Cluster headaches occur behind one eye and are grouped. Headaches associated with hypertension occur mainly on awakening. A sudden onset and nuchal rigidity may indicate a subarachnoid hemorrhage.

28. **(2)** Bell's palsy is typically preceded or accompanied by pain in the ear on the paralyzed side. The paralysis is confined to the face, and there is no bowel involvement.

29. **(3)** Clients who are under stress have periods of hyperventilation in which they "blow off" more carbon dioxide (CO_2) than necessary. They experience numbness and tingling in their hands and faces and may experience syncope. Breathing into a paper bag increases CO_2 level and relieves the symptoms of respiratory alkalosis.

30. **(2)** The differentiating feature between the two tremors is that the essential tremor occurs with purposeful movements. Handwriting may be affected with both tremors. The tremor with Parkinson's disease occurs at rest. Essential tremors improve with beta-blockers as well as alcohol.

31. **(2)** Micrographia is a classic manifestation of Parkinson's disease. The client has impairment of rapid successive movements and loss of automatic movements, such as swinging the arms while walking.

32. **(4)** The most common cause of bacterial meningitis in the first month of life is the group B streptococci. *Streptococcus pneumoniae* and *Neisseria meningitides* are usually associated with meningitis after age 1 month in areas where the conjugate Hib vaccines are used.

33. **(2)** Multiple sclerosis (MS) is characterized by exacerbations and remissions of the symptoms. Only 10% of MS clients have a progressive form of the disease from the onset. Many clients (35%–40%) have problems of optic neuritis, sensory loss, and weakness and do respond to corticosteroids.

34. **(4)** Nuchal rigidity is a stiff neck; the child cannot move his head forward and cannot bring his chin in contact with his chest. Movement of the head from side to side does not elicit nuchal rigidity.

35. **(3)** This accurately fits the description of a petit mal or absence seizure, which is a type of generalized seizure that begins in childhood and usually ends in early adulthood (30s). There is usually impairment of consciousness, automatic symptoms, and mild tonic-clonic symptoms. Classically, "staring off into space" is the reporting symptom.

36. **(4)** Increase in the pulse pressure and decrease in pulse rate are indications of increasing cerebral edema and intracranial pressure and would necessitate immediate intervention. A child's urine output should be 20–30 ml/hr.

37. **(2)** Tourette's syndrome is a hereditary, chronic neuromuscular disorder consisting of various motor and vocal tics. Tics are sudden, involuntary, brief, repetitive, motor movements that often begin in childhood and change over time. ADHD frequently occurs concomitantly with Tourette's syndrome.

38. **(1)** Involvement of more than one CNS area, age 15–60 years, two or more separate episodes of symptoms involving different sites, or gradual progression over at least 6 months meets the criteria for multiple sclerosis.

39. **(2)** A formal hearing acuity test is most important in a child with a history of bacterial meningitis because of the ototoxic medications used to treat the disease. A vision test should be done on all children but is not specific for a child with a history of meningitis. A lumbar puncture or ECG would not be appropriate.

40. **(3)** The most likely causes of seizures in adolescents and young adults are idiopathic disease, trauma, and substance abuse. Congenital abnormalities are the likely cause of seizures in newborns. In children under 6 years old, metabolic causes, CNS infection, and fever can cause seizures. Trauma, malignant tumor, and CVA are likely causes for seizures in elderly clients.

41. **(2)** The recommended dose for acetaminophen is no more than 4 gm/day. This client may be experiencing analgesic rebound headache. Appropriate prophylactic medications for migraine include beta-blockers (propranolol), tricyclic antidepressants (amitriptyline), selective serotonin reuptake inhibitors (paroxetine), anticonvulsants (topiramate), and calcium channel blockers (verapamil). It is not necessary to order expensive tests for clients with migraine or tension headache. Usually a careful, thorough history is sufficient.

42. **(3)** The most common finding in children with meningococcemia (71%) is fever and a purpuric rash. The rash of rubella, Lyme disease, and roseola is finer, and none of these problems is life threatening, unlike with meningococcemia, which makes it a "do not miss" diagnosis.

43. **(4)** This is a common complaint of the client with subarachnoid hemorrhage headache. This client should be immediately referred to a neurologic surgeon.

44. **(3)** The speech center (Broca's area) is most often located in the left hemisphere. The client would experience weakness of the right side of the body and a right-sided visual deficit as well.

45. **(4)** Options #1, #2, and #3 all precipitate the development of an embolus that can result in an embolic stroke ("brain accident"). Diabetes will precipitate occlusive disease of the cerebral arteries and the possible development of a thrombotic stroke, not an embolic stroke.

46. **(2)** A simple partial seizure is characterized by unilateral paresthesia, numbness and tingling, and spastic movement of the extremities ("jacksonian" seizure). The client has no loss of consciousness or incontinence of the bowel or bladder.

47. **(3)** The characteristics of a benign tremor are a fine to coarse rhythmic tremors of the hands and feet that increase with activity and may be absent at rest. Frequently the voice is also involved. An ingestion of a small amount of alcohol may decrease symptoms.

48. **(1)** The description is that of a petit mal or absence seizure. Although the etiology of the majority of seizures is unclear, the client should be referred for neurologic evaluation to determine if an underlying abnormality is present.

49. **(2)** It is important to determine first if the client has stayed on his medication schedule. The symptoms may be the result of missed medication or overmedication, especially with pyridostigmine (Mestinon). The symptoms may also be exacerbated by exercise and heat.

50. **(1)** The clinical presentation is classic for Horner's syndrome, especially the lack of sweating (anhidrosis) on the ipsilateral (same) side of the face and neck as the eye symptoms. The client needs to be referred for further neurologic workup.

51. **(4)** Homonymous hemianopia is the loss of the vision in one half of the visual field. Either the right or left field of vision may be affected. It is most often caused by a lesion or pathology in the optic tract or occipital lobe.

Pharmacology

52. **(3)** Neuropathic pain is traditionally treated with a variety of medications, including anticonvulsants, tricyclic antidepressants, and opioids. Sympathetic blockade may be used in recalcitrant cases. NSAIDs are not generally considered first-line treatment.

53. **(2)** Although most medication is discontinued after 4 years of no seizure activity, a confirmatory EEG should be obtained. Not all seizure clients require medication; referral to and monitoring by a neurologist are appropriate.

54. **(3)** Scopolamine patches placed behind the ear and provide medication for 3 days. The correct dose for meclizine (Antivert) is 12.5–25 mg PO tid to qid; for dimenhydrinate (Dramamine) 50 mg tid or qid; and for prochlorperazine (Compazine) 5–10 mg q4h prn.

55. **(2)** The correct dose is ergotamine (Ergostat) 2 mg sublingually (SL). Sumatriptan (lmitrex) is given subcutaneously (SC), or 100 mg PO, and the ketorolac dose is 30–60 mg intramuscularly (IM). Amitriptyline (Elavil) is not used for abortive therapy.

56. **(2)** Hyperplasia of the gums is a common side effect of phenytoin (Dilantin). The child should have regular dental prophylactic hygiene to deal with the problem.

57. **(3)** Carbidopa/levodopa (Sinemet) induces a number of adverse reactions, including hypotension, GI upset, psychosis, and motor complications. For best absorption, it should not be given around meals, despite GI side effects. It exerts no known effect on slowing disease progression.

58. **(3)** Onset of drug action and relief of trigeminal neuralgia symptoms occur in 24 hours, usually in 4–6 hours. Laboratory tests are usually monitored based on the specific medication, not a peak and trough. These medications may be given to treat seizures.

12

Physical Examination & Diagnostic Tests

1. The nurse practitioner is preparing to examine the abdomen of a client. What is the correct sequence in which to conduct the examination?

   1. Inspection, palpation, percussion, auscultation.

   2. Palpation, percussion, auscultation, inspection.

   3. Percussion, palpation, auscultation, inspection.

   4. Inspection, auscultation, percussion, palpation.

2. When obtaining a history from a young female adult client with abdominal pain, which of the following priority areas must be assessed:

   1. Food preferences and dislikes.

   2. Location of the pain and associated symptoms.

   3. Past medical history and medication history.

   4. First day of last menstrual period.

3. To test for a positive obturator sign in a client with abdominal pain, the nurse practitioner:

   1. Passively internally rotates the right hip from the 90-degree hip/knee flexion position. *obturator sign = appendicitis*

   2. Asks the client to take a deep breath while applying pressure in the area of the gallbladder.

   3. Percusses over the costovertebral angles.

   4. Percusses at the right midclavicular line directly below the umbilicus and continues upward.

4. Diagnosis of acute hepatitis B includes the following results:

   1. Positive HBsAg, anti-HBc, HBeAg, IgM anti-HBc.

   2. HbeAg positive, HbsAg positive.

   3. HbeAg negative, HbsAg negative.

   4. IgM anti-HBc (high titer), HBsAg negative.

5. The nurse practitioner is performing the initial physical examination on a 51-year-old man. The history reveals that the client's father died of colon cancer, but the client is asymptomatic. What priority diagnostic tests are used to screen this client?

   1. Barium enema and upper gastrointestinal (GI) series.

   2. Carcinoembryonic antigen (CEA) titer and sigmoidoscopy.

   3. Proctoscopy, biopsy, and colonoscopy.

   4. Fecal occult blood testing and flexible sigmoidoscopy.

6. The anti-HCV test indicates that the client has:

   1. Acute hepatitis C.

   2. Chronic hepatitis C.

   3. Resolved hepatitis C.

   4. Acute, chronic, or resolved hepatitis C.

7. The diagnosis of early acute pancreatitis would be considered by the nurse practitioner based on physical findings and which of the following laboratory results?

   1. White blood cell (WBC) count of 10,300/mm^3.

   2. Serum amylase of 75 U/L.

   3. Serum amylase of 300 U/L.

   4. Serum lipase of 75 U/L.

8. An overweight middle-aged woman has right upper quadrant pain that radiates to her right subscapular area and is severe and persistent. She is also experiencing anorexia, nausea, and a fever. Her most recent meal was a double quarter-pound hamburger with cheese, French fries, and a vanilla shake. Based on this information, the nurse practitioner examines the abdomen and percusses for costovertebral angle tenderness. The abdomen is tender in the right upper quadrant. Which of the following signs, if positive, corresponds to the correct diagnosis?

   1. Obturator sign; client has appendicitis.

   2. Costovertebral angle tenderness; client has a urinary tract infection.

   3. Murphy's sign; client has cholecystitis.

   4. McBurney's sign; client has a strangulated hernia.

9. The nurse practitioner reviews laboratory results for a patient that reveals a positive *Helicobacter pylori* test. The nurse practitioner interprets this finding as an infection associated with:

   1. Gastroesophageal reflux disease.

   2. Irritable bowel syndrome.

   3. Duodenal ulcer.

   4. Infectious esophagitis.

10. When assessing a client with a complaint of severe abdominal pain, the nurse practitioner notes a firm flat abdomen, no bowel sounds, and positive guarding by the client. What diagnostic study should be ordered immediately?

    1. CBC and differential.

    2. Serum electrolytes.

    3. Hemoglobin S.

    4. Coombs antiglobulin test.

Disorders

11. Diarrhea is often associated with:

    1. Infectious gastroenteritis, inflammatory bowel disease, and diverticulitis.

    2. Diseases of the colon or rectum.

    3. Fever and abdominal pain in sexually transmitted diseases.

    4. Dysuria and flank pain in urinary tract infections.

12. Esophageal pain may radiate to the:

    1. Infrascapular area.

    2. Right shoulder.

    3. Neck and left arm.

    4. Periumbilical area.

13. The viral gastroenteritis seen in older children and adults has a short incubation (18–72 hours) and short duration (24–48 hours), is characterized by abrupt onset of nausea and abdominal cramps followed by vomiting and diarrhea, and is often accompanied by headache and myalgia. What causes this disorder?

    1. Enteric adenovirus.

2. Enteric calicivirus (Norwalk).

3. Rotavirus.

4. Cytomegalovirus.

14. The nurse practitioner suspects peritonitis in a client. The best action is to:

    1. Percuss over the costovertebral angle and watch for signs of pain.

    2. Perform a rectal examination and test the stool for blood.

    3. Auscultate the abdomen for decreased bowel sounds.

    4. Palpate for a tense, hard abdomen and check for a positive obturator sign.

15. Which of the following suggests an emergent condition?

    1. Pain in an adolescent that is rated as 5 on a scale of 1–10 and is relieved by having a bowel movement.

    2. Localized pain that steadily increases for more than 6 hours with rebound tenderness and guarding.

    3. Pain in an adolescent girl that is sudden in onset and localized in the right lower quadrant and lasts 14–36 hours.

    4. Pain that follows the onset of vomiting and diarrhea.

16. Peptic ulcer disease (PUD) should be treated empirically before diagnostic studies are done when the client's ulcer pain:

    1. Occurs with blood in the stool.

    2. Can be relieved by food, antacids, or vomiting.

    3. Is accompanied by weight loss.

    4. Is atypical or occurs with anemia.

17. A careful history of a client with a chief complaint of diarrhea reveals that this adult has recurrent abdominal pain and diarrhea that alternates with constipation. The most likely diagnosis is:

    1. Drug-induced diarrhea.

    2. Inflammatory bowel disease.

    3. Giardiasis.

    4. Irritable bowel syndrome.

18. What are assessment characteristics of clients with dysphagia caused by motility disorders?.

    1. Usually have more difficulty swallowing solids than liquids.

    2. May have a stricture due to esophagitis after long history of reflux disorder.

    3. Have dysphagia for both solids and liquids.

    4. May have marked weight loss.

19. The pathogenesis of gastroesophageal reflux disease (GERD) is:

    1. Frequent and excessive retrograde movement of stomach contents into the esophagus due to abnormal lower esophageal sphincter (LES) function.

    2. Hiatal hernia that leads to esophageal irritation and inflammation.

    3. Reflux of gastric contents after meals when client is in upright position, often after vigorous exercise.

    4. Initiated by erosion of the gastrointestinal mucosa into LES, decreasing LES pressure and causing a burning sensation in the stomach.

20. A client comes to the emergency department concerned about pain and swelling in his groin. He tells the nurse practitioner that his doctor said he has an incarcerated hernia. The examination of the client reveals a hernia that:

    1. Easily moves back and forth across the abdominal wall.

    2. Protrudes from the groin area and cannot be reduced into the abdomen.

    3. Is very painful to palpation with significant abdominal swelling.

    4. Decreases in size when the client increases intraabdominal pressure.

21. Which finding indicates a need for endoscopy in clients with PUD?

    1. All new cases of dyspepsià.

    2. Symptoms persisting after 8–12 weeks of therapy.

    3. All clients with dyspepsia who smoke and use alcohol.

    4. Good response to empiric treatment after 7–10 days.

22. The nurse practitioner understands that the following principle would be helpful in educating clients with GERD:

    1. A hiatal hernia is always a coexisting and major contributing factor.

    2. The lower esophageal sphincter (LES) has become a poor antireflux barrier.

    3. The amount of acid reflux depends on a familial tendency for GERD.

    4. Overeating and use of caffeine and alcohol cause GERD.

23. Inflammatory toxigenic gastrointestinal illness is characterized by:

    1. No fecal leukocytes, secretory diarrhea, affects colon.

    2. No fecal leukocytes, watery diarrhea, affects distal small bowel.

    3. Fecal leukocytes, secretory diarrhea, affects colon.

    4. Fecal leukocytes, watery diarrhea, affects colon.

24. Irritable bowel syndrome (IBS) affects:

    1. Men more than women.

    2. Children more than young adults.

    3. Women more than men.

    4. Elderly persons more than young adults.

25. The nurse practitioner understands that hepatitis B can be transmitted in blood and blood products. Another common mode of transmission of hepatitis B is:

    1. Respiratory contact.

    2. Contaminated fluid.

    3. Fecal-oral route.

    4. Perinatal exposure.

26. A young adult presents to the office with a chief complaint of intermittent heartburn that becomes worse after eating and at night and that is relieved temporarily by antacids. The client states he has regurgitated very bitter-tasting material into the mouth several times in the last 14 days. The physical examination is unremarkable. The most likely diagnosis is:

    1. Viral esophagitis.

    2. Irritable bowel syndrome.

    3. Gastroesophageal reflux disease.

    4. Carcinoma of the esophagus.

27. Which two forms of viral hepatitis are primarily transmitted by the fecal-oral route?

    1. Hepatitis A and B.

    2. Hepatitis B and C.

    3. Hepatitis A and D.

    4. Hepatitis A and E.

28. An indirect inguinal hernia:

    1. Is a portion of the bowel or omentum that protrudes directly through floor of inguinal canal and exits through external inguinal ring.

    2. Occurs mainly in middle and later years.

    3. Is caused by a weakness in the abdominal structure.

    4. Passes through internal abdominal ring, traverses spermatic cord through inguinal canal, and exits at external inguinal ring.

29. Which is true about enterobiasis?

    1. The parasite is in the soil and enters the body through the feet. It can cause anemia.

    2. The parasite causes pruritus around the anus because the gravid females exit through the anus at night and lay eggs on the skin. The human is the only host of this parasite.

    3. The eggs of this parasite enter the body by ingestion of dirt (pica) or dirt on unwashed vegetables that contain the eggs, or through water containing eggs.

    4. This parasite is a protozoan. The source is usually contaminated water, but it is spread from person to person by fecal-oral contamination.

30. The therapeutic diet modification in GERD consists of which type of diet?

    1. Low energy and low calorie.

    2. Energy controlled and high calorie.

3. High energy and hemodynamically stabilized.

4. No acidic or fatty foods, chocolate, or peppermint.

31. Nonpharmacologic management of GERD includes which of the following?

1. Weight reduction and sleep with head of bed elevated 4–6 inches with blocks.

2. Lying down and resting after meals and weight reduction.

3. Drinking large amounts of fluids with meals and avoiding alcohol.

4. Avoiding mint, orange juice, milk, and high-energy diet.

32. An organism associated with etiology of peptic ulcer disease (PUD) is:

1. *Streptococcus pneumoniae.*

2. *Helicobacter pylori.*

3. *Moraxella catarrhalis.*

4. *Staphylococcus aureus.*

33. The most common cause of cirrhosis is:

1. Hepatitis A and hepatitis B.

2. Hepatitis B and Wilson's disease.

3. Hepatitis D and congestive heart failure.

4. Chronic hepatitis B and C and alcohol.

34. Prolapse of a vascular anal cushion through the anal canal with resultant entrapment by the internal anal sphincter describes:

1. Prolapse of the rectal mucosa.

2. Hemorrhoid.

3. Tumor.

4. Inguinal hernia.

35. An acute febrile illness with jaundice, anorexia, malaise, and an incubation period of 45–160 days; having a chronic and an acute form; and transmitted by parenteral, sexual, and perinatal routes describes:

1. Hepatitis A.

2. Hepatitis B.

3. Hepatitis C.

4. Hepatitis D.

36. A client with a history of cholelithiasis presents to the office complaining of increased pain. The nurse practitioner would arrange immediate hospital admission for possible prompt intervention if the history also showed that the client is:

1. Human immunodeficiency virus (HIV) positive.

2. 75 years old and diabetic.

3. 5 weeks pregnant.

4. Vomiting with a slight fever.

37. An older adult male presents to the nurse practitioner for evaluation of "heartburn" and recent significant weight loss. He states that taking antacids and an oral histamine (H_2) blocker for 4 weeks has not relieved his symptoms, and that after eating it feels like his stomach has a problem with digestion of solid food. He also gives a history of being a cigarette smoker and drinks alcohol daily. What differential diagnosis must the nurse practitioner consider first?

1. Gastric ulcer.

2. Acid reflux.

3. Esophageal tumor.

4. Lung tumor.

38. An adult client presents to the nurse practitioner complaining of weakness and vomiting. He gives a history of "several" drinks per day for the past 12 years and cirrhosis. The nurse practitioner observes that the client's lips appear to have dark blood on them. What emergent condition does the nurse practitioner suspect?

1. Seizure disorder.

2. Cerebral hemorrhage.

3. Pancreatitis.

4. Esophageal varices.

39. What usually benign diagnosis can result in small bowel obstruction and infarction and requires immediate referral to a surgeon?

1. Gastric ulcer.

2. Endometriosis.

3. Hernia.

4. Ectopic pregnancy.

40. A young adult female presents to the nurse practitioner for evaluation of 2 days of increasing crampy abdominal pain. She states that she also has some mild nausea, anorexia, and a low-grade fever. The client states that the pain is periumbilical. Her STAT complete blood count (CBC) reveals a slightly elevated white count but is otherwise normal. What is the nurse practitioner's next step in the care of this client?

    1. Refer to a gynecologist for evaluation of possible ectopic pregnancy.

    2. Refer to surgeon for evaluation of possible appendicitis.

    3. Observe overnight and reassess the next day.

    4. Place on a clear liquid diet and have client watch for increasing symptoms.

41. The nurse practitioner's adult client has early alcoholic cirrhosis diagnosed by liver biopsy. In teaching the client about her disease, it is important that the nurse practitioner inform her that the disease is most likely irreversible at this point, but that the following will generally halt the progression of the disease:

    1. Vitamin B supplements.

    2. Long term, low dose corticosteroids.

    3. Abstinence from alcohol.

    4. Maintenance of a nutritious diet.

42. An elderly client presents with fever, leukocytosis, lower left quadrant pain, and diarrhea alternating with constipation. The nurse practitioner would make the diagnosis of:

    1. Appendicitis.

    2. Diverticulitis.

    3. Irritable bowel syndrome.

    4. Pancreatitis.

43. Which clients would be at **lowest** risk for developing diverticular disease?

    1. Vegetarians with high-fiber diets.

    2. Obese clients with high-cholesterol diets.

    3. Elderly clients on small meal diets.

    4. Fad dieters on low-sugar diets.

44. The nurse practitioner knows that the following symptom is characteristic of left-sided colon cancer:

    1. Anemia.

    2. Tenesmus.

    3. Bright-red rectal bleeding.

    4. Change in bowel habits.

45. The nurse practitioner knows that in clients with ulcerative colitis and disease proximal to the sigmoid colon, careful surveillance is required because of an increased risk of:

    1. Colon cancer.

    2. Peptic ulcer disease.

    3. Depression.

    4. Perforation.

46. Which is true of PUD in elderly clients?

    1. Smoking does not increase the risk of PUD.

    2. Duodenal ulcers are more common in elderly persons.

    3. Perforation is a rare complication.

    4. Weight loss and anorexia are often the only symptoms.

47. Which is true of early cancer of the esophagus in the elderly client?

    1. Alcoholism and smoking increase the risk for cancer of the esophagus.

    2. It is usually an adenocarcinoma.

    3. Dysphagia for liquids, cough, and hoarseness are early symptoms.

    4. Boring-type midchest pain indicates mediastinal involvement and requires immediate surgery.

48. A client has a history of colon polyps. The nurse practitioner knows:

    1. Polyps of the cecum are most likely to be malignant.

    2. Polyps <1 cm are more suspicious for malignancy.

    3. Villous polyps are rarely malignant.

    4. Sessile polyps are more likely to be malignant than pedunculated polyps.

49. The nurse practitioner is interpreting the notation of "string sign" on an upper GI series performed on an infant. This is associated with a diagnosis of:

    1. Intussusception.
    2. Hirschsprung's disease.
    3. Pyloric stenosis.
    4. Gastroesophageal reflux.

50. The nurse practitioner identifies the following condition as most conducive to the development of metabolic alkalosis in a child:

    1. Severe anxiety resulting in hyperventilation.
    2. Excessive vomiting related to gastroenteritis.
    3. Depressed respirations from excessive narcotics ingestion.
    4. Decreased renal function with glomerular damage.

51. The nurse practitioner in the emergency department examines a child with severe diarrhea and vomiting resulting in dehydration. One of the orders is to start an intravenous (IV) line of 500 ml normal saline with 10 mEq potassium to run at 23 ml/hr. The child is NPO. What would be a priority action before initiating the IV fluid with potassium?

    1. Weigh the child.
    2. Obtain serum electrolyte values.
    3. Make sure the child is voiding adequately.
    4. Determine amount of previous fluid loss.

52. A young child is brought to the clinic by her mother complaining of abrupt onset of vomiting followed by more than 10 liquid stools with mucus for the past 48 hours. The temperature is 100°F orally. The stool smear by the nurse practitioner is negative for WBCs. What is the most likely etiologic pathogen for this young child's gastroenteritis?

    1. Rotavirus.
    2. *Shigella dysenteriae.*
    3. *Campylobacter jejuni.*
    4. *Salmonella.*

53. The symptoms of abdominal discomfort after meals, diarrhea or constipation, anorexia, weight loss, failure to grow, and failure to develop sexually are most often associated with:

    1. Ulcerative colitis.
    2. Irritable bowel syndrome.
    3. Carcinoma of the colon.
    4. Crohn's disease.

54. What are the most consistent clinical findings in children with acute appendicitis?

    1. An elevated WBC count and pyuria.
    2. High fever and tenderness around the umbilicus.
    3. Low-grade fever and periumbilical abdominal pain.
    4. Nausea, vomiting, and diarrhea.

55. What question by the nurse practitioner would be appropriate to ask the parents of an infant suspected of intussusception?

    1. "Does the infant have clay-colored stools?"
    2. "Does the infant have projectile vomiting?"
    3. "Does the infant have constant abdominal pain?"
    4. "Does the infant have red currant jelly stools?"

56. The major symptom of reflux in infants is:

    1. Vomiting or regurgitation, especially after feeding.
    2. Poor weight gain in infants.
    3. Hyperirritability and refusal of feeding.
    4. Fever and diarrhea.

57. Optimal medical therapy for young infants with vomiting or regurgitation of GERD consists of:

    1. Frequent small feedings and burping after each feeding.
    2. Placing the infant prone after frequent feedings.
    3. Placing the infant supine after feedings.
    4. Thickening the feedings and using proton pump inhibitors.

58. What is true regarding the management of an infant born to an HBsAg-positive mother?

    1. No prophylaxis against hepatitis B is required because the infant is not at risk for the development of hepatitis B based on exposure to mother.

    2. One dose of hepatitis B immunoglobulin should be administered by 36 hours after birth.

    3. The nurse practitioner should administer one dose of hepatitis B vaccine.

    4. One dose of hepatitis B immunoglobulin should be administered within 12 hours of birth and a complete three-dose immunization of hepatitis B vaccine administered at the usual recommended intervals.

59. What physical findings would lead the nurse practitioner to suspect Hirschsprung's disease in a 6-month-old infant?

    1. Rectal bleeding, diarrhea, and prolonged jaundice at birth.

    2. History of constipation and current abdominal distention.

    3. Irritability, vomiting, and dehydration.

    4. History of colic, bloody diarrhea, and nausea.

60. A common cause of acute abdominal pain in children under 5 years old is:

    1. Appendicitis.

    2. Intussusception.

    3. Incarcerated hernias.

    4. Gastroenteritis.

61. The nurse practitioner understands that common causes of recurrent abdominal pain in children are:

    1. Intussusception, gastroenteritis, and right lower lobe pneumonia.

    2. Psychogenic pain, trauma, and urinary tract infection.

    3. Parasitic infestation, musculoskeletal pain, and chronic stool retention.

    4. Incarcerated hernia, appendicitis, inflammatory bowel disease.

62. A mother brings her adolescent son the nurse practitioner for evaluation after a dirt-bike accident. The client states that the bike flipped over and struck him on the abdomen. He has a hematoma just below the left anterior rib area. The nurse practitioner must be particularly aware of which possibility?

    1. Ruptured bowel due to blunt trauma.

    2. Bladder trauma.

    3. Hypovolemia due to ruptured spleen.

    4. Arrhythmias.

63. A 2-year-old Asian American comes to the clinic with her parents and infant brother. The chief complaint is abdominal pain and flatulence and diarrhea after eating. Until 3 months ago, she had continued to be breast-fed twice a day. The nurse practitioner would suspect:

    1. Irritable bowel syndrome.

    2. Hirschsprung's disease.

    3. Lactose intolerance.

    4. Food allergy.

64. A 10-year-old girl comes to the clinic with complaints of nausea, vomiting, and right upper quadrant pain during vigorous play. She is also more tired than usual. Serologic tests for immunoglobulin M (IgM) antibodies are ordered to rule out:

    1. Cholecystitis.

    2. Hepatitis A.

    3. Infectious mononucleosis.

    4. Hepatitis B.

65. A 5-year-old presents to the clinic with diffuse abdominal pain, irritability, and a low-grade fever. The mother states the toddler has not had a bowel movement since the previous morning. Physical examination reveals umbilical tenderness, guarding, and hypoactive bowel sounds. The nurse practitioner's next step is to:

    1. Refer to physician/surgeon for further evaluation.

    2. Assess for rebound tenderness and do a rectal exam.

3. Prescribe pediatric Fleet enemas.

4. Assess dietary intake for past 24 hours.

66. A 2-year-old child is seen for a foreign body in the GI tract. The nurse practitioner pays particular attention to the size of the object, knowing that passing the ligament of Treitz is difficult with objects larger than:

1. 5 cm.

2. 8 cm.

3. 10 cm.

4. 12 cm.

67. A 2-month-old infant presents with coughing that results in emesis that occurs when laid supine after eating. The infant has lost 1.3 lb since birth, with a birth weight of 7.5 lb. The nurse practitioner focuses the assessment toward the possibility of:

1. Suck-swallow incoordination.

2. Gastroesophageal reflux.

3. Tracheoesophageal fistula.

4. Infantile colic.

Pharmacology

68. A 28-year-old male has been diagnosed with hepatitis C and is started on ribavirin therapy. The nurse would:

1. Instruct client to take acetaminophen (Tylenol) 30 minutes before each treatment.

2. Emphasize that client must not father children during and for 6 months after therapy.

3. Encourage client to use herbal therapy with gingko to decrease feelings of depression.

4. Instruct client to eat three well-balanced high-calorie meals daily.

69. An adult client has been treated intermittently for PUD for the past 12 years. He has always responded quickly to ranitidine (Zantac) and antacids. He continues to smoke. He presents to the clinic with severe epigastric pain, weakness, and lightheadedness. Stool guaiac testing is pos-

itive, and his hemoglobin is 11.2 gm/dl. His weight has decreased slowly over the past 6 months for unknown reasons. Based on this information, what should the nurse practitioner do next?

1. Refill his medications.

2. Give medications and refer to smoking cessation clinic.

3. Discontinue cimetidine and start omeprazole (Prilosec).

4. Consult with physician.

70. The nurse practitioner is examining a 30-year-old obese man complaining of indigestion and heartburn with a strong acid taste in the mouth about an hour after meals. The history is negative for chronic illnesses. A diagnosis of GERD is made. What is the best initial treatment for this client?

1. Eat five small meals daily and lie down after meals.

2. Take propantheline (Pro-Banthine) 15 mg tid 30 minutes before eating.

3. Decrease weight and take ranitidine (Zantac) 150 mg bid.

4. Take omeprazole (Prilosec) 40 mg qd and antacids.

71. Which of the following would be prescribed as initial treatment for uncomplicated PUD?

1. Clarithromycin 500 mg bid.

2. Doxepin (Sinequan) 25 mg hs.

3. Omeprazole (Prilosec) 20 mg qd.

4. Pirenzepine 50 mg tid.

72. Which drug would be most useful for the nurse practitioner to prescribe for an adult client to prevent ulcers due to nonsteroidal antiinflammatory drugs (NSAIDs)?

1. Celecoxib (Celebrex).

2. Cimetidine (Tagamet).

3. Doxepin (Sinequan).

4. Pirenzepine.

73. After percutaneous or permucosal exposure to an HBsAg-positive source, what is the appropriate treatment for the client?

    1. In an unvaccinated client, begin the hepatitis B series.

    2. In a known hepatitis B responder with an adequate response, no treatment is necessary.

    3. In a known hepatitis B responder with inadequate anti–hepatitis B surface antigen, give hepatitis B immune globulin (HBIG) and initiate a new hepatitis B vaccine series.

    4. In an unknown hepatitis B responder who completed the entire hepatitis B vaccine series, give a hepatitis B booster.

74. *Helicobacter pylori* has been found to be a causative factor in many cases of PUD. Successful treatment for an adult client requires therapy with which regimen?

    1. Clarithromycin, amoxicillin, and omeprazole (Prilosec).

    2. Pepto-Bismol, cephalexin (Keflex), and metronidazole (Flagyl).

    3. Lifestyle changes, Pepto-Bismol, and cimetidine (Tagamet).

    4. H$_2$ blocker, amoxicillin (Amoxil), and antacid.

75. A primary therapy for clients with mild ulcerative colitis is:

    1. Metronidazole (Flagyl).

    2. Sulfasalazine (Azulfidine).

    3. Amoxicillin (Amoxil).

    4. Cephalexin (Keflex).

76. The stepwise approach to management of GERD for an adult client includes life style changes and what medications?

    1. Antacids prn and cimetidine (Tagamet) 800 mg hs.

    2. Antacids prn and ranitidine (Zantac) 150 mg bid.

    3. Antacids prn and omeprazole (Prilosec) 20 mg qd.

    4. Cisapride (Propulsid) 10 mg 15 minutes before meals and hs.

77. For a client exposed to household or sexual contacts with hepatitis A, the nurse practitioner would:

    1. Give immunoglobulin 0.02 mg/kg as soon as possible but no later than 2 weeks after exposure.

    2. Give one dose of HBIG and immunoglobulin 0.02 mg/kg as soon as possible.

    3. Give immunoglobulin 0.02 mg/kg and two doses of HBIG.

    4. Understand that no injections are needed.

78. Shigellosis is treated by:

    1. No medication intervention, careful toileting and bathroom sanitation, and keeping the perineal area clean.

    2. Symptomatic treatment and antidiarrheal agent (loperamide) as needed.

    3. Symptomatic treatment and trimethoprim-sulfamethoxazole (TMP-SMX) dosed for age and weight bid × 7–10 days.

    4. Boiling water and quinacrine 100 mg PO tid × 5 days.

79. Pharmacologic management of nausea and vomiting includes:

    1. Emetrol 15–30 ml PO in adults.

    2. Promethazine (Phenergan) 25 mg for adults and children over 6 years.

    3. Hydroxyzine (Vistaril) 1 mg IM for adults and children 12 years and older.

    4. Trimethobenzamide (Tigan) 10 mg PO prn for adults.

80. The two major factors that lead to disruption of the gastrointestinal (GI) mucosa with subsequent development of an ulceration are:

    1. Alcohol consumption and NSAIDs.

    2. NSAIDs and smoking.

    3. NSAIDs and *Helicobacter pylori*.

    4. *Helicobacter pylori* and smoking.

81. A young woman presents with a history of recent unprotected sexual activity with a partner now diagnosed with hepatitis B. She is currently asymptomatic and does not recall having

a vaccine in the past. What is the best action for the nurse practitioner?

1. Draw a hepatitis B e antibody test (anti-HBe).

2. Administer one dose of HBIG.

3. Administer two doses of HBIG and initiate vaccination.

4. Administer one dose of HBIG and initiate vaccination.

82. What condition is a contraindication for the administration of the hepatitis B vaccine?

1. Pregnancy.

2. Lactation.

3. Severe hypersensitivity.

4. Age >60 years.

83. A 78-year-old client is diagnosed with enterocolitis, and the physician prescribes vancomycin (Vancocin) 125 mg PO qid. In following this client's progress, the nurse practitioner would monitor which of the following in regard to medication tolerance?

1. CBC, platelet count, clotting studies.

2. Serum creatinine, blood urea nitrogen (BUN), hearing changes.

3. Serum electrolytes, urinalysis, ataxia.

4. Changes in bowel habits, diarrhea, electrocardiographic changes.

84. A client with PUD is treated with a regimen that includes bismuth subsalicylate (Pepto-Bismol), tetracycline, and metronidazole (Flagyl). The client calls the nurse practitioner to report that his stools are unusually dark. He is not experiencing any gastric discomfort, orthostatic hypotension, or increased lethargy. How would the nurse practitioner interpret this information?

1. He is probably bleeding and should come in immediately.

2. He ate something to affect the color of his stool.

3. His stools are dark secondary to Pepto-Bismol.

4. The stool discoloration is caused by metronidazole.

85. A 3-year-old child is seen in the clinic for chronic, relapsing diarrhea. A stool for ova and parasites is obtained and is positive for *Giardia*. What is the most appropriate pharmacologic intervention?

1. Ampicillin (Omnipen).

2. Erythromycin (E-Mycin).

3. Metronidazole (Flagyl).

4. Tetracycline (Achromycin).

86. A patient with a history of arthritis and gastric ulcers comes to the clinic complaining of severe GI distress. The client has been taking ranitidine (Zantac) 150 mg bid. Although the nurse practitioner would ask all the following questions, which would be considered the most important?

1. "Are you taking the Zantac with food?"

2. "Are you taking the Zantac with water?"

3. "Have you changed your eating habits recently?"

4. "What medication are you using for the arthritis?"

87. When teaching a client with hepatitis C who is receiving interferon and ribavirin therapy, the nurse would encourage the client to eat:

1. Small frequent meals high in carbohydrate.

2. Small frequent meals high in protein.

3. Three well-balanced high-calorie meals daily.

4. Three well-balanced meals daily with minimal fluid intake.

Answers & Rationales

Physical Examination & Diagnostic Tests

1. **(4)** Inspection and auscultation should be conducted first in order to prevent undue guarding. The nurse practitioner should auscultate and listen to the abdomen before percussing and palpating it, because palpation may alter the frequency of bowel sounds. If the examination is painful initially, the client will be uncomfortable allowing the examiner to continue.

2. **(4)** Although all the information is important in determining the cause of abdominal pain, for a young female client of childbearing age, ascertaining whether or not the client is pregnant is a priority. The nurse practitioner should obtain a gynecologic history, including dates of last two normal menstrual periods, condom use, whether sexually active, and timing of last sexual intercourse. The location and character may help identify the origin of the pain. Abrupt onset of pain usually has a different etiology than pain that develops over hours. Whether or not the pain has changed since onset can help in determining if a larger area of the abdomen is becoming involved or if the pain is subsiding. Both visceral and parietal pain can be referred to remote sites along shared nerve pathways. Aggravating and alleviating factors can provide clues as to the origin of the pain. Past medical history and medication history can give clues to known conditions and to medications that may be causing the symptoms or are being used for conditions that can cause abdominal pain. For example, a client taking ranitidine (Zantac) may fail to mention a history of gastroesophageal reflux disease (GERD).

3. **(1)** If abdominal pain results from passive internal rotation of the right hip from the 90-degree hip/knee flexion position, the client has a positive obturator sign, which suggests appendicitis. In a positive Murphy's sign (Option #2), pain and a brief inspiratory arrest result when a client takes a deep breath while the examiner applies pressure over the gallbladder, suggestive of cholecystitis. Percussion over the costovertebral angles that elicit pain is positive for costovertebral angle tenderness, suggestive of pyelonephritis. Percussion over the right midclavicular line below the umbilicus and continuing upward is a technique for locating the liver.

4. **(1)** Hepatitis B surface antigen (HBsAg) is found in active or chronic hepatitis B disease. In acute illness, the two factors in serum are HBsAg and antibody to the hepatitis B core antigen (anti-HBc). When the client has made a recovery, HBsAg usually is negative and evidence of surface antibody (anti-HBs) is found. Hepatitis B e antigen (HBeAg) indicates active replication of the virus. Immunoglobulin M (IgM) anti-HBc negative results indicate chronic disease. Positive HBsAg indicates chronic disease. Negative HBsAg indicates prior exposure.

5. **(4)** These are standard diagnostic tests used for screening a client with a high risk of colon cancer. CEA is used more to determine recurrence of cancer; barium enema, upper GI series, and proctoscopy do not provide sufficiently reliable information for detecting the malignancy. The earliest marker of colon carcinoma is a guaiac stool from Hemoccult

testing. The fecal occult blood test is a protocol for collecting and testing six samples from three consecutive stools at the client's home. Flexible sigmoidoscopy allows direct visual examination of the distal portion of the colorectal area by a trained examiner using a flexible endoscope after cleansing of the descending and sigmoid colon and rectum. This procedure identifies 80% of neoplasms in the colorectal area. The American Cancer Society (2001) guidelines recommend fecal occult testing annually and sigmoidoscopy every 5 years for adults over age 50. All positive tests should be followed up with a colonoscopy. A colonoscopy is a procedure that allows direct visual examination of the entire colorectal area using a colonoscope.

6. **(4)** This is the surface marker for hepatitis C. At present there is no way to differentiate the diffuse forms of hepatitis C because the viremia level is well below the threshold of most assays.

7. **(3)** Options #2 and #3 are almost identical. (NOTE: *Use the testing strategy that both are wrong or one is the correct answer.*) In acute pancreatitis the serum amylase increases within 3–6 hours of onset. The serum lipase elevates after the increase in amylase. (In adults, normal level for serum amylase is 50–180 U/L and for serum lipase 55–417 U/L.)

8. **(3)** The history, right upper quadrant pain that radiates to the right subscapular area, and positive Murphy's sign are all associated with cholecystitis. A positive obturator sign at McBurney's point is a sign associated with appendicitis. Clients with strangulated hernias have colicky abdominal pain, nausea, vomiting, abdominal distention, and hyperperistalsis. Those with reducible hernias are asymptomatic or have only mild pain.

9. **(3)** *Helicobacter pylori* appears to be associated with the majority of duodenal and gastric ulcers not attributed to chronic NSAID use. Prevalence of *H. pylori* infection in clients with duodenal ulcers is about 70%–75%. Factors that contribute to GERD include incompetent lower esophageal sphincter and abnormal esophageal clearance. The most common pathogens for clients with infectious esophagitis are *Candida albicans*, herpes simpex, and cytomegalovirus. Infectious esophagitis is usually seen in immunosuppressed clients. Irritable bowel syndrome is a chronic functional disorder

without structural or biochemical abnormalities.

10. **(1)** The client is demonstrating symptoms classic for appendicitis. The nurse practitioner would want to obtain a complete blood cell (CBC) count with differential. Hemoglobin S is specific for sickle cell. Coombs antiglobulin test shows the presence of antigen-antibody complexes.

Disorders

11. **(1)** Diarrhea is a common symptom in infectious gastroenteritis, inflammatory bowel disease, diverticulitis, and early intestinal obstruction. Colorectal diseases are often associated with constipation that clearly precedes the onset of abdominal pain. With sexually transmitted diseases, abdominal pain can often occur with vaginal discharge or bleeding and sometimes irregular menses. Dysuria, flank pain, hematuria, and urinary frequency are common signs and symptoms of upper or lower urinary tract infections or ureteral calculi.

12. **(3)** Esophageal pain may radiate to the neck and left arm. Gallbladder pain can radiate to the infrascapular area, diaphragm pain to the right shoulder, and the pain of appendicitis to the periumbilical area.

13. **(2)** Gastroenteritis is a common cause of abdominal pain in children. Symptoms vary depending on the type of viral infection. Rotavirus mainly affects infants 3–15 months of age in the winter months, causing voluminous watery diarrhea without leukocytes. Enteric adenoviruses are the second most common viral infection in infants, with symptoms similar to rotavirus except the duration of illness may be longer. Enteric calicivirus (Norwalk) mainly causes vomiting but also diarrhea in older children and adults. Duration of symptoms is short, usually 24-48 hours. Cytomegalovirus rarely causes diarrhea and is common after bone marrow transplants and in late stages of HIV infection.

14. **(4)** Tense hard abdomen, verbal refusal or severe pain when asked to jump, and positive obturator sign suggest peritonitis. Costovertebral angle tenderness is a sign of a

renal disorder. Stool for occult blood is not a test for peritonitis. Decreased bowel sounds could be present in appendicitis or bowel obstruction but are not a peritoneal sign.

15. **(2)** Localized pain that steadily increases for 6 hours or more with rebound tenderness and guarding could be caused by an emergent condition, such as appendicitis or ruptured ectopic pregnancy. Pain in an adolescent girl that is relieved by having a bowel movement could be constipation. Pain that is sudden in onset in the right lower quadrant and lasts 14–36 hours could be mittelschmerz if the girl is midway through her menstrual cycle. Pain that follows the onset of vomiting and diarrhea usually occurs in gastroenteritis.

16. **(2)** Pain that awakens a client early in the morning from sleep or is relieved or worsened by food ingestion is typical of peptic ulcer pain. Atypical pain or pain that occurs with anemia or weight loss could be caused by a disorder other than peptic ulcer, such as gastric cancer. Anemia may also indicate acute blood loss from a bleeding ulcer or less often, chronic blood loss. The client's ulcer could be bleeding, indicated by blood in the stool.

17. **(4)** Irritable bowel syndrome (IBS) presents with abdominal pain and altered bowel habits. These symptoms can be aggravated by psychological stresses. Symptoms disappear while sleeping. Bacterial or viral gastroenteritis presents as abdominal pain with diarrhea and vomiting of abrupt onset. Drug-induced diarrhea follows initiation of drug therapy; there is no mention of previous drug therapy with this client. In inflammatory bowel disease, nocturnal diarrhea and abdominal pain are often accompanied by rectal fistula, fever, and skin lesions. Diarrhea occurring with giardiasis is malodorous. Weight loss occurs over weeks.

18. **(3)** Clients with dysphagia due to a motility disorder report dysphagia for both liquids and solids and repeated swallowing or performing a rapid Valsalva maneuver to help food or liquid pass into the stomach. It is episodic, nonprogressive, and unpredictable. Those with dysphagia due to obstruction have more difficulty swallowing solids than liquids, may have a stricture due to esophagitis, may have progressive dysphagia and chronic heartburn, and may report marked weight loss if esophageal cancer is present.

19. **(1)** Esophageal inflammation caused by excessive reflux that overpowers the normal mucosal defense mechanism leads to symptoms of reflux. Persons with and without hiatal hernia can experience gastroesophageal reflux. Physiologic or normal reflux occurs in most people after eating when they are in an upright position, especially during vigorous exercise, but its low frequency and small volume do not lead to symptoms. Symptoms of PUD are initiated by erosion of the gastrointestinal mucosa.

20. **(2)** The most common hernia is an inguinal hernia, protruding at the inguinal canal. Incarcerated means the hernia cannot be reduced or returned to the abdominal cavity. A reducible hernia easily moves across the abdominal wall. There should be no abdominal swelling, and if the hernia is particularly painful and associated with nausea and vomiting, strangulation should be considered.

21. **(2)** All cases of recurrent, not new, dyspepsia indicate a need for endoscopy. Endoscopy is reserved for clients with no response to empiric therapy after 7–10 days and symptoms persisting after 8–12 weeks of therapy. Dyspepsia may be characterized by fullness, belching, and regurgitation and may include PUD and gastroesophageal reflux. Smoking should be discontinued and alcohol intake decreased to a moderate level in PUD and GERD, but endoscopy is not indicated for these clients.

22. **(2)** The factor contributing most to reflux is an incompetent lower esophageal sphincter (LES), the antireflux barrier. Hiatal hernia is not believed to be an important factor in the etiology of reflux. Hiatal hernias usually cause no symptoms, but they may be associated with greater reflux and delayed esophageal acid clearance in clients with reflux. Reflux occurs postprandially in the upright position and may be exacerbated by meals, but overeating is not a direct cause. Alcohol and excessive use of caffeine may affect the LES pressure.

23. **(3)** The etiologic agents that produce inflammation and cause diarrhea are characterized by positive fecal leukocytes. Viral diarrhea is free of pus, so no fecal leukocytes would be found on the smear. Noninflammatory diarrhea is usually caused by rotavirus. Toxigenic bacteria cause diarrhea by elaborating toxins released after bacterial

growth in the intestine. The term indicates colonic involvement by invasive bacteria or parasites or toxin production that affects the large bowel. These poisonous substances result in secretory diarrhea.

24. **(3)** The female/male ratio for IBS is 4:1. A disease of young and middle-aged adults, IBS frequently appears at age 20–25.

25. **(4)** A common means of hepatitis B transmission is from mother to baby, perinatally. Other mechanisms of transmission are by infected body fluids, sexual contact, and parenterally. Hepatitis E virus is spread in contaminated water. Hepatitis A spreads by fecal-oral and person-to-person transmission.

26. **(3)** The client is presenting with the most reliable symptoms of GERD. GERD is most often related to inappropriate relaxation of the LES, which allows reflux of gastric acid and pepsin into the distal esophagus. Common presentations of IBS are differentiated by cramping, abdominal pain, or altered bowel habits predominating. Clients with esophagitis complain of the acute onset of chest pain, dysphagia, and odynophagia. Bleeding is associated with carcinoma.

27. **(4)** Hepatitis A and E are transmitted by the fecal-oral route. Hepatitis A spreads rapidly in households and day care centers for children. Risk is higher in day care centers with young children who wear diapers. Outbreaks can also occur from contaminated food and water infected with human sewage. Hepatitis B is transmitted by blood transfusion, needle sharing, sexual contact, and vertical (perinatal) transmission. Hepatitis B is not primarily transmitted by the fecal-oral route. Hepatitis C is primarily transmitted through parenteral exposure to blood or blood products. Hepatitis D occurs as a coinfection with hepatitis B; mode of transmission is via blood or blood products, sexually (with hepatitis B also present), or injection drugs.

28. **(4)** Because indirect hernias are caused by a congenital defect in which the processus vaginalis remains patent, they occur more often in younger persons. A portion of the bowel or omentum comes through the internal abdominal ring, traverses the spermatic cord through the inguinal canal, and exits at the external inguinal ring. In a direct hernia the omentum or bowel protrudes directly through the floor of the inguinal canal and exits through the external inguinal ring. Because a weakness in the abdominal structures is the cause, direct hernia occurs more often in middle and later years of life.

29. **(2)** Enterobiasis parasites reside in the intestine. Females lay eggs on the skin outside the anus, resulting in extreme pruritus. The only host is humans. Hookwoom larvae reside in the soil, enter the body through the feet, and can cause anemia. When dirt containing roundworm eggs is ingested through pica or unwashed vegetables, or if contaminated water is consumed, an intestinal infestation occurs. Giardiasis results from ingestion of the protozoan *Giardia lamblia* through contaminated water or oral-fecal transmission.

30. **(4)** Certain acidic and fatty foods, such as chocolate, peppermint, and orange, juice should be avoided. Low-energy diets are used in obesity for weight loss. Energy-controlled diets are used for clients with diabetes mellitus for increased glucose tolerance. High-energy and hemodynamically stabilized diets are used for clients with anorexia for increased weight and fat. Severe cases may require parenteral feeding.

31. **(1)** A high-energy diet is used for clients with anorexia. The major nonpharmacologic intervention for GERD is to advise the client not to lie down within 3 hours after meals, the period of greatest reflux. Clients with GERD also should reduce weight, avoid large meals and exercise after meals, and elevate the head of the bed. Certain drinks (alcohol, mint, orange juice) should be avoided because they delay gastric emptying. Acidic foods (tomato products, spicy foods) may cause symptoms of heartburn and should be avoided. The client should be taught to avoid bending after meals. Drinking large amounts of fluid with meals does not influence GERD.

32. **(2)** *Helicobacter pylori* has been implicated in the etiology of PUD. The three main causes of PUD are use of NSAIDs, chronic *H. pylori*, and acid secretory states (e.g., Zollinger-Ellison syndrome). The other organisms listed are implicated in other types of infections (e.g., acute otitis media, skin infections). *Streptococcus pneumoniae* and *Moraxella catarrhalis* have been implicated as causative agents in pneumonia.

33. **(4)** Chronic hepatitis B and C and alcohol are the most important causes of cirrhosis in the United States. Especially in men, one six-pack of beer or four to six glasses of wine daily significantly increases the risk for long-term hepatic injury leading to cirrhosis, with women at risk from half that amount. Hepatitis A is a self-limited infection without a known chronic state. Hepatitis D acute infections do not directly result in a high incidence of cirrhosis. Wilson's disease is a rare autosomal metabolic disease that may lead to cirrhosis, but the incidence is lower than alcohol and hepatitis B and C. The disease usually occurs between ages 10 and 30 years and is characterized by excessive deposition of copper in the liver. In advanced cirrhosis, hemochromatosis may be associated with congestive heart failure.

34. **(2)** A hemorrhoid results when a vascular anal cushion prolapses through the anal canal and is entrapped by the internal anal sphincter. In a rectal mucosa prolapse the wall of the rectum prolapses. A tumor is not a vascular anal cushion. An inguinal hernia is a result of trapped peritoneal fluid in the tunica vaginalis of the testis. When the vaginalis is open, an abdominal structure may be forced into it, resulting in an inguinal hernia. Hemorrhoids become symptomatic as a result of activities that increase venous pressure, such as prolonged sitting, straining on stool, and pregnancy.

35. **(2)** These characteristics describe hepatitis B, which is prevalent among intravenous drug users and homosexuals. Hepatitis A has similar symptoms but can usually be transmitted by the fecal-oral route and has an incubation period of 15–50 days (average 30 days) and no chronic form. Hepatitis C infection rarely causes jaundice. It is transmitted parenterally and has an incubation period of 14–140 days (average 42–49 days) and a chronic form. Hepatitis D coexists with hepatitis B, is transmitted parenterally, and can also become chronic. Hepatitis E is characterized by oral-fecal transmission associated with contaminated food and water and has an incubation period of 14–60 days and no chronic disease state.

36. **(2)** Although most clients need eventual intervention, those who are elderly and diabetic are at increased risk and should be hospitalized for prompt diagnosis, intravenous fluids, pain control, and surgical consultation.

Clients with diabetes mellitus and cirrhosis have an increased of cholelithiasis.

37. **(3)** Clients with esophageal tumor typically describe dysphagia for solid food. The symptom of heartburn caused by either gastric ulcer or acid reflux should be controlled with an H_2 blocker or proton pump inhibitor. Weight loss and progressive solid food dysphagia are clinical findings of esophageal cancer. Esophageal cancer usually develops in men (men/women ratio 3:1) age 50–70 years. Chronic tobacco and alcohol use increases the risk. Solid food dysphagia is present in more than 90% of clients. Clients with PUD have a history of NSAID use, smoking, and nonspecific epigastric pain. Alcohol does not appear to cause ulcers. Clinical manifestations of lung cancer include cough, hemoptysis, dyspnea, chest pain, and weight loss.

38. **(4)** Esophageal varices are dilated submucosal veins that may result in upper GI bleeding. One-third of clients develop upper GI bleeding. Clients with a history of heavy alcohol intake are at increased risk for cirrhosis and portal hypertension, which may result in variceal bleeding. These clients often present clinically with bleeding, spontaneous "coffee grounds" or bright-red blood, hypotension, and eventual shock. Esophageal varices are found in half of clients with cirrhosis. Clients with seizure disorders have seizures for 30–90 seconds, history of head trauma, and eye deviation during the seizures. Pancreatitis usually presents with abdominal pain in the epigastrium. Clients with cerebral hemorrhage have neurologic deficits that gradually progress in stepwise fashion.

39. **(3)** A strangulated hernia is irreducible, and the blood supply to the trapped bowel is compromised, resulting in bowel infarction. Ulcers, endometriosis, and ectopic pregnancy may cause abdominal pain and may be surgical emergencies but do not cause bowel obstruction.

40. **(2)** Increasing crampy abdominal pain that starts as periumbilical pain, anorexia, and fever are classic symptoms of appendicitis. A surgeon should evaluate the client to decrease the risk of rupture. Although ectopic pregnancy should always be a consideration in young females with abdominal pain, the characteristics of the pain and other symptoms are not typical of an ectopic pregnancy.

41. **(3)** Abstinence from alcohol, the most important treatment for cirrhosis, will stop its progression. The client's diet should be nutritious with adequate protein and calories. Salt should be restricted if the client has fluid retention. Vitamin supplementation is needed, but an adequate amount is obtained through diet and multivitamins without extra vitamin B supplements. Ferrous sulfate is given for iron deficiency anemia. Dietary protein should be restricted during acute client episodes. Long-term corticosteroids are not used in chronic disease management. For selected clients, liver transplantation is indicated.

42. **(2)** Diverticular disease presents with change in bowel habits (diarrhea alternating with constipation or both) and blood in the stool; if diverticulitis develops, flatus, low-grade fever, and leukocytosis may be present. Clients with diverticulitis have a range of mild to severe disease. Abdominal pain in the left lower quadrant ranges from mild to moderate with frequent nausea and vomiting. Appendicitis may present with pain in the right lower quadrant and may not be severe until perforation occurs. Other signs, including nausea and vomiting, leukocytosis, and fever, may or may not be present. IBS may present with aching or cramping periumbilical or lower abdominal pain, often precipitated by meals and relieved by defecation. Pain may radiate to the left chest or arm. There may be alternating episodes of diarrhea and constipation. Clients with pancreatitis may present with epigastric pain or tenderness that lasts for hours and may radiate to the back. They also may have fever, nausea/vomiting, mental confusion, and jaundice.

43. **(1)** A high-fiber diet is the treatment for diverticular disease, and vegetarians who eat increased amounts of fruits, vegetables, grains, and cereals are in the lowest risk category. Options #2, #3, and #4 clients are at higher risk. Low-sugar diets and high-cholesterol diets do not influence the incidence of diverticular disease.

44. **(4)** Colorectal cancer occurs most often in individuals over age 50. A change in bowel habit, with reduced caliber of stool and blood mixed with the stool, are characteristic of left-sided colon cancer, which is the most common site. Anemia is found with right-sided lesions. Bright-red rectal bleeding and tenesmus are characteristic of rectal cancer.

45. **(1)** Colon cancer risk in ulcerative colitis clients increases by 0.5%–1% per year after the tenth year of diagnosis. Folic acid 1 mg/day assists in decreasing the risk. Colonoscopy every 1–2 years is recommended 8–10 years after diagnosis. PUD is associated with NSAID use, *H. pylori* infection, and acid hypersecretory states. Perforation is associated with diverticulitis and intraabdominal infection resulting from perforation of a colonic diverticulum. Risk factors for depression include genetic factors, developmental problems, and social stresses.

46. **(4)** PUD in elderly clients often does not cause the usual pain and indigestion associated with PUD in younger clients. Smoking does increase the risk, and, without the pain, perforation is common. Gastric ulcers are more common in elderly clients; perforation may occur.

47. **(1)** Cancer of the esophagus is found primarily in elderly men. Alcoholism and smoking are the primary risk factors for esophageal cancer. The cell type is usually squamous cell. Dysphagia for liquids, cough, and hoarseness as well as midchest pain indicate late disease, which does not usually respond to treatment, including surgery.

48. **(4)** Flexible sigmoidoscopy and colonoscopy are screening tools for colorectal cancer recommended after age 50. They are useful for identifying adenomatous polyps, which are considered premalignant. Sessile or flat polyps are more suspicious for malignancy. Polyps of the cecum and polyps <1 cm are less likely to be malignant, and villous polyps are often malignant.

49. **(3)** The string sign is indicative of a narrow pyloric channel and is associated with pyloric stenosis. Intussusception would be evaluated by a barium enema. Hirschsprung's disease (congenital aganglionic megacolon) can be diagnosed with a Wagenstein-Rice series (air rises in the inflated colon). Gastroesophageal reflux is usually diagnosed by clinical findings in infants. Barium swallow will reveal free regurgitation of barium from stomach to esophagus. An upper GI series would be performed to rule out causes of vomiting.

50. **(2)** Excessive vomiting with loss of acid and gastric juice is the most common cause of metabolic alkalosis. Respiratory problems do not precipitate primary metabolic acid-base

imbalance, and renal disease most often causes metabolic acidosis. Severe anxiety resulting in hyperventilation results in respiratory alkalosis. Hyperventilation results in an increase in pH.

51. **(3)** It is critical that a child be voiding before starting an IV solution with potassium. The problem with renal compromise is always a possibility, and adequate output should be established before initiating fluid therapy. Options #2, #3, and #4 are important but not the priority in this situation. Clinical evaluation of the child client with dehydration should be prioritized as the volume of fluid intake, urine output, fever, and underlying medical conditions. Weight is also important in estimating dehydration but needs to be compared to prior weights. Important laboratory values include urine specific gravity, BUN, creatinine, hematocrit, and serum albumin.

52. **(1)** Rotavirus is the most frequent cause of gastroenteritis in children 6 months to 2 years of age. The Norwalk virus is more predominant in school-age children. Up to 58% of diarrhea in children results from viral infections, causing vomiting and then diarrhea. The stool smear is negative for WBCs in viral causes and positive in bacterial causes (Options #2, #3, and #4). In viral diarrhea the fever is mild, and diarrhea is watery and nonbloody.

53. **(4)** Clinical features of Crohn's disease include severe weight loss, abdominal pain, growth failure, and weight loss. In IBS, abdominal pain predominates. Altered bowel habits with either diarrhea or constipation are also seen. Clinical findings associated with carcinoma of the colon include mild occult blood loss with intermittent episodes of acute bleeding. Ulcerative colitis clinical features include diarrhea, rectal bleeding, and moderate weight loss.

54. **(3)** Appendicitis usually begins as periumbilical abdominal pain accompanied by anorexia and nausea, but not necessarily vomiting or diarrhea. Within hours the client may develop a low-grade fever. Most laboratory tests are normal. A WBC count >15,000/mm^3 is often noted but neither confirms nor excludes the diagnosis of appendicitis. Pyuria is not indicative of appendicitis and suggests renal disease.

55. **(4)** Red currant jelly stools are seen in intussusception and are caused by a mixture of stool, mucus, and blood. Clay-colored stools are seen with hepatitis. Projectile vomiting is associated with pyloric stenosis. Infants with intussusception usually have periods of severe pain followed by intervals in which they appear comfortable. Constant or recurrent abdominal pain is experienced by about 10% of healthy children 5–15 years of age. School phobia may be associated with the etiology of the pain. An organic etiology is found in less than 10% of clients.

56. **(1)** The major symptom of reflux is vomiting or regurgitation. It may occur during sleep, and frequently after feeding. Poor weight gain, hyperirritability, and refusal of feeding may be signs in some infants but are not the major symptoms. Fever or diarrhea may be present in clients with acute otitis media, gastroenteritis, or urinary tract infections.

57. **(1)** The optimal therapy for GERD should include frequent small feedings, burping after each feeding, and placing the baby on an inclined surface at 30 degrees. The prone position is not advocated because it allows gravity to promote reflux and sudden infant death syndrome (SIDS). The supine position leads to more reflux compared with the prone position. The effectiveness of thickened feedings has not been demonstrated because it is believed to delay gastric emptying and thus promotes reflux. Proton pump inhibitors are useful in controlling esophagitis, but long-term effects in infants are not defined. Pharmacologic therapy in young infants has received scant justification in the research literature.

58. **(4)** The recommendations for an infant born to an HBsAg-positive mother are that the baby should have one dose of hepatitis B immunoglobulin (by 12 hours after birth) and a complete three-dose immunization of hepatitis B vaccine. The vaccine will stimulate the newborn's active immunity.

59. **(2)** Classic signs and symptoms of Hirschsprung's disease in later infancy include alternating diarrhea and constipation and abdominal distention. The stools are offensive and ribbon-like, the abdomen is enlarged, and the veins are prominent. The other listed physical findings are not usually found in Hirschsprung's disease but are prevalent in other GI disorders.

60. **(4)** Gastroenteritis is the most common cause of abdominal pain in all age groups. The incidence of appendicitis increases after age 5 and peaks between 15 and 30 years. Intussusception and incarcerated hernias are uncommon and certainly occur less often than gastroenteritis in children.

61. **(3)** Parasitic infestations cause recurrent episodes of abdominal pain, often with diarrhea, nausea, and vomiting, depending on the type of infestation. Musculoskeletal pain is usually sharp and recurs with various activities or body movements that trigger the pain. Chronic stool retention occurs in a child with a history of ineffective toilet training. There is often a family history of constipation. All the other conditions present with acute symptoms, except for psychogenic pain that is recurrent, which is a diagnosis of exclusion.

62. **(3)** The location of the injury suggests a ruptured spleen. Although bowel and bladder problems are possible with blunt trauma to the abdomen, the upper abdominal location makes a spleen injury more likely. Older children may complain of dizziness, fatigue, chest pain, and palpitations due to arrhythmias, but hematomas are not usually present.

63. **(3)** Lactose intolerance is common among Asian clients. The primary symptoms are bloating, flatulence, abdominal cramps, and diarrhea 2 hours after eating food containing lactose. Symptoms of irritable bowel syndrome (IBS) include abdominal pain and diarrhea alternating with constipation. IBS is more common during late adolescence. Hirschsprung's disease is four times more common in boys than girls; 10%–15% of clients have Down syndrome. Food allergies are common in children under age 3 years. Clinical findings occur minutes to 2 hours after ingestion of the food. Clinical findings include hives, facial angioedema, flushing, and throat itching.

64. **(2)** Right upper quadrant pain during exercise, malaise, nausea, and vomiting are early signs of hepatitis A. Elevated IgM antibodies indicate a recent or current infection. Clinical findings of cholecystitis include colicky pain in the right upper quadrant with radiation to the flanks after a large meal. Mononucleosis, common in college-age adults and young children, has the classic triad of fever, exudative pharyngitis, and adenopathy (particularly posterior cervical). Hepatitis B causes symptoms ranging from asymptomatic seroconversion to acute illness with malaise, anorexia, and nausea to fatal hepatitis.

65. **(2)** To rule out appendicitis (although rare, it can occur in young children), further physical examination is necessary, as well as diagnostic testing and assessment for lactose intolerance, urinary tract infection, or extraabdominal causes. Assessment of dietary intake and prescribing pediatric Fleet enemas would not be appropriate if surgery is indicated.

66. **(1)** Objects 5 cm or larger have difficulty passing the ligament of Treitz and other points of narrowing, such as the gastroesophageal junction. Ingested foreign bodies tend to lodge in areas of natural constriction.

67. **(2)** Increased abdominal pressure after eating with the infant in a supine position can result in passage of gastric contents into the esophagus, which often be aspirated during sleep, resulting in the forceful coughing, resultant emesis, and esophageal reflux. Suck-swallow incoordination can cause the same problems regardless of position, as can tracheoesophageal fistula. Colic is characterized by severe crying for more than 3 hours a day, but in healthy well-fed infants.

Pharmacology

68. **(2)** Ribavirin has been associated with birth defects. Acetaminophen is not recommended because it can be hepatotoxic. Ginko is not recommended because it decreases platelet aggregation. The client should eat frequent small meals due to the nausea.

69. **(4)** For clients with recurring symptoms after a course of treatment for PUD, the nurse practitioner should consult the physician. The client is having symptoms of active bleeding, and endoscopy may be indicated at this point. The physician should be consulted regarding the next step. Omeprazole, a proton pump inhibitor that inhibits acid secretion, is useful for hypergastrinemia, and may be useful in PUD clients not controlled by H_2 antagonists in the absence of active bleeding.

70. **(3)** H$_2$ blockers, changes in diet, and weight reduction are the first-line treatments for GERD. The client should be advised to sit up after meals and sleep with his head elevated. Anticholinergics (propantheline) may increase the problem by lowering the LES pressure. Omeprazole is not recommended for the first phase of treatment and is indicated for clients whose symptoms persist after 6 weeks of standard doses of H$_2$ receptor antagonist therapy.

71. **(3)** Goals of PUD treatment include relief of pain, healing of ulcer, and cost-effectiveness. The proton pump inhibitors heal 90% of duodenal ulcers after 4 weeks and 90% of gastric ulcers after 8 weeks. Proton pump inhibitors such as omeprazole are recommended for ulcers because these drugs provide faster pain relief and more rapid healing than H$_2$ antagonists. Anticholinergics (doxepin, pirenzepine) are useful when used with the H$_2$ receptors but are limited by side effects and used only in Canada and Europe at this time. Clarithromycin is used in eradication therapy for 10–14 days against active *H. pylori*–associated ulcer.

72. **(1)** Therapy with a cyclooxygenase (COX-2) selective agent (celecoxib, rofecoxib) is recommended for the majority of clients at high risk of NSAID-induced complications. Prostaglandins such as isoprostol are also used to decrease recurrent ulcerations in clients requiring NSAIDs but have not been shown to increase ulcer healing. Cimetidine has been shown to increase healing. Doxepin and pirenzepine are not currently prescribed in the United States.

73. **(2)** If a person exposed to a client known to be positive for hepatitis B has sufficient immunity to hepatitis B, no treatment is necessary. If this same person had not been vaccinated, in addition to initiation of the hepatitis B vaccine series, HBIG 0.06 ml/kg IM is also administered. If an exposed person has had an inadequate immune response to the hepatitis B vaccine series, a hepatitis B booster should be given. There is no need to repeat the series. If the response to the hepatitis B vaccine series is unknown, test the exposed person's HBsAg level and decide which intervention, if any, is needed.

74. **(1)** Clients with refractory ulcers due to *H. pylori* are successfully treated with the triple-drug therapy of omeprazole, amoxicillin (or metronidazole if penicillin allergic), and clarithromycin. An H$_2$ receptor may be substituted for the proton pump inhibitor (omeprazole) for less expensive therapy. Treatment should be given for 10–14 days. After completion of *H. pylori* eradication therapy, treatment should continue with a proton pump inhibitor or H$_2$ receptor antagonist for 4–8 weeks to promote healing of the ulcer. Cephalosporins are not recommended.

75. **(2)** Sulfasalazine therapy for clients with mild ulcerative colitis results in symptomatic improvement in 50%–75% of cases. If no response is seen after 2–4 weeks, the addition of prednisone is recommended. This drug prevents relapse of ulcerative colitis once remission is induced. The other drugs listed are not recommended as first-line treatment.

76. **(2)** Since 25% of clients are effectively treated with lifestyle changes, therapy should begin with use of these measures. If these are not completely effective, an H$_2$ receptor antagonist can be added; twice-daily dosing is recommended. Omeprazole is recommended only for refractory cases after 6 weeks of standard doses of H$_2$ receptor antagonists. Cisapride is not recommended due to possible cardiac side effects. Lifestyle changes and antacids as needed are recommended as initial therapy.

77. **(1)** To minimize the risk of a contact developing hepatitis A, immunoglobulin 0.02 ml/kg should be given as soon as possible after exposure. It has not been shown to be effective if administered more than 2 weeks after exposure.

78. **(3)** Treatment with TMP-SMX shortens the course and prevents further spread of the organism. Prevention of dehydration that can result from the diarrhea is accomplished through symptomatic treatment (clear liquids for 24–48 hours, no dairy products, electrolyte-rich sports drinks, advance diet as tolerated). Antidiarrheal medications are not recommended because intestinal motility is important in recovery. Option #4 would be appropriate treatment for nonpregnant adults who have giardiasis.

79. **(1)** The Emetrol dose for adults is 15–30 ml. Promethazine 25 mg can be given to children over 12 years old (not 6 years old) and adults. The older child and adult dose for hydroxyzine is 25–100 mg. Trimethobenzamide is dosed at 200 mg, not 10 mg.

80. **(3)** NSAIDs are more often associated with mucosal disruptions causing gastric ulcers. *H. pylori* is associated with mucosal disruption that leads to PUD. Alcohol and smoking are not causes of GI mucosal disruption.

81. **(4)** For unvaccinated clients with exposure to hepatitis B, one dose of hepatitis B immune globulin (HBIG) is administered and the HBV vaccine series initiated. HBIG may be protective or may attenuate the severity of the illness if given within 7 days of exposure (adult dose of 0.06 ml/kg). If the client thinks the individual may have been vaccinated but does not know if there was a response, the nurse practitioner may have prevaccination antibody testing done. The HBe antibody is drawn to determine the potential for transmission; it generally appears about 3 months after onset of infection.

82. **(3)** The only contraindication to the hepatitis B vaccine is prior anaphylaxis or severe hypersensitivity to the vaccine or components of the vaccine.

83. **(2)** Vancomycin causes problems with nephrotoxicity and ototoxicity (eighth cranial nerve). Renal function should be monitored regularly with laboratory tests and the client evaluated frequently for hearing loss. The geriatric client is particularly susceptible.

84. **(3)** This is a common observation for a client taking Pepto-Bismol. He may also experience a problem with discoloration of his tongue. The stool discoloration is not related to bleeding or metronidazole.

85. **(3)** The drug of choice for treating *Giardia* is metronidazole 5 mg/kg (up to 250 mg) tid × 5 days (80%–95% effective). This drug is well tolerated in children. Metronidazole has a disulfiram-like effect and should not be used in children or adolescents receiving ethanol-containing medications. All the other drugs are ineffective for *Giardia*. Tetracycline should not be prescribed to children under age 8 for any reason.

86. **(4)** H$_2$ blockers are not effective in preventing ulcerations from NSAIDs. If the client is using NSAIDs to control the pain from arthritis, the nurse practitioners should consider changing to a prostaglandin (misoprostol) or proton pump inhibitor (omeprazole) to prevent NSAID-induced ulcer.

87. **(1)** Small frequent meals are recommended due to drug side effects of nausea, vomiting, and fatigue.

13

Hematology

Physical Examination & Diagnostic Tests

1. On physical examination a palpable, firm, non-tender supraclavicular lymph node is noted on the left side of the body. This finding is consistent with a diagnosis of:

   1. Bacterial infection draining from the internal jugular chain.

   2. Thoracic or abdominal malignancy.

   3. Inflammation of the tonsils and adenoids.

   4. Non-Hodgkin's lymphoma.

2. Which test is most important for diagnosing iron deficiency anemia?

   1. Direct Coombs.

   2. Serum folate level.

   3. Serum ferritin.

   4. Red blood cell (RBC) count.

3. The term *shotty* is often used to describe lymph nodes that are:

   1. Tender, mobile, and >5 mm.

   2. Small and pellet-like.

   3. Discrete and cystic.

   4. Irregular, soft, and fixed to surrounding tissue.

4. A macrocytic, normochromic anemia is diagnosed in an elderly male client. What should be the next test(s) ordered?

   1. Serum iron and total iron-binding capacity (TIBC) levels.

   2. Bone marrow biopsy.

   3. Colonoscopy.

   4. Vitamin B_{12} and RBC/folate levels.

5. The nurse practitioner would suspect dissemi- nated intravascular coagulation (DIC) if the client's laboratory results, including prothrom- bin time (PT), indicated:

   1. Increased PT, decreased platelet count, and decreased fibrinogen.

   2. Decreased PT, increased hematocrit, and increased fibrinogen.

   3. Increased platelet count, decreased hemat- ocrit, and increased PT.

   4. Increased platelet count, increased hemat- ocrit, and decreased PT.

6. In the examination of lymph nodes the nurse practitioner understands:

   1. Children are more likely to develop general- ized lymphadenopathy than adults in response to a mild infection.

   2. Older adults frequently have enlarged, non- tender supraclavicular and epitrochlear lymph nodes due to aging.

   3. Lymphadenopathy in an adult indicates acute or chronic infection and rarely malig- nancy.

   4. Enlarged neck lymph nodes in children with no other physical findings are highly suspi- cious of Burkitt's lymphoma.

7. After confirming the diagnosis of iron deficiency anemia in an adult client based on complete blood count (CBC), peripheral smear, serum iron, TIBC, and serum ferritin, what would be the next essential test for the nurse practitioner to order?

   1. Stool guaiac ×3.

   2. Prothrombin time/partial thromboplastin time (PT/PTT).

   3. Liver function tests.

   4. Endoscopy.

8. Evaluation of an elderly male client reveals a macrocytic, normochromic anemia. Subsequent testing shows normal folate level and decreased vitamin B_{12} level. Further evaluation could include:

   1. Referral to a hematologist for a bone marrow biopsy.

   2. Schilling's test.

   3. Upper gastrointestinal (GI) series.

   4. No tests are indicated at this time.

9. The most sensitive test for the diagnosis of sickle cell anemia is:

   1. CBC with a peripheral smear.

   2. Bone marrow biopsy and aspiration.

   3. Hemoglobin electrophoresis.

   4. Hemoglobin and hematocrit.

10. A mother brings her school-age child to the clinic and reports a recent history of easy fati- gability ("he can't keep up with his brother any more"), unexplained bruising, and multiple courses of antibiotics for symptoms of upper res- piratory infection (URI) during the past 6 months. Physical examination reveals scattered bruising in no apparent pattern, pallor, and cer- vical lymphadenopathy. What should be the first step of the diagnostic workup for this child?

    1. Chest x-ray and electrocardiogram (ECG).

    2. Liver function tests and abdominal ultrasound.

    3. PT/PTT.

    4. CBC with differential and platelet count.

11. In evaluating the laboratory findings for a child with iron deficiency anemia, the nurse practi- tioner expects:

    1. Mean corpuscular volume (MCV) 80 (μm^3) and low reticulocyte count.

    2. MCV 120 and hemoglobin 12 gm.

    3. MCV 99 and hematocrit 34%.

    4. MCV 96 and normal reticulocyte count.

12. The nurse practitioner explains a bone marrow aspiration procedure to a 4-year-old child. Which behavior of the child would reflect effec- tive teaching?

    1. Appears calm as the nurse takes her for the procedure.

    2. Asks if she can have ice cream after the pro- cedure.

    3. States that her blood is bad and "the doctor will make it better."

    4. Points at her doll and says, "They have to put a needle here to look at my blood."

13. An elderly male client presents to the office with complaints of fatigue, dizziness, decreased activity tolerance, and occasional bounding heart rate. Physical examination reveals pallor (including mucous membranes), tachycardia, and general appearance of lethargy. The nurse practitioner orders CBC with differential, peripheral smear, serum iron, TIBC, and serum ferritin because there is a high index of suspicion for:

    1. Sideroblastic anemia.

    2. Pernicious anemia.

    3. Folic acid deficiency anemia.

    4. Iron deficiency anemia.

14. Anemia of chronic disease would reveal which of the following laboratory findings?

    1. Decreased iron, decreased TIBC, and decreased serum ferritin.

    2. Decreased iron, decreased TIBC, and increased serum ferritin.

    3. Decreased iron, increased TIBC, and decreased serum ferritin.

    4. Decreased iron, increased TIBC, and increased serum ferritin.

15. Which of the following statements is true concerning the leukemias?

    1. Liver function studies are decreased in the later stages of the disease process.

    2. Initial white blood cell (WBC) count is the most important predictor of prognosis.

    3. Thrombocytopenia is rarely present.

    4. The prognosis is better if a child is younger than 2 years.

Disorders

16. Which of the following signs and symptoms are associated with a diagnosis of childhood acute lymphocytic leukemia (ALL)?

    1. Splenomegaly, facial rash, and cough.

    2. Expiratory wheezing, bleeding, and hepatomagaly.

    3. Bleeding, fever, and pain.

    4. Bone pain, fever, and night sweats.

17. Sickle cell anemia is caused by:

    1. Exposure to ionizing radiation.

    2. Genetically induced production of abnormal hemoglobin S.

    3. Deficiency of dietary folic acid.

    4. Long-term use of thiazide diuretics.

18. An adult client presents to the nurse practitioner with a history of erythrocytosis. One common complaint that could cause a serious complication for this client is:

    1. A laceration.

    2. Vomiting and diarrhea.

    3. Coughing.

    4. Dizziness.

19. A client has a folic acid deficiency anemia. The nurse practitioner teaches the client to eat foods rich in folic acid, such as:

    1. Green leafy vegetables, nuts, and liver.

    2. Carrots, salmon, and avocados.

    3. Cottage cheese, yogurt, and skim milk.

    4. Lima beans, brussels sprouts, and potatoes.

20. Which of the changes occur in the RBC indices for pernicious anemia?

    1. Microcytic, normochromic.

    2. Microcytic, hypochromic.

    3. Normocytic, normochromic.

    4. Macrocytic, normochromic.

21. Which statement is true concerning thalessemia?

    1. It is characterized by defective lymphocyte synthesis.

    2. Thalessemia minor does not require pharmacologic treatment.

    3. Thalessemia major is associated with high RBC counts and elevated serum iron.

    4. It is characterized with an acute onset of symptoms leading to leukocytosis.

22. Iron deficiency anemia is an example of:

    1. Macrocytic, normochromic anemia.

    2. Macrocytic, hypochromic anemia.

    3. Microcytic, hypochromic anemia.

    4. Normocytic, normochromic anemia.

23. An adult client with pernicious anemia may present with which signs and symptoms?

    1. Paresthesias, unsteady gait, lethargy, and fatigue.

    2. Hepatomegaly, jaundice, and right upper quadrant pain.

    3. Hypertension, angina, and peripheral edema.

    4. Blurred vision, diplopia, and decreased visual acuity.

24. Anemia of chronic disease is a:

    1. Normochromic, normocytic anemia.

    2. Normochromic, microcytic anemia.

    3. Hypochromic, microcytic anemia.

    4. Hypochromic, macrocytic anemia.

25. A young adult presents to the clinic for a routine checkup. History is unremarkable, but on physical examination the nurse practitioner palpates an enlarged (2-cm) mobile, nontender, rubbery lymph node on the left posterior cervical chain. What is the practitioner's next step?

    1. Order a throat culture and monospot test.

    2. Refer to a surgeon for a lymph node biopsy.

    3. Order a STAT chest x-ray.

    4. No intervention is necessary at this time.

26. The nurse practitioner understands that "B" symptoms associated with non-Hodgkin's lymphoma (NHL) include:

    1. Bruising and bleeding.

    2. Peripheral edema, shortness of breath, and ascites.

    3. Fever, night sweats, and unexplained weight loss (>10% of body weight).

    4. Headache, fatigue, and weakness.

27. In teaching a client with anemia to include foods rich in iron in the diet, the nurse practitioner encourages the client to eat:

    1. Cheese, milk, and yogurt.

    2. Red beans, whole-grain bread, and bran cereal.

    3. Tomatoes, cabbage, and citrus fruits.

    4. Beef, spinach, and peanut butter.

28. Anemia of chronic disease is associated with:

    1. Malnutrition and vitamin B_{12} deficiency.

    2. Infections, inflammation, and neoplasms.

    3. Traumatic injuries and folate deficiency.

    4. Excessive menstrual flow, trauma, and heredity.

29. The nurse practitioner is concerned about the development of which complication in a young child with a diagnosis of iron deficiency anemia?

    1. Crohn's disease.

    2. Pernicious anemia.

    3. Impaired cognitive development.

    4. Hepatic and spleen dysfunction.

30. The nurse practitioner is counseling a client who has a child with sickle cell disease. The client asks, "If my child has sickle cell disease, does that mean that I'm at an increased risk for developing the same problems?" The nurse practitioner's response would be based on which principle of sickle cell disease?

    1. The mother is at an increased risk because the condition is inherited; she probably has the condition and has not had an active episode.

    2. The mother is not at risk for developing the condition because males are carriers of the trait.

    3. The mother has a 25% chance of being affected by the disease, especially during times of stress.

    4. Both parents are carriers of the trait but do not have active disease; each child has a 25% chance of having the condition.

31. During a clinic visit, the nurse practitioner notes that an 11-month-old infant is pale. The physical examination reveals pulse 170, height 25th percentile, and weight 95th percentile. The nurse questions the mother about the infant's diet. The mother states that the infant eats mostly pureed fruits and whole milk. The nurse practitioner expects which diagnostic finding?

    1. Normal hemoglobin.
    2. Elevated MCV.
    3. Low serum ferritin level.
    4. Macrocytic, hyperchromic anemia.

32. The nurse practitioner knows that an infant who is exclusively breast-fed is at risk for developing iron deficiency anemia at age:

    1. 1 month.
    2. 2 months.
    3. 4 months.
    4. 6 months.

33. The nurse practitioner understands that most adult clients with Hodgkin's disease present with:

    1. Nausea, vomiting, and diarrhea.
    2. Night sweats, weight loss, and fever.
    3. Painless, movable mass in the neck, axilla, or groin.
    4. Hepatosplenomegaly with a painful mass in the mediastinum.

34. What is the most common leukemia found in the older adult, typically asymptomatic and characterized by median survival of about 10 years?

    1. Acute myelogenous.
    2. Chronic myelogenous.
    3. Acute lymphocytic.
    4. Chronic lymphocytic.

35. Folic acid deficiency most often results from:

    1. Lead exposure.
    2. Poor dietary habits.

    3. Gastrointestinal bleeding.
    4. Genetic defect.

Pharmacology

36. The nurse practitioner determines that an adult male client has an iron deficiency anemia, and has ruled out gastrointestinal (GI) bleeding as the cause. The nurse practitioner:

    1. Refers the client to a hematologist.
    2. Administer iron dextran 50 mg IM weekly for 4 weeks.
    3. Prescribes ferrous sulfate 300 mg PO tid and schedules the client return in 1 month for a repeat CBC, serum iron, and TIBC.
    4. Schedules the client return in 6 months for additional stool guaiac testing.

37. What information would the nurse practitioner include in teaching a client about the treatment of vitamin B_{12} deficiency?

    1. The client will be taking vitamin B_{12} tablets twice daily for 1 year.
    2. The client will be taking oral folic acid supplements daily for life.
    3. The client will receive monthly cyanocobalamin (vitamin B_{12}) injections for life (after being given weekly injections for the first month).
    4. The client will require iron supplementation and monthly blood transfusions until the deficiency is corrected.

38. Treatment of anemia of chronic disease should include:

    1. Folic acid supplement 1 mg PO qd.
    2. Iron sulfate ($FeSO_4$) supplement 300 mg PO tid.
    3. Treatment of the underlying condition.
    4. Weekly epoetin alfa (Epogen) injections.

39. The nurse practitioner has prescribed elemental iron 6 mg/kg/day in three divided doses for a toddler diagnosed with iron deficiency anemia. What instructions would the nurse include for the parents?

    1. Give the iron with food to increase the absorption of the medication.

    2. Give the medication through a straw to decrease the staining of the teeth.

    3. Avoid foods containing ascorbic acid, which decreases absorption of the medication.

    4. If a dose is missed, double up on the next two doses.

40. After initiating vitamin B_{12} therapy, the nurse practitioner would expect which of the following at a 2-week follow-up visit to the clinic?

    1. Ferritin level of 40 ng/ml.

    2. Reduced RBCs, WBCs, and platelets.

    3. Increased macrocytosis and anisocytosis.

    4. Increased hemoglobin/hematocrit and reticulocyte count.

41. It is recommended to administer a 0.5 ml (25 mg) test dose of which medication?

    1. Nascobol (intranasal B_{12} gel).

    2. Folic acid.

    3. Iron dextran.

    4. Ferrous sulfate (Feosol).

42. What is the prophylactic treatment regimen for adult clients without infection or fever who have neutropenia?

    1. Trimethoprim-sulfamethoxazole 100 mg 2 tabs PO bid twice weekly, acyclovir (Zovirax) 400 mg PO bid, and fluconazole (Diflucan) 100 mg PO qd.

    2. Azithromycin (Zithromax pack) and fluconazole (Diflucan) 100 mg PO qd.

    3. Trimethoprim-sulfamethoxazole 100 mg 2 tabs PO bid qd and dexamethosone (Decadron 5–12 pack).

    4. No medication needed with clients who do not have a fever or infection.

Answers & Rationales

Physical Examination & Diagnostic Tests

1. **(2)** A Virchow's node in the left supraclavicular region is of concern due to the high correlation with abdominal or thoracic malignancy. Infections and inflammatory conditions produce tender, inflamed lymph nodes.

2. **(3)** The serum ferritin correlates with total body iron stores because it is the major iron storage protein. Its value is reduced in iron deficiency anemia. Direct Coombs measures in vivo RBC coating by immunoglobulins and is positive in autoimmune hemolytic anemia, blood transfusion reactions, and drug-induced hemolysis. Serum folate measures the folic acid level in the blood.

3. **(2)** "Shotty," or small and pellet-like, lymph nodes that are movable, cool, nontender, discrete, and up to 3 mm in diameter are usually considered normal.

4. **(4)** It is important to determine the type of macrocytic anemia so that the appropriate therapy can be ordered. Therefore the vitamin B_{12} and RBC/folate levels would be ordered. These tests would determine if the client has a pernicious anemia (the most common type) or a folate deficiency (also common in elderly clients). Serum iron and TIBC would be ordered if an iron deficiency anemia was suspected (not in this case because this is a microcytic anemia). There is no indication for a colonoscopy. It would be premature to order a bone marrow biopsy without performing initial testing and potentially overlooking an easily treated condition (e.g., pernicious anemia, folate deficiency anemia).

5. **(1)** DIC is a complication of infection, malignancy, and sometimes trauma. DIC is the inappropriate accelerated systemic activation of the coagulation cascade, resulting in simultaneous hemorrhage and thrombosis. Laboratory results would show increased PT and decreased platelet count and fibrinogen in response to the hemorrhage and clotting.

6. **(1)** Children often have generalized lymphadenopathy in response to mild infections of the skin or respiratory tract. Palpable lymph nodes are generally not present in healthy individuals, but some may have small, discrete, nontender nodes that are not clinically significant. Enlarged lymph nodes may indicate infection, inflammation, and malignancy in both children and adults. Painless, firm supraclavicular or cervical lymph node is a common sign of Hodgkin's disease in children, not Burkitt's lymphoma, in which the child has other associated symptoms depending on the system affected.

7. **(1)** Stool guaiac testing would identify blood loss from the gastrointestinal tract—the most common cause of iron deficiency anemia. The other tests should be done if the stool guaiac results are positive. Finding the cause of the iron deficiency is paramount, and the stool guaiac test is an easy, noninvasive method of ruling out bleeding as the cause.

8. **(2)** Schilling's test will determine the cause of the vitamin B_{12} deficiency. It will distinguish between inadequate intake (an intrinsic factor deficiency) or a malabsorption problem. This will allow the practitioner to prescribe the

most appropriate therapy for the client. A bone marrow biopsy and an upper GI series are not indicated at this time.

9. **(3)** Normal and abnormal hemoglobin can be detected by electrophoresis, which matches hemolyzed RBC material against standard bands for the various known hemoglobins, including hemoglobin S, the abnormal hemoglobin associated with sickle cell anemia. CBC with peripheral smear and hemoglobin/hematocrit would not yield enough information to diagnose sickle cell anemia. Bone marrow biopsy would not be necessary and would not indicate the presence of hemoglobin S.

10. **(4)** This clinical presentation would make the practitioner consider the diagnosis of leukemia, necessitating a workup. CBC with differential, along with platelet count (indicators of bone marrow function), is the diagnostic approach for leukemia. Further testing may be necessary, but the workup should always include a CBC.

11. **(1)** The findings associated with iron deficiency anemia include low MCV (<90), decreased hemoglobin/hematocrit, and low reticulocyte count. Elevated MCV is associated with macrocytic anemias (e.g., pernicious anemia).

12. **(4)** Dolls and puppets are effective teaching tools for the preschool child. Using the doll reflects the child's understanding of the procedure. Children will often withdraw and appear calm when they have feelings of anxiety.

13. **(4)** This client's clinical picture is a classic presentation for anemia. Further testing would be needed to determine the type of anemia involved. The most common cause in elderly men is GI bleeding, which would cause an iron deficiency anemia. The tests that were ordered would confirm or rule out this diagnosis; the peripheral smear is especially important in diagnosing the specific type of anemia. If the smear ruled out the diagnosis of iron deficiency anemia, it would lead the practitioner to other diagnoses (including the remaining choices) and the appropriate laboratory tests required for confirmation.

14. **(2)** Normal to increased iron stores (serum ferritin) with concurrent low serum iron is the hallmark finding of anemia of chronic disease.

Serum iron is decreased along with TIBC. Options #1 and #4 contain incorrect information for the anemias. Option #3 contains the findings for iron deficiency anemia.

15. **(2)** The client is at higher risk if initial WBC count >50,000 cells/mm^3. Liver function studies and uric acid levels are increased. Approximately 75% of clients have marked thrombocytopenia with platelets <100,000 cells/mm^3. Prognosis is poor for children <2 years and >10 years of age. The most likely diagnosis in children is acute lymphocytic (ALL), then acute myelogenous (AML) leukemia. For adults the most likely diagnosis is chronic myelogenous (CML), then chronic lymphocytic (CLL) leukemia.

Disorders

16. **(3)** Early presenting symptoms of ALL include pallor, bleeding, pain, and fever associated with infiltration of the bone marrow of proliferative lymphocytic cells, which ultimately leads to bone marrow failure. The symptoms listed in Options #1 and #2 are often found in juvenile chronic myelogenous leukemia (CML). Option #4 symptoms are often noted in CML.

17. **(2)** Sickle cell anemia is a genetic disorder characterized by the production of hemoglobin S, an anemia secondary to shortened erythrocyte survival, microvascular occlusion by sickle-shaped erythrocytes, and increased susceptibility to certain infections. Exposure to ionizing radiation has been associated with the development of certain malignancies, especially leukemia. A deficiency of dietary folic acid does not cause sickle cell anemia, although folic acid is used in the treatment of these clients to help increase hematopoiesis and aid in recovery from aplastic events. Long-term use of thiazide diuretics has been implicated in the development of hemolytic or aplastic anemias in rare cases.

18. **(2)** Erythrocytosis (or polycythemia) can be worsened by dehydration from any cause. Coughing and dizziness will have no effect on the condition, and a laceration may actually improve the symptoms because of the blood loss.

19. **(1)** Green leafy vegetables, nuts, and liver are excellent sources of folic acid. Also, cereals and breads are now fortified with folic acid. The other foods are not significant sources of folic acid.

20. **(4)** A macrocytic (MCV >100), normochromic anemia resulting from atrophic gastric mucosa not secreting intrinsic factor is the definition of pernicious anemia. These indices could also include folic acid deficiency anemia. Options #1 and #2 could include iron deficiency anemia or anemia of chronic disease. Option #3 could also include anemia of chronic disease.

21. **(2)** Thalessemias are chronic, inherited anemias characterized by defective hemoglobin synthesis leading to a decreased RBC count, profound microcytosis, normal serum iron, and normal RBC distribution width (RDW) in thalessemia minor, which does not require pharmacologic treatment. Clients with thalessemia minor should not be given iron supplements to resolve anemia. Clients with thalessemia major are usually managed by a hematologist.

22. **(3)** Iron deficiency anemia is a microcytic, hypochromic anemia. The RBCs are smaller (microcytic) due to the decrease in hemoglobin production caused by inadequate amounts of iron, which also makes the cell appear pale (hypochromic). The other selections describe other types of anemia, which would be determined by the peripheral smear.

23. **(1)** Vitamin B_{12} deficiency may result in neurologic signs and symptoms, including paresthesias, unsteady gait, lethargy, and fatigue. These findings are specific to pernicious anemia and must be assessed in all clients who present with anemia. The other signs and symptoms are not characteristic of pernicious anemia.

24. **(1)** Anemia of chronic disease is a chronic normochromic, normocytic anemia. There is normal production of hemoglobin, along with normal maturation of RBCs.

25. **(2)** Lymphadenopathy as described, without evidence of infection, should always be referred to a surgeon for biopsy, the only definitive test to rule out a malignancy (a frequent cause of lymphadenopathy not caused by infectious processes). No signs or symptoms suggest the need for a throat culture, monospot test, or chest x-ray. Not intervening is inappropriate because the cause of lymphadenopathy needs to be determined.

26. **(3)** This constellation of symptoms (fever, night sweats, weight loss) is used in the staging of NHL, the presence of which is considered to be a poor prognostic indicator. The other symptoms may occur depending on the amount of disease involvement, but they are not considered "B" symptoms, also known as constitutional symptoms.

27. **(4)** Beef, spinach, and peanut butter are iron-rich foods. Options #1, #2, and #3 are examples of foods rich in calcium, fiber, and vitamin C, respectively.

28. **(2)** Anemia or chronic disease is associated with infections (e.g., tuberculosis), chronic inflammatory conditions (e.g., systemic lupus erythematosus, rheumatoid arthritis), and malignancies. Excessive blood loss from menstrual flow or traumatic injuries would more likely cause an iron deficiency anemia. Malnutrition can contribute to iron, vitamin B_{12}, and folate deficiencies.

29. **(3)** With iron deficiency anemia the amount of oxygen-carrying hemoglobin is reduced. Long-term oxygen deprivation can lead to impaired cognitive and motor development. Pernicious anemia is associated with lack of intrinsic factor. Crohn's disease has a familial incidence and leads to diarrhea-related problems. The liver and spleen are both involved in RBC production.

30. **(4)** Sickle cell disease is transmitted by both parents, who have the sickle cell trait but do not show symptoms of disease. Each pregnancy carries a 25% chance of sickle cell disease and a 25% chance of the child carrying the trait.

31. **(3)** Iron deficiency anemia is often found in this age group, especially in infants who do not eat a balanced diet that includes foods rich in iron (e.g., iron-fortified cereals). This is a microcytic, hypochromic anemia with a decrease in serum iron (ferritin). MCV would be decreased (<90).

32. **(4)** The normal, full-term infant is born with sufficient iron stores to prevent iron deficiency for the first 6 months of life.

33. **(3)** Most clients present with a painless, movable mass in the neck, axilla, or groin. Older clients may present with fatigue, weight loss, persistent fever, and night sweats. Often the client has pain in diseased areas after consuming alcohol (an unexplained finding). Hepatosplenomegaly presents with advanced disease.

34. **(4)** Chronic lymphocytic leukemia (CLL) is found primarily in middle-aged and older adults (<10% of clients under age 50). Acute myelogenous leukemia (AML) incidence increases with age (about 50% of clients under age 50). Chronic myelogenous leukemia (CML) occurs at a median age of 45 years. Acute lymphocytic leukemia (ALL) is most common in children and gradually increases in frequency in later life.

35. **(2)** Folic acid deficiency most often results from dietary deficits and frequently affects elderly, chronically ill, and alcoholic clients and food faddists. Pregnancy requires an increase in folic acid, as do disease states such as cancer, chronic inflammation, Crohn's disease, rheumatoid arthritis, and malabsorption syndromes.

Pharmacology

36. **(3)** Treatment with iron orally for at least 6 months is necessary to correct both the anemia and the depleted body iron stores. Iron dextran may be used if the client is unable to take PO medications. The client should have hemoglobin/hematocrit, iron, and TIBC rechecked after 1 month on iron supplementation. If there is no improvement in all parameters, most notably a rise in the hemoglobin by 1 gm/dl, the client should be referred to a hematologist. Referral to a GI specialist or repeat of stool guaiac testing is unnecessary because there is no indication that this client's condition is caused by bleeding.

37. **(3)** If the deficiency is not caused by inadequate intake, the client will require lifetime supplementation of vitamin B_{12}. It must be given as an intramuscular or subcutaneous injection to ensure absorption.

Oral folic acid, iron, and blood transfusions would not treat the cause of the deficiency, and therefore the resulting anemia would not be corrected.

38. **(3)** Treatment of the underlying condition leads to resolution of the anemia of chronic disease. Folic acid and iron supplements are indicated for folate and iron deficiency anemias, respectively. Epoetin alfa injections are indicated for conditions that affect erythropoiesis, including chronic renal failure, chemotherapy-induced anemia, and acquired immunodeficiency syndrome (AIDS). Clients with underlying iron deficiency anemia **and** anemia of chronic disease may benefit from a trial of iron therapy.

39. **(2)** Iron medications can cause staining of the teeth, so it is a good practice to give the medication through a straw. It is best to give iron on an empty stomach (if tolerable) to increase absorption. Ascorbic acid increases absorption of iron. If a dose is missed, it is best to give the dose when it is remembered as long as it is not too close to the next dose. The next two doses would not be increased.

40. **(4)** In addition to a sense of well-being, improved appetite, and decreased neurologic symptoms (gait disturbances, paresthesias, numbness/tingling in fingers, extreme weakness), the hemoglobin/hematocrit and reticulocyte count should increase with vitamin B_{12} therapy.

41. **(3)** The use of IM or IV iron dextran is for clients who cannot tolerate oral supplementation or who have GI disease that limits oral absorption. Therapy should be initiated with a test dose of 0.5 ml (25 mg) to observe for anaphylaxis.

42. **(1)** Adult clients with neutropenia should be treated with prophylactic antibiotics, antivirals, and an antifungal when they have no infection or fever. Broad-spectrum antibiotic treatment is ordered for clients with neutropenic fever and a suspect culture. After blood cultures are obtained, a regimen is started that includes cephalosporin, an aminoglycoside, and extended-spectrum penicillin.

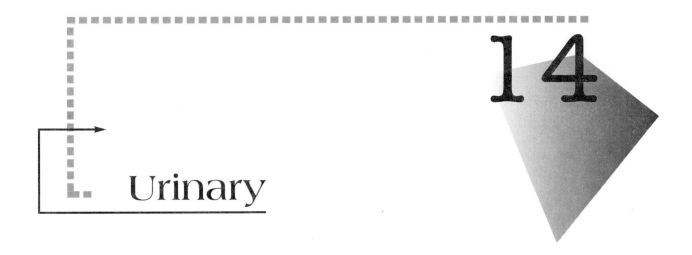

Urinary

Physical Examination & Diagnostic Tests

1. Which urinalysis (UA) findings suggest a urinary tract infection (UTI)?

   1. Protein only.

   2. Alkaline pH and positive nitrite and leukocyte esterase.

   3. Hematuria and pyuria only.

   4. Red color without presence of red blood cells (RBCs).

2. What do intravenous urography and voiding cystourethrography assist in diagnosing?

   1. Congenital anomalies, stone formation, and foreign bodies.

   2. Renal size and presence of a stone.

   3. Problem in the urethra, prostate, or bladder.

   4. Visualization of the ureter and renal pelvis.

3. Physical examination for a child reveals 2+ proteinuria. What would be the next step in the differential diagnosis?

   1. Quantify protein excretion.

   2. Evaluate for orthostatic proteinuria.

   3. Reassure patient and follow up in 6 months.

   4. Evaluate for nephritis.

4. According to the Agency for Health Care Policy and Research (AHCPR) Guideline Panel, the basic continence evaluation done by the primary care provider should include:

   1. History, physical examination, postvoid residual volume, and urinalysis (UA).

   2. Postvoid residual volume, blood urea nitrogen (BUN), serum creatinine, and UA.

   3. History, physical examination, serum glucose, BUN, serum creatinine, and UA.

   4. Urodynamic/endoscopic/imaging tests, UA, and serum creatinine.

5. Which of the following clients would be a good candidate for urodynamic studies (UDS)?

   1. Client with history of stress incontinence and urge incontinence.

   2. Client with recent surgery for bladder suspension.

   3. Client with initial incontinence episode after total knee replacement.

   4. Elderly man with residual volume of 45 ml after 250-ml voiding.

6. The nurse practitioner is evaluating serum blood studies on a client who is experiencing a slight increase in blood pressure (BP). She has no previous history of high BP or other chronic disease. Which serum laboratory value would be of most concern to the practitioner?

   1. Serum creatinine 5.2 mg/dl.

   2. BUN 30 mg/dl.

   3. Serum potassium 4.5 mEq/L.

   4. Serum osmolarity 290 mOsm/kg.

7. When taking a history on voiding patterns in adults, the nurse practitioner knows:

   1. Adults normally void q2–3h in a 24-hour period (8–12 times a day).

   2. First sensation to void occurs when the bladder fills to 200–300 ml.

   3. Normally, 15–20 minutes pass between first urge to void and reaching functional capacity.

   4. Adults typically reach functional (comfortable) capacity at 200–300 ml and may experience some leakage if voiding is delayed.

8. The nurse practitioner expects which findings on examination of an older client with dehydration?

   1. Tongue furrows and skin tenting on forehead.

   2. Specific gravity of urine 1.004.

   3. Pulse rate 58 (strong, regular) and BP 100/62.

   4. Geographic tongue and reduced saliva pool.

9. Which diagnostic test is considered **essential** in the preliminary workup of a client with incontinence?

   1. UA with culture and sensitivity (C&S).

   2. Bedside urodynamic studies.

   3. Intravenous and retrograde pyelography.

   4. Renal sonography.

Disorders

10. A young woman explains to the nurse practitioner that she has been having frequent and painful urination. The nurse practitioner orders a clean-catch urine specimen for routine UA with C&S. Laboratory results show 10^5/ml *Escherichia coli* and 10^4/ml *Staphylococcus epidermidis*. The nurse practitioner would:

    1. Treat the *E. coli.*

    2. Order penicillin (amoxicillin)

    3. Treat the *S. epidermidis.*

    4. Encourage citric fruit juices.

11. An elderly woman is incontinent of urine. Her perineal area is red and excoriated. What would the nurse practitioner advise the family caregiver to **avoid** using on the skin in the perineal area?

    1. Petrolatum.

    2. Moisture-barrier films.

    3. Mild soap and water.

    4. Zinc oxide ointment.

12. A young adult comes to the student health clinic complaining of severe abdominal discomfort and bloody urine. A priority in the diagnostic workup would include:

    1. Intravenous pyelography to rule out a kidney stone.

    2. Straining all urine.

    3. Microscopic urine examination.

    4. 24-hour urine culture.

13. Which plan would be most appropriate for an older client with functional incontinence?

    1. Evaluate need for pads.

    2. Limit fluid intake in the evenings.

3. Perform Credé's maneuver.

4. Provide a bedside commode.

14. A 60-year-old man presents with recurrent urinary tract infections (UTIs). What is the most likely cause?

1. Balanitis.

2. Epididymitis.

3. Chronic bacterial prostatitis.

4. Benign prostatic hypertrophy.

15. What is a possible cause of transient and reversible urinary incontinence?

1. Poor pelvic support causing hypermobility of the base of the female bladder.

2. Lower urinary tract problems, such as carcinoma.

3. Cystocele or uterine prolapse in women.

4. Ingestion of certain medications, such as sedatives, diuretics, anticholinergics, and α-adrenergic agents.

16. Which statement characterizes functional incontinence?

1. Leakage of urine during activities that increase abdominal pressure, such as coughing, sneezing, and laughing.

2. Mainly caused by factors outside the urinary tract, especially immobility, that prohibit proper toileting habits.

3. Characterized by the inability to delay urination, with an abrupt and strong desire to void.

4. Occurrence of incontinence with overdistention of bladder.

17. What are the two most common pathogens in community-acquired UTIs?

1. *Klebsiella pneumoniae* and *Proteus mirabilis*.

2. *Staphylococcus saprophyticus* and *Escherichia coli*.

3. *Proteus mirabilis* and *Staphylococcus saprophyticus*.

4. *Escherichia coli* and *Proteus mirabilis*.

18. What is the usual clinical presentation of an adult client with cystitis?

1. No symptoms noted.

2. Acute onset of chills, fever, flank pain, headache, malaise, and costovertebral angle tenderness.

3. Complaints of dysuria, urgency, frequency, nocturia, and suprapubic heaviness.

4. Signs and symptoms of fever, irritability, decreased appetite, vomiting, diarrhea, constipation, dehydration, and jaundice.

19. In children, hypertension and history of a sore throat may indicate which disorder?

1. Congestive heart failure.

2. Glomerulonephritis.

3. Vasculitis.

4. Cushing's syndrome.

20. Recurrent UTIs in women are caused by relapse or reinfection. The nurse practitioner understands which of the following about relapse?

1. Is less common than reinfection and occurs within 2 weeks of completing drug therapy for the infection.

2. Is responsible for most recurrent UTIs in women.

3. May result from residual urine after voiding due to prolapsed uterus or bladder or lack of estrogen.

4. Can be treated with the same medication regimen used for the original infection.

21. The nurse practitioner understands that the treatment of pyelonephritis:

1. Suggests a structural problem in female clients.

2. Requires hospitalization, parenteral antibiotic therapy, and intravenous voiding pyelography in male clients.

3. Requires hospitalization, parenteral antibiotic therapy, and intravenous voiding pyelography in female clients.

4. Requires no follow-up.

22. When assessing a child with glomerulonephritis, what symptoms would the nurse practitioner expect to be present?

    1. Fever >102°F and bilateral flank pain.

    2. Periorbital edema and increased blood pressure.

    3. Anorexia and complaints of dysuria.

    4. Oliguria with strong concentrated urine.

23. When instructing the parents regarding the course of poststreptococcal glomerulonephritis in their child, the nurse practitioner would tell them to expect bloody urine for how long after onset of diuresis?

    1. 1 week. ✓

    2. 1–2 weeks.

    3. 2–3 weeks.

    4. 4–7 days.

24. What is the term given to the type of urinary incontinence associated with conditions such as Parkinson's disease, Alzheimer's disease, and stroke?

    1. Stress incontinence.

    2. Urge incontinence.

    3. Functional incontinence.

    4. Overflow incontinence.

25. A 40-year-old white man presents to the clinic with a history of uric acid renal calculi. Knowing that the alkaline-ash, low-purine diet is difficult for clients to adhere to, which other option should the nurse practitioner consider?

    1. Monitor the client for another episode.

    2. Discuss the alkaline-ash, low-purine diet in detail with the client.

    3. Start the client on allopurinol (Zyloprim) and monitor serum uric acid level.

    4. Refer the client to a urologist.

26. A mother brings in her 3-year-old daughter to the clinic, stating that she noticed a swelling in the child's abdominal area just below the rib cage on the left side. The nurse practitioner observes a bulging of the area, and the child does not want to be touched due to abdominal tenderness. What is the best action for the nurse practitioner at this visit?

    1. Immediately contact a pediatrician for consultation.

    2. Schedule a referral with a pediatrician in the near future.

    3. Perform UA and draw blood for creatinine and potassium.

    4. Explain to the child that it is necessary to examine the abdomen.

27. A male client presents with complaints of blood in his urine; it is painless and he has no difficulty with urination. The nurse practitioner obtains UA to confirm presence of blood, and no bacteria are present. What is the priority diagnosis that must be ruled out on this client?

    1. Cancer of the prostate.

    2. Prerenal failure.

    3. Renal calculi.

    4. Cancer of the bladder.

28. The nurse practitioner is taking the history of a client who has been diagnosed with renal calculi. What information in the history would the nurse practitioner identify as a precipitating factor in the development of renal calculi?

    1. Increased incidence of UTIs over the past 3 years.

    2. Drinking 6–8 oz of milk daily.

    3. History of fractured femur and prolonged bed rest.

    4. High intake of citrus fruit and high-fiber carbohydrates.

29. A client is diagnosed with renal failure, thought to be postrenal in origin. What would the nurse practitioner identify as a possible precipitating cause of this client's renal failure?

    1. History of myocardial infarction (MI) with severe hypotensive episode.

    2. Advanced prostatic hypertrophy with hematuria.

    3. Renal vascular changes secondary to long history of diabetes.

    4. Exposure to carbon tetrachloride at the job site.

30. A nurse practitioner recognizes which factor as contributing to the development of prerenal failure?

    1. History of an anaphylactic reaction that rendered the client unconscious.

    2. Extended treatment of an infection with gentamicin (Garamycin).

    3. Acute pyelonephritis with subsequent glomerulonephritis.

    4. Renal vascular changes secondary to atherosclerotic disease.

31. The nurse practitioner teaching a female client about bladder health would include all the following guidelines **except**:

    1. Drink at least six to eight glasses of water per day.

    2. Avoid doing Kegel's exercises.

    3. Avoid constipation.

    4. Consider estrogen replacement after menopause.

32. A 75-year-old white woman presents to the clinic with her husband, her primary caregiver. She has a history of multi-infarct dementia (MID), likely from a long history of untreated hypertension. Her husband reports that for the past 2 days she has been agitated and increasingly confused, and he has not been able to redirect her. He denies the addition of new medications or over-the-counter herbal supplements. What would the nurse practitioner suspect?

    1. New infarct.

    2. Worsening of dementia.

    3. Urinary tract infection.

    4. Underlying stress to caregiver.

Pharmacology

33. A client is diagnosed with benign prostatic hypertrophy. Which medication should be recognized by the nurse practitioner as likely to aggravate this condition?

    1. Glyburide (DiaBeta).

    2. Oral buspirone (Buspar).

    3. Inhaled ipratropium (Atrovent).

    4. Ophthalmic timolol (Timoptic).

34. Which of the following agents can be useful for stress incontinence?

    1. Propantheline (Pro-Banthine) 7.5–30 mg three to five times a day.

    2. Oxybutynin (Ditropan) 2.5–5 mg tid to qid.

    3. Doxepin (Sinequan) 10–25 mg qd/bid/tid initially to maximum total daily dose of 25–100 mg.

    4. Conjugated estrogen (Premarin) 0.3–1.25 mg/day orally or vaginally, medroxyprogesterone (progestin) 2.5–10 mg/day continuously or intermittently.

35. To decrease the production of uric acid stones, the nurse practitioner orders which medication?

    1. Allopurinol (Zyloprim).

    2. Potassium citrate (Urocit-K).

    3. Bethanechol (Urecholine).

    4. Phenazopyridine (Pyridium).

36. A 70-year-old woman is treated with oxybutynin (Ditropan) for her urinary frequency and urgency. The nurse practitioner would explain to the client she will probably experience:

    1. Increased sensitivity to sunlight.

    2. Dizziness on standing.

    3. Dry mouth and increased thirst.

    4. Increased bruising.

37. A mother brings her 6-year-old daughter to the clinic. The child is complaining of burning on urination, and the urine is cloudy. A dipstick test of the urine is positive for leukocyte esterase. The mother states the child had a fever with nausea and vomiting the last time she took Gantrisin (sulfisoxazole). An appropriate medication for this client is:

    1. Nitrofurantoin (Macrodantin) 50 mg PO qid × 7 days.

    2. Trimethoprim-sulfamethoxazole (Septra DS) 1 tab PO bid × 10 days.

    3. Ciprofloxacin (Cipro) 200 mg PO bid × 10 days.

    4. Clarithromycin (Biaxin) 250 mg PO bid × 10 days.

38. All the following medications can cause urinary incontinence in the older adult **except**:

    1. Hypnotics.

    2. Antibiotics.

    3. Sedatives.

    4. Antidepressants.

39. The nurse practitioner has selected nitrofurantoin (Macrodantin) for treatment of a chronic UTI in a female geriatric client. Which parameter should the nurse evaluate before administration of this medication?

    1. Creatinine clearance (>50 ml/min).

    2. Levels of serum alanine aminotransferase (ALT).

    3. Current medications that include anticoagulants.

    4. History of allergic reactions to sulfa-based medications.

40. A 46-year-old man with a history of renal calculi presents with complaints of severe flank pain radiating to his groin area. He is also experiencing nausea and vomiting, and his temperature is 99°F. What is the best initial therapy that the nurse practitioner can provide?

    1. Morphine sulfate 10 mg SC.

    2. Ibuprofen (Advil) 600 mg PO q6h.

    3. Increase fluid intake and strain all urine.

    4. Trimethobenzamide (Tigan) 250 mg PO.

41. The nurse practitioner is prescribing nitrofurantoin (Macrodantin) for a woman who is experiencing problems with UTIs. What specific directions should the nurse give this client regarding administration of nitrofurantoin?

    1. Take with food and expect brownish discoloration to urine.

    2. Do not take with milk products; take on empty stomach for better absorption.

    3. Take four times a day until symptoms have subsided for at least 24 hours.

    4. Do not take acetaminophen (Tylenol) or ibuprofen (Advil) with nitrofurantoin.

42. A young woman presents with complaints of burning on urination, frequency, and urgency. Phenazopyridine (Pyridium) is prescribed. What specific directions should the nurse practitioner provide for this client regarding phenazopyridine?

    1. May discolor contact lenses; if sclerae begin to turn yellow, return to the office.

    2. Always take on an empty stomach to increase absorption.

    3. Do not take any medication containing aspirin or salicylate.

    4. May interfere with effectiveness of mini-pill for birth control.

43. When prescribing oxybutynin (Ditropan) for the client with overactive bladder symptoms, which disorder in the client's medical history must the nurse practitioner consider before prescribing?

    1. Diabetes.

    2. Cough.

    3. Narrow-angle glaucoma.

    4. Gallstones.

44. Angiotensin-converting enzyme (ACE) inhibitors are recommended for slowing the progression of chronic renal disease but are contraindicated in the following disorder:

    1. Cardiovascular disease.

    2. Hypertension.

    3. Diabetes.

    4. Renal artery stenosis.

14 ▸ Answers & Rationales

Physical Examination & Diagnostic Tests

1. **(2)** Alkaline pH and positive nitrite and leukocyte esterase are the test results indicating the presence of UTI. Proteinuria alone suggests glomerulonephritis. Hematuria and pyuria without bacteria may indicate chlamydia, gonorrhea, viral infection, or less often tuberculosis. If a dipstick test is negative for RBCs but the urine is red, a substance that can change the color of urine is likely the cause.

2. **(1)** Intravenous urography and voiding cystourethrography can help identify congenital anomalies, stone formation, and foreign bodies. Renal size and the presence of stones can be seen in flat plate and upright films of the abdomen. Cystoscopy can visualize the urethra, prostate, and bladder. Urethroscopy can visualize the ureter and renal pelvis.

3. **(2)** In children, 25%–60% of proteinuria is orthostatic in nature and must be evaluated first.

4. **(1)** The 1996 AHCPR Guideline Panel encouraged primary health care providers to initiate the basic evaluation of urinary incontinence by performing a history and physical examination, measurement of postvoid residual volume, and UA. The other tests may be performed based on the findings from the initial evaluation.

5. **(1)** The optimal clients for UDS include those who have not had prior incontinence surgery or who have clear symptoms of stress or urge incontinence. Postvoid residual may be seen in an elderly male client.

6. **(1)** The primary concern in this client is the greatly elevate serum creatinine of 5.2 mg/dl. All the other serum values are within normal limits. This client should be referred to a nephrologist immediately because she is approaching the range considered for dialysis (6.0 mg/dl). The nurse practitioner should order whole parathyroid hormone level, liver function tests, lipid and renal panels, and magnesium/calcium levels. Having these laboratory tests completed will assist the nephrologist in determining the cause of the client's renal failure. A complete review of the client's medications should be initiated to determine if she is taking any medication that may cause renal failure, including ACE inhibitors (e.g., captopril)). The client's family history may be reviewed to rule out familial kidney disorders (e.g., Alport's syndrome).

7. **(2)** Adults normally void four to six times in a 24-hour period (q4–6h). Most adults usually do not awaken to void at night unless they have a medical problem (e.g., benign prostatic hypertrophy, urge incontinence, diuretic therapy). The feeling of the bladder filling occurs at about 90–150 ml, with the first urge at 200–300 ml. Normally, 1–2 hours pass between the first urge to void and reaching functional capacity. Adults typically reach functional (comfortable) capacity at 300–600 ml and should *never* experience leakage if voiding is delayed.

8. **(1)** Signs of dehydration in the older adult are skin tenting on the forehead, concentrated urine (specific gravity >1.025), oliguria, sunken eyes, lack of axillary moisture, orthostatic BP

changes, tachycardia, dry mucous membranes of mouth and nose, and absent or small saliva pool. In the obese elderly client who has lost weight, tenting of the forehead is not always a reliable clinical sign due to excessive loss of subcutaneous fat. As the older client becomes dehydrated, aqueous humor of the eye also decreases. Gentle palpation of the eyeball will reveal a boggy versus a firm eyeball, a useful assessment tool in these clients. It is important to examine the mouth because it reveals reliable assessment data in the older adult suspected of dehydration. A geographic tongue (patchy papillary loss causing a maplike appearance) should not be confused with tongue furrows and tongue coating.

9. **(1)** UA with C&S is essential to an incontinence workup and can be done in the primary care office before more discriminating tests to evaluate bladder storage and emptying. A symptomatic or asymptomatic UTI can cause symptoms of urgency and frequency, which are associated with incontinence.

Disorders

10. **(1)** *E. coli* is the most common organism causing UTI in young women, and counts of 10^5 are diagnostic. *E. coli* will likely respond to trimethoprim-sulfamethoxazole (Septra DS) or any suitable, sensitive antiinfective agent, and the client should also be treated for the UTI. *S. epidermidis* is normal skin flora and is likely a contaminant due to inappropriate clean-catch specimen collection technique.

11. **(2)** Although effective in protecting healthy skin from urine, moisture-barrier films contain alcohol and can burn and irritate denuded skin and therefore should be used sparingly. If the perineal area is already red and excoriated, using a moisture-barrier film is contraindicated. Each time the client is changed, the caregiver should cleanse the perineal area with mild soap and water and then apply a thin layer of petrolatum or zinc oxide to treat the irritant dermatitis. The addition of vitamin C 250 mg and zinc 220 mg daily will aid the healing process. Once the perineal area is healed, vitamin C and zinc should be discontinued.

12. **(3)** The nurse practitioner suspects UTI and needs to confirm the diagnosis with microscopic urine examination to identify white blood cells (WBCs) and bacteria. If no WBCs or bacteria are seen, an abdominal radiograph should be ordered to rule out a kidney stone, which is also part of the differential diagnosis.

13. **(4)** Functional incontinence is the inability to toilet appropriately due to impaired mobility. Ensuring that the client has the appropriate equipment in the home (bedside commode, walker, wheelchair, accessible bathroom, clothing that is easily removed) will assist the client in maintaining independence. Discussing the use of pads (e.g., Depends) may provide a sense of independence while on outings. This client may also benefit from scheduled toileting every 2 hours to reduce "accidents." Often these clients become socially isolated and depressed because of their concern about an accident in public. The nurse practitioner should explore all options available. Evaluating the need for pads is effective with stress incontinence. Limiting fluid intake in the evenings to reduce nocturnal incontinence is appropriate for urge incontinence. Performing Credé's maneuver is appropriate for overflow incontinence.

14. **(3)** This client likely has chronic bacterial prostatitis, which is difficult to treat because the bacteria reside in prostatic calculi and corpora amylacea. Chronic bacterial prostatitis requires 3–4 months of therapy with trimethoprim-sulfamethoxazole (Septra DS), or a quinolone (e.g., ciprofloxacin) may be necessary to prevent urinary symptoms.

15. **(4)** Sedative-hypnotics, diuretics, anticholinergics, α-adrenergic agents, and calcium channel blockers can cause reversible transient urinary incontinence. Poor pelvic support is a possible cause of stress incontinence. Urge incontinence, or the inability to delay urination with a sudden and powerful urge to void, is a possible result of lower urinary tract problems. A prolapsed uterus or bladder can cause overflow incontinence with overdistention of the bladder.

16. **(2)** Functional incontinence is the inability to toilet appropriately due to impaired mobility. Stress incontinence is leakage from the bladder during activities that increase intraabdominal pressure and therefore pressure on the bladder,

forcing urine leakage. Urge incontinence is an inability to delay urination, with a strong abrupt urge to void, caused by bladder hyperactivity or hypersensitive bladder. The client often has little warning before urine passes out of the bladder. Incontinence with overdistention of the bladder is called overflow incontinence, caused by an underactive or noncontracting detrusor muscle or by bladder outlet or urethral obstruction. It is characterized by frequent urination in small amounts.

17. **(2)** *E. coli* is the pathogen in 80%–90% of community-acquired UTIs. Gram-positive *S. saprophyticus* is the second most common pathogen. *K. pneumoniae* and *P. mirabilis* are also possible pathogens. In hospital settings, *E. coli* is less prevalent.

18. **(3)** Cystitis in adults usually presents with dysuria, urgency, frequency, nocturia, and suprapubic heaviness. Acute onset of chills, fever, flank pain, headache, malaise, and costovertebral angle tenderness are common in pyelonephritis in adults. Infants with cystitis may exhibit fever, irritability, decreased appetite, vomiting, diarrhea, constipation, dehydration, and jaundice.

19. **(2)** Acute hypertension in children and adolescents is usually caused by an identifiable secondary cause, such as glomerulonephritis due to streptococcal infection.

20. **(1)** Relapse is an uncommon cause of recurrent UTI in women and occurs within 2 weeks of completion of antibiotic therapy. It may need to be treated for 2–12 weeks. Reinfection is the cause of most UTIs in women and may be caused by residual urine resulting from a prolapsed uterus or bladder or by lack of estrogen in perimenopausal women. If the client has up to two UTIs a year, single-dose or 3-day antibiotic therapy may be used.

21. **(2)** Pyelonephritis in men suggests a structural abnormality and is usually an indication for hospitalization, parenteral antibiotics, and an intraveneous voiding pyelogram. Pyelonephritis in women is usually a result of invasion of the urinary tract by bacteria that have ascended the urethra from the introitus of the urethra. If bacteremia is suspected, women need to be hospitalized as well. Suggested follow-up is by telephone contact within 12–24 hours of initiation of antibiotic therapy and at 2 weeks and 3 months for posttreatment urine cultures.

22. **(2)** The facial edema and increased BP are common. Generally, the child does not have a high fever, and the urine is not concentrated but it may be decreased in amount.

23. **(2)** Gross hematuria may occur for 1–2 weeks after the diuresis and microscopic hematuria for up to 2 years. It is essential that parents be educated about poststreptococcal glomerulonephritis to ensure they know what to expect and to ensure that they know what is considered abnormal. Appropriate education will ensure that the parent will know when to notify a health care professional.

24. **(2)** Urge incontinence is associated with conditions such as Parkinson's disease, Alzheimer's disease, and stroke that involve the central nervous system, causing detrusor motor and/or sensory instability.

25. **(3)** Although discussing the alkaline-ash, low-purine diet with the client is appropriate, most clients, when they learn how difficult the diet is to follow, will be noncompliant with the diet even though they realize they risk developing another uric acid renal calculi. Starting the client on allopurinol (Zyloprim) 100 mg qd PO and monitoring to ensure that the serum uric acid level remains at normal levels will control the incidence of uric acid stones while allowing the client freedom without such strict dietary restrictions. Monitoring the client for another episode is inappropriate because the serum uric acid is likely elevated and a repeat incident is likely imminent. Referral to a urologist is inappropriate at this time because there is no acute episode.

26. **(1)** The nurse practitioner should contact the pediatrician immediately; this is frequently the first sign of a Wilms' tumor, which can be malignant. Because Wilms' tumor is very fragile, the abdomen should not be examined. The nurse practitioner should not wait for a referral because the child may not be seen immediately. The practitioner should contact the pediatrician by telephone to discuss the clinical findings and to arrange for an emergency appointment. UA and blood testing can be done, but often these tests are negative.

27. **(4)** Painless hematuria is the most common presenting symptom in the client with bladder cancer. Painless hematuria often occurs early in the course of bladder cancer and is often the only symptom the client will exhibit. There is no evidence of renal failure (oliguria, edema). Renal calculi would be characterized by both hematuria and flank pain. Prostate cancer often presents with the other symptoms of benign prostatic hypertrophy.

28. **(3)** A sedentary lifestyle or episodes of immobilization can predispose a client to the development of renal calculi. UTIs usually do not precipitate problems with renal calculi; however, the presence of renal calculi will predispose the client to UTIs. Milk intake of 6–8 oz daily is not excessive and will not predispose a client to renal calculi, and increased intake of citrus and high-fiber carbohydrates is good for the client's dietary needs.

29. **(2)** Postrenal failure results from development of an obstructive problem distal to the kidney, as seen in advanced prostatic hypertrophy with hematuria. A severe hypotensive episode, often seen after acute MI, is considered prerenal. The vascular changes resulting from diabetes and the exposure to nephrotoxic chemicals are considered intrarenal.

30. **(1)** The precipitating factor in prerenal failure is most often an incident that precipitated renal ischemia, such as a shock situation (anaphylactic reaction). Treatment with nephrotoxic medications such as gentamicin (Garamycin), pyelonephritis, and renal vascular changes are causes of intrarenal failure.

31. **(2)** Routinely performing Kegel's (pelvic floor) exercises assists in maintaining strong pelvic floor musculature. Weak pelvic floor musculature may contribute to urinary incontinence, especially with activity. The nurse practitioner should include teaching about avoiding dietary substances that can irritate the bladder, such as caffeine, alcohol, and spicy foods.

32. **(3)** Acute onset of increased confusion, inability to redirect, and increased agitation indicate an infection, likely a UTI, in the elderly client with dementia. The nurse practitioner should obtain a UA and empirically treat for UTI until the UA results are received. Because the client has no neurologic symptoms (e.g., weakness, flaccidity), a new infarct is unlikely. Acute confusion is not a sign of worsening dementia because dementia is gradual process. The caregiver bringing the client with this acute problem would not indicate underlying caregiver stress, which usually presents when persons complain of stress to their own primary care provider.

Pharmacology

33. **(3)** Benign prostatic hypertrophy is a common cause of urinary retention in older men. Inhaled ipratropium is an atropine-like bronchodilator used to treat chronic bronchitis, and its anticholinergic agent may aggravate urinary retention. Neither glyburide (oral antihyperglycemic) nor buspirone (oral antianxiety agent) has an effect on the urinary system. Timolol is a topical agent used to treat glaucoma and does not have a systemic effect.

34. **(4)** Combination hormone replacement therapy using conjugated estrogen (Premarin) 0.3–1.25 mg/day orally or vaginally, medroxyprogesterone (progestin) 2.5–10 mg/day continuously or intermittently can be useful for management of stress incontinence. Propantheline and oxybutynin may be useful in urge incontinence; research is limited on their use for urge incontinence. Doxepin (Sinequan) is a tricyclic antidepressant and is used infrequently.

35. **(1)** To decrease the formation of uric acid stones, a urinary alkylating agent such as allopurinol is frequently used. As standard practice, the nurse practitioner should check the client's serum uric acid level monthly for 3 months to ensure the levels are decreasing to normal ranges, then annually once serum uric acid levels are normalized.

36. **(3)** Oxybutynin produces anticholinergic effects, and dry mouth is a common side effect. Because this client is elderly, the nurse practitioner should review the client's list of medications to verify that no other medications will exacerbate dry mouth. If another medication will increase this side effect (e.g., diuretic), the practitioner should advise the client of methods to relieve the dry mouth, such as hard candy or chewing gum. The client

may also be taking other medications with anticholinergic side effects, which could be increased with the addition of oxybutynin to the point the client could be at risk for falls. Careful review of the client's medication list is essential before adding a new drug. The other reactions are not consistent with oxybutynin administration.

37. **(1)** The clinical presentation indicates UTI. The dipstick is positive for bacteria. The child may have had a reaction to sulfisoxazole, so it would be best to avoid sulfa drugs at this time. Another appropriate medication for UTI in children is amoxicillin. Ciprofloxacin is not recommended for children under 18 years old, and clarithromycin is not a first-line drug for UTI.

38. **(2)** Sedatives and hypnotics lead to sedation and muscle relaxation in all groups but particularly in the elderly population; central nervous system (CNS) changes from aging may lead to increased muscle relaxation, with the addition of a sedative-hypnotic leading to urinary incontinence. Antidepressants have anticholinergic effects and lead to sedation; CNS changes and the addition of antidepressants with anticholinergic side effects will increase muscle relaxation in the elderly client and contribute to urinary incontinence. Antibiotics have not been implicated in the development of urinary incontinence in older clients.

39. **(1)** Nitrofurantoin is contraindicated if renal function is impaired, antibacterial concentration in the urine is inadequate, or risk of toxicity is increased. To treat chronic UTI, the nurse practitioner would consider nitrofurantoin 100 mg PO hs as prophylactic treatment. Using this dose in the elderly client should not cause serum or tissue accumulation of the drug. Liver function studies may be indicated if the client experiences adverse reactions to the medication. Anticoagulants and sulfa-based drugs are not reported to cause significant drug interactions.

40. **(1)** The severe pain of renal calculi should be addressed before other treatments or diagnostics. The severe pain needs to be treated as soon as possible with morphine sulfate 10 mg SC or meperidine (Demerol). Ibuprofen may be used for beginning pain. Trimethobenzamide can be used, but only after initiation of pain relief.

41. **(1)** The most important side effects of nitrofurantoin are gastrointestinal upset, which can be decreased if the medication is taken with food or milk, and discoloration of the urine. The client should continue taking nitrofurantoin for at least 3 days after sterile urine is obtained. If applicable to this client, the drug may interfere with the efficacy of oral contraceptives.

42. **(1)** The nurse practitioner should advise the client that if she experiences yellow discoloration of the sclerae while taking phenazopyridine, she is to return to the office immediately. This may indicate poor renal excretion and requires a renal workup (renal panel, parathyroid and thyroid-stimulating hormone, serum magnesium/calcium, 24-hour urine for creatinine clearance) and possible referral to a nephrologist. Phenazopyridine should be administered with food, and no drug interactions occur with aspirin or oral contraceptives.

43. **(3)** Oxybutynin is contraindicated in clients with narrow-angle glaucoma. Clients with open-angle glaucoma may take this medication.

44. **(4)** Angiotensin-converting enzyme (ACE) inhibitors increase pressure within the kidney in renal artery stenosis, causing an increase in serum creatinine and potassium. ACE inhibitors have protective properties for clients with cardiovascular disease, hypertension, and diabetes.

15

Male Reproductive

Physical Examination & Diagnostic Tests

1. Which organ is **not** palpable on physical examination of a male client?

   1. Vas deferens.

   2. Testes.

   3. Epididymis.

   4. Cowper's glands.

2. Review of a laboratory report indicating elevated serum gonadotropin would raise suspicion of which disorder?

   1. Seminal vesiculitis.

   2. Vas deferens disease.

   3. Testicular disease.

   4. Benign prostatic hypertrophy (BPH).

3. Which of the following structures can be palpated during an external examination of a male client?

   1. Epididymis.

   2. Cowper's ducts.

   3. Seminal vesicles.

   4. Ejaculatory ducts.

4. What would be most helpful in diagnosing gynecomastia?

   1. History and physical examination.

   2. Liver function test.

   3. Thyroid function test.

   4. Mammogram.

5. The correct position in which to place a healthy adult male client to examine the rectum and prostate is:

   1. Left lateral Sims' position with right knee flexed and left leg extended.

   2. Supine position with hips and legs flexed and feet positioned on the examining table.

   3. Modified knee-chest position with client prone and knees flexed under hips.

   4. Leaning over the examination table with chest and shoulders resting on the table.

6. Which test is a tumor marker used to diagnose advanced prostatic cancer?

    1. Alpha-fetoprotein (AFP).

    2. Prostate-specific antigen (PSA).

    3. Prostatic acid phosphatase (PAP).

    4. Human chorionic gonadotropin (hCG).

7. Which statement is correct about the prostate-specific antigen (PSA) test?

    1. PSA can be elevated in clients with benign prostatic hypertrophy (BPH).

    2. PSA is not elevated in clients with prostatitis.

    3. Prostatic massage will not elevate PSA levels.

    4. PSA does not increase in recurrence of prostate cancer.

8. Which procedure is used in screening males (age 40) for prostate cancer, but is not diagnostic?

    1. Prostate-specific antigen (PSA) test.

    2. Digital-rectal examination (DRE).

    3. Urinalysis (UA) and complete blood count (CBC).

    4. PSA test and DRE.

9. When examining the scrotum of an adult Hispanic male, a normal finding is:

    1. Symmetric scrotal sac with two movable testes.

    2. Smooth, rubbery, saclike surface that is sensitive to gentle compression.

    3. Asymmetric sac with left side lower than right side. ✓

    4. Reddish color that is darker than body skin with sebaceous cysts.

Disorders

10. A 49-year-old male smoker presents to the clinic with complaints of painless gross hematuria. What is the most serious problem that needs to be considered by the nurse practitioner?

    1. Bladder cancer.

    2. Benign prostatic hypertrophy (BPH).

    3. Erectile dysfunction (ED).

    4. Urinary tract infection (UTI).

11. What finding is indicative of testicular torsion?

    1. Scrotal swelling with tenderness that occurs only after age 40.

    2. Sudden onset of pain with a firm, tender mass in the scrotum.

    3. Positive Prehn's sign.

    4. Cremasteric reflex.

12. On a routine physical examination a client expresses concern over the observation that one side of his scrotum is larger than the other side. He states that it has been getting larger for the past few months and that the scrotum is smaller in the morning and enlarges through the day. He has felt a heaviness in the scrotum, denies any acute pain, but does confirm some discomfort in his lower back. He reports no history of trauma to the scrotal area. On examination the nurse practitioner confirms the enlargement. Further examination reveals that the scrotum will transilluminate and that manual manipulation of the scrotum does not cause pain. What is the initial diagnosis for this client?

    1. Hydrocele.

    2. Orchitis.

    3. Epididymitis.

    4. Traumatic injury.

13. Which statement is correct concerning circumcision?

    1. Circumcision is helpful in preventing phimosis.

    2. Circumcision is a cause of paraphimosis.

    3. Balanoposthitis is the direct result of circumcision in older men.

    4. Circumcision increases the incidence of cancer of the penis.

14. Acute epididymitis is characterized by:

    1. Absence of dysuria.

    2. Nonenlarged scrotum.

3. Tenderness over epididymis.

4. Lack of abdominal pain.

15. Which of the following is true about hypogonadism?

1. Usually presents with impotence.

2. May cause an increased libido.

3. Is not associated with gynecomastia.

4. Does not contribute to infertility.

16. Which of the following is true about impotence?

1. Can be caused by antihypertensives.

2. Is caused by infections only.

3. Is not the result of multicausal factors.

4. Is not the result of vascular problems.

17. Circumcision can prevent which of the following?

1. Paraphimosis.

2. Epididymitis.

3. Sexually transmitted disease.

4. Prostatitis.

18. Which action is true about the prostate?

1. Secretes fluid that is acidic.

2. Secretes fluid that is alkaline.

3. Secretes androgens.

4. Produces sperm.

19. An elderly man presents to the clinic with complaints of difficulty voiding and hematuria. The rectal examination reveals a firm prostate about 5 cm in diameter, asymmetric, with firm nodules. The PSA level is 14. The next action is to:

1. Medicate with finasteride (Proscar) 5 mg PO daily and reevaluate in 3 months.

2. Advise client to avoid caffeine, alcohol, and over-the-counter decongestants.

3. Obtain a urinalysis to determine presence of infection and amount of hematuria.

4. Refer to urologist for biopsy and diagnostic evaluation for prostatic cancer.

20. A 15-year-old male presents with complaints of severe scrotal pain for the past 2 hours. The scrotum is swollen and extremely tender; palpation of the epididymis is not possible. What does the nurse practitioner recognize as the immediate treatment?

1. Narcotic analgesics and bed rest.

2. Warm packs and scrotal support.

3. Antibiotics, ice packs, and analgesics.

4. Referral to a surgeon for exploration.

21. A 20-year-old male client presents with scrotal pain. A suspected diagnosis that requires immediate referral is:

1. Testicular torsion.

2. Hydrocele.

3. Epididymitis.

4. Inguinal hernia.

22. An adult male client is being evaluated for dysuria, fever, and perineal pain. The physical examination by the nurse practitioner reveals a distended bladder. Further examination should **not** include:

1. Urine culture.

2. Prostate massage.

3. Cultures for gonorrhea and chlamydia.

4. Blood urea nitrogen (BUN) and creatinine.

23. An older adult male presents with a history of burning on urination and difficulty urinating that has been increasing over the past few days. A STAT urinalysis (UA) reveals the presence of leukocytes and bacteria. What is the primary diagnosis considered by the nurse practitioner?

1. Bladder cancer.

2. Testicular torsion.

3. Benign prostatic hypertrophy.

4. Renal failure.

24. The client with localized prostate cancer will exhibit which symptoms?

1. Hesitancy, frequency, and dysuria.

2. Fatigue, severe constipation, and dysuria.

3. Hematuria, nocturia, and weight loss.

4. Myalgia, confusion, and lethargy.

25. A young client presents with a complaint of a feeling of fullness in the scrotum. Physical examination reveals a round, soft, nontender, nonadherent, bluish testicular mass resembling a "bag of worms." No variation in size occurs with respiration or Valsalva maneuver. The mass transilluminates and is located anterior to the testes. The most likely diagnosis is:

    1. Varicocele.

    2. Hernia.

    3. Tumor.

    4. Spermatocele.

26. An uncircumcised client presents with a complaint of not being able to retract the foreskin over the glans penis. What is the most likely diagnosis?

    1. Lateral phimosis.

    2. Phimosis.

    3. Peyronie's disease.

    4. Paraphimosis.

27. A middle-aged client complains of a tight band causing a lateral curvature of the penis during erection and painful intercourse. What is the most likely diagnosis?

    1. Phimosis.

    2. Lateral phimosis.

    3. Lateral paraphimosis.

    4. Peyronie's disease.

28. A middle-aged uncircumcised client presents with red pinpoint pustules and papules on the prepuce and glans. The most likely diagnosis is:

    1. Peyronie's disease.

    2. Balanitis.

    3. Phimosis.

    4. Paraphimosis.

29. A male client is diagnosed with balanitis. The most likely cause is:

    1. Candidiasis.

    2. Herpes genitalis.

    3. Lichen planus.

    4. Psoriasis.

30. A male client presents with a complaint of sexual dysfunction. The nurse practitioner understands that sexual dysfunction is impairment of:

    1. Erection only.

    2. Emission only.

    3. Ejaculation only.

    4. Erection, emission, or ejaculation.

31. A man presents with a complaint of dysuria, enlarged scrotal tenderness over the epididymis, and abdominal pain. What is the most likely diagnosis for this client?

    1. Testicular torsion.

    2. Vas deferens inflammation.

    3. Epididymitis.

    4. Balanitis.

32. The nurse practitioner knows that erectile dysfunction is:

    1. Primarily psychological in origin.

    2. Primarily associated with men over age 70 years.

    3. The persistent inability to achieve and maintain an erection adequate for sexual intercourse.

    4. The physiologic dysfunction when smooth muscle contracts, causing a lack of adequate amount of blood in the penis to render a rigid, larger penis.

33. Priapism is classified as which type of sexual dysfunction?

    1. Erection.

    2. Emission.

    3. Ejaculation.

    4. None of the above.

34. Which of the following is correct in response to a client's question concerning a possible cause of prostate cancer?

    1. Syphilis.

    2. Gonorrhea.

    3. Cryptorchidism.

    4. Balanitis.

35. A male client complains of impotence. Which of the following may be a contributing factor?

    1. Antihypertensive drugs.

    2. Sexual intercourse.

    3. Smoking cigarettes.

    4. Frequent masturbation.

36. A young male presents for a sports physical examination. In addition to examining for hernias, it would be appropriate for the nurse practitioner to do which of the following?

    1. Teach testicular self-examination.

    2. Perform PSA test.

    3. Examine for prostate cancer.

    4. Perform PSA test and DRE.

37. An older male presents with gynecomastia. The most likely cause is:

    1. Cirrhosis.

    2. Diabetes mellitus.

    3. Hypergonadism.

    4. Peptic ulcer disease.

38. Concerning the male breast, which is a correct statement?

    1. Gynecomastia is the result of low estrogen and normal levels of testosterone.

    2. Most breast cancers in men are estrogen-receptor positive.

    3. Breast cancer in males is very common.

    4. Gynecomastia is a nonhormonal or tissue alteration.

39. Which is true of prostate cancer?

    1. Rarely diagnosed in men >50 years of age.

    2. Soft, indiscrete, symmetric nodules of the prostate.

    3. Obstructive symptoms rarely present.

    4. Asymmetric, discrete, hard nodules of the prostate.

40. Which symptoms would be a concern about a possible diagnosis of prostate cancer in a male over 50 years of age?

    1. Hesitancy, dribbling, and urgency.

    2. Decreased force of urine stream.

    3. Pain and feeling of a full bladder.

    4. Rapid onset of obstructive symptoms of urine output.

41. Which statement is correct concerning testicular cancer?

    1. It is a common problem in men over age 50.

    2. It is directly related to testicular trauma.

    3. It presents suddenly with pain.

    4. It is primarily found in young men.

42. Which of the following is true about acute bacterial prostatitis?

    1. Characterized by recurrent urinary tract infections.

    2. Involves an ascending infection of the urinary tract.

    3. Always occurs in men under age 30.

    4. Usually treated with 12-week course of antibiotics.

43. Which finding is indicative of orchitis?

    1. Extremely painful scrotum.

    2. No history of parotitis.

    3. No evidence of systemic viral infection.

    4. Decreased serum amylase.

44. A client has nongonococcal urethritis (NGU). The nurse practitioner understands that:

    1. No related problems occur if NGU is untreated.

    2. Clients with NGU are often asymptomatic.

    3. NGU is easily differentiated from gonococcal urethritis on physical examination.

    4. There is a very purulent discharge with a foul odor.

45. What organism is the most common cause of NGU in men?

    1. *Chlamydia trachomatis.*

    2. *Neisseria gonorrhoeae.*

    3. *Escherichia coli.*

    4. *Streptococcus faecalis.*

46. Cryptorchidism is defined as:

    1. Testicular underdevelopment.

    2. Imbalance of estrogen/androgen ratio.

    3. Undescended testicles.

    4. Absence of spermatogenesis.

47. Which test is a useful tumor marker for testicular cancer?

    1. Alpha-fetoprotein (AFP).

    2. Prostate-specific antigen (PSA).

    3. Prostatic acid phosphatase (PAP).

    4. Alkaline phosphatase (ALP).

48. The most common causative agent of orchitis is:

    1. Arbovirus.

    2. Echovirus.

    3. Mumps.

    4. Rubeola.

49. What are common symptoms of benign prostatic hypertrophy (BPH)?

    1. Dribbling, hesitancy, loss of stream volume and force, and recurrent urinary tract infections.

    2. Dysuria, urgency, frequency, nocturia, and suprapubic heaviness or discomfort.

    3. Obstructive symptoms, such as a weak urine stream, abdominal straining to void, hesitancy, incomplete bladder emptying, and terminal dribbling.

    4. Acute onset of fever, chills, flank pain, headache, malaise, costovertebral angle tenderness, and possibly hematuria.

50. A 14-year-old boy comes into the clinic from school with complaints of sudden, severe scrotal pain radiating inguinally. He has no difficulty voiding and has some nausea but no vomiting.

Examination reveals scrotal edema and erythema. The scrotum on the affected side is slightly higher than the unaffected side, and the cremasteric reflex is negative. What would the nurse practitioner determine as the best treatment for this client?

    1. Bed rest with ice pack and scrotal elevation.

    2. Warm scrotal pack and return to clinic the next day.

    3. Immediate referral to a urologist.

    4. Schedule for an ultrasound in the morning.

51. A 25-year-old client with a history of sickle cell disease complains of a sudden problem with erections that are not sexually oriented. He is currently experiencing a painful erection and he is unable to void. The nurse practitioner determines the treatment of choice is:

    1. Meperidine (Demerol) and bed rest.

    2. Immediate referral to a urologist.

    3. Increased hydration for sickle cell crisis.

    4. Determination of PSA level.

52. The nurse practitioner is speaking with a group of male teenagers who are most concerned about symptoms associated with gonorrhea. Which of the following would the nurse practitioner include in the discussion?

    1. Reddish lesions may appear on the palms of the hands and soles of the feet.

    2. Men may observe a rash over the body of the penis.

    3. Urinary dribbling may result from irritation of the urinary tract.

    4. Painful urination results from inflammation of the urethra.

53. A 65-year-old uncircumcised man presents to the clinic with complaints of penile tenderness, inability to retract the foreskin, and serosanguineous drainage from beneath the foreskin. The nurse practitioner must first consider a possible diagnosis of:

    1. Balanitis.

    2. Penile cancer.

    3. Herpes.

    4. Penile trauma.

54. What is considered a major contributing factors in erectile dysfunction?

    1. Diet high in vitamin C.

    2. Diabetes mellitus.

    3. Allergies.

    4. Low-sodium diet.

Pharmacology

55. A client has been taking doxazosin (Cardura) 2 mg PO daily for 3 weeks for treatment of BPH. He returns to the clinic and is complaining of feeling dizzy when he stands up. Which action would the nurse practitioner take?

    1. Determine blood pressure (BP) with client lying down, standing, and sitting.

    2. Order urinalysis (UA) to determine hematuria and presence of bacteria.

    3. Review with client his symptoms over the past 3 weeks.

    4. Perform rectal examination to determine if prostate is smaller than previously noted.

56. In planning treatment for a client with balanitis, the nurse practitioner orders:

    1. Rest, ice, and elevation.

    2. Massage therapy.

    3. Antifungal agents.

    4. Emergency circumcision.

57. A 28-year-old man presents with complaints of fever, low back pain, perineal pain, and intense pain on voiding. Rectal examination reveals a tender, swollen, firm, warm prostate. Based on the client's symptoms, the treatment of choice is:

    1. Trimethoprim-sulfamethoxazole (TMP-SMX; Septra DS) 1 tab bid × 30 days.

    2. Tetracycline (Achromycin) 250 mg qid × 10 days.

    3. Amoxicillin (Amoxil) 500 mg tid × 14 days.

    4. Erythromycin (Ilosone) 250 mg q6h × 24 days.

58. A 70-year-old man complains of scrotal pain with dysuria and frequency that has been increasing over the past 2 weeks. Physical examination reveals extreme scrotal tenderness and swelling, urethral discharge, and testes normal in size and position. UA reveals pyuria. What is the treatment of choice for this client?

    1. Nitrofurantoin (Macrodantin) 100 mg PO qid × 14 days.

    2. TMP-SMX (Septra DS) 1 tab PO bid × 10 days.

    3. Doxazosin (Cardura) 1 mg PO qd × 10 days.

    4. Oxbutynin (Ditropan) 5 mg PO tid × 10 days.

59. Finasteride (Proscar) is prescribed for a 50-year-old man who is experiencing a problem with urination secondary to an enlarged prostate. The nurse practitioner would teach this client that while he is taking this medication, it is important to:

    1. Increase his fluid intake.

    2. Restrain from sexual activity.

    3. Use contraceptives during intercourse.

    4. Increase intake of folic acid.

60. A 75-year-old client is diagnosed with chronic bacterial prostatitis and the nurse practitioner selects TMP-SMX (Septra DS) as the treatment. How should the TMP-SMX be prescribed for this client?

    1. 2 tabs bid × 10 weeks.

    2. 1 tab tid × 3 days, then 2 tabs × 10 days.

    3. 2 tabs qid × 2 days, then 1 tab bid × 14 days.

    4. 1 tab bid × 30 days.

61. Which of the following would be considered an initial treatment for Peyronie's disease?

    1. Surgery.

    2. Trial of vitamin E 400 IU bid.

    3. Circumcision.

    4. Oxybutynin (Ditropan).

Answers & Rationales

Physical Examination & Diagnostic Tests

1. **(4)** Cowper's glands (bulbourethral glands) are located near the prostate and beside the urethra near the base of the penis. These glands are part of the nonpalpable internal genitalia, consisting of glands and ducts. The testes, vas deferens, and epididymis are part of the external genitalia.

2. **(3)** Gonadotropin is elevated in testicular disease, whereas PSA is elevated in disease of the prostate, such as BPH.

3. **(1)** The epididymis is part of the external genitalia, whereas the ducts and glands are part of the internal genitalia. The comma-shaped epididymis is palpated on the posterolateral surface of each testis. The seminal vesicles (pair of glands) lie behind the urinary bladder in front of the rectum. These vesicles join the ampulla of the vas deferens to form the ejaculatory duct.

4. **(1)** A complete history and physical examination usually provide the cause of gynecomastia without further testing, since it can be caused by medication, starving and refeeding, or lack of androgen production (atrophying testes), which changes the estrogen/androgen ratio.

5. **(4)** For client comfort and ease of examination, the healthy ambulatory adult is asked to lean over the examination table with his chest and upper body resting on the table. Although Option #1 is correct, it is the position used for examining a client who is confined to bed.

6. **(3)** PAP is an enzyme marker. An increased value is the result of increased metabolism and catabolism of cancer cells of the prostate; in three fourths of clients the cancer arises in the posterior lobe of the prostate. PAP is also used to monitor therapy with antineoplastic drugs and cancer metastatic to bone (osteoblastic lesions). AFP (oncofetal antigen) is produced by fetal liver, yolk sac, and intestinal epithelium and disappears from blood soon after birth; it is not present in healthy individuals. AFP is increased in primary hepatocellular cancer, embryonal cell (nonseminomatous germ cell) cancer, testicular tumors, and others. PSA (protein marker), which is more sensitive than PAP, increases in prostate cancer and in BPH. Human CG (hormone marker), produced by placental syncytiotrophoblasts, is not usually found in sera of healthy nonpregnant women but increases in seminomatous and nonseminomatous testicular cancer.

7. **(1)** PSA can be elevated in clients with BPH and those with prostatitis, as well as after prostate gland massage. PSA does increase with the increasing burden of the tumor, as in recurrent prostate cancer.

8. **(2)** Recommended screening for prostate cancer should begin at age 40 with DRE, with PSA testing to begin at age 50 if there are no risk factors or symptoms. UA and CBC are used in an annual physical examination as screening procedures but are not indicated in screening for prostate cancer. PSA test and DRE are indicated for men over age 50.

9. **(3)** The scrotal sac is asymmetric, darker than body skin, and often appears reddened in red-haired men (abnormal finding if found in clients without red hair). The scrotal surface may be coarse with small lumps on the skin, which are sebaceous or epidermoid cysts that may have an oily discharge.

Disorders

10. **(1)** Gross hematuria in a client over 40 years old should be considered possible bladder cancer until proven otherwise. Smoking increases the client's risk of bladder cancer.

11. **(2)** The sudden pain in testicular torsion is not relieved when the involved testicle is elevated to relieve pressure. Prehn's sign, passive elevation of the testes, is associated with epididymitis. The cremasteric reflex is absent. Testicular torsion is most common among neonates and adolescents, with the highest incidence during puberty.

12. **(1)** The lack of pain, increase in size of scrotal contents, and transillumination are characteristic of hydrocele. Orchitis and epididymitis are usually characterized by pain; orchitis is most often associated with parotitis or mumps. There is no history of injury, and the scrotum would be tender to palpation.

13. **(1)** Circumcision is helpful in preventing phimosis and paraphimosis because both are a retraction dysfunction of the prepuce. In phimosis the foreskin is too tight to be retracted backward over the glans penis. In paraphimosis, once the foreskin has been retracted behind the glans penis, it is too constricted to return to a position of covering the glans penis.

14. **(3)** Acute epididymitis is characterized by an acute scrotal pain, dysuria, and enlarged unilateral scrotum with abdominal pain. Scrotal pain is relieved when the involved testicle is elevated.

15. **(1)** A man will present with impotence and decreased libido. These same men will often have gynecomastia due to the low or absent production of gonadotropin. Males with Klinefelter's syndrome (chromosomal abnormality with karyotype of 47,XXY–47,XXXXY) is the most common cause of male hypogonadism, with failure of both spermatic function and virilization.

16. **(1)** Impotence can be caused by antihypertensives such as propranolol (Inderal LA). The nonselective beta-blockers are believed to decrease vascular resistance and central effect. Erectile dysfunction is reported to begin at doses of 120 mg/day. Other causes of impotence are infections, trauma, and vascular and psychological disorders.

17. **(1)** Paraphimosis is a retraction disorder related to a constricted prepuce that can be relieved through circumcision.

18. **(2)** The prostate secretes an alkaline fluid that helps sperm survive in the acidic environment of the female reproductive tract. Androgens are produced by Leydig's cells of the testes. Sperm are produced in the seminiferous tubules of the testes.

19. **(4)** The DRE and levels of PSA are the primary indicators of prostatic cancer and should be thoroughly evaluated by a urologist. The other options are directed toward treatment of BPH and should be considered only after prostatic cancer has been ruled out.

20. **(4)** This involves the differential diagnosis between epididymitis and testicular torsion. Irreversible damage will be done to the testicles if torsion is not released in 3–4 hours. Time should not be wasted with other treatments if torsion is strongly suspected.

21. **(1)** Testicular torsion and testicular cancer are considerations that may be curable but must be treated early. Hydrocele, epididymitis, and inguinal hernias also require referral but do not require immediate attention.

22. **(2)** In suspected acute prostatitis, only a rectal exam should be performed, if at all. Vigorous massage must be avoided because of the risk of inducing bacteremia. Urine culture, urethral cultures for gonorrhea and chlamydia, and blood collection for BUN and creatinine are indicated to help make the diagnosis.

23. **(3)** BPH is often seen in men over age 50. Bladder cancer should be ruled out as a diagnosis.

24. **(1)** All the symptoms listed can be found in the client with prostate cancer, but only the symptoms listed in Option #1 are localized. The client often is asymptomatic.

25. **(1)** Varicocele presents as described, whereas a hernia may transilluminate, and bowel sounds sometimes can be auscultated in the scrotum. Hernias vary in size with Valsalva maneuver. Tumors do not transilluminate.

26. **(2)** Phimosis is a retraction disorder of the penile foreskin or prepuce. It can occur at any age and is usually the result of poor hygiene and chronic infection (the foreskin cannot be retracted back over the glans penis). Paraphimosis is the inability to retract the foreskin from behind the glans penis.

27. **(4)** Peyronie's disease is a fibrotic condition that causes lateral curvature of the penis during erection.

28. **(2)** Inflammation of the glans penis and prepuce (balanitis) is associated with poor hygiene and usually found in men with poorly controlled diabetes and candidiasis.

29. **(1)** Candidiasis is the usual cause of balanitis (see previous rationale).

30. **(4)** In sexual dysfunction, erection, emission, or ejaculation may not be functioning due to multifactorial causes, such as vascular disorder, neuropathy, and trauma. Peyronie's disease and priapism are examples of erection dysfunction.

31. **(3)** Epididymitis presents as described, and on palpation the epididymis often "feels like a bag of worms" in the scrotal sac rather than a fairly smooth cord.

32. **(3)** This is the correct definition of erectile dysfunction (ED), which may be experienced by 40% of 40-year-old men and 70% of men over age 70. It involves a dysfunction in the hemodynamic mechanism of smooth muscle relaxation that increases blood flow in the penis and ultimately causes venous trapping (compression of subtunical venules) and rigidity.

33. **(1)** Priapism is a condition of prolonged penile erection related to venous obstruction and unrelated to sexual arousal.

34. **(3)** Clients with undescended testicles are more prone to developing prostate cancer. The other conditions listed are not causes of prostate cancer.

35. **(1)** Antihypertensive drugs such as propranolol (Inderal LA) can cause impotence.

36. **(1)** This is the age group (15–35) that is affected by testicular cancer, and self-examination can be valuable in securing early diagnosis and treatment. PSA testing is recommended at age 50 and DRE at age 40.

37. **(1)** Cirrhosis and diseases of the hepatic system are often a cause of gynecomastia. It is thought that cirrhosis and other hepatic disease alter the estrogen/androgen ratio. None of the other diseases has been implicated in gynecomastia.

38. **(2)** Gynecomastia is the result of an increased estrogen/androgen ratio in men, and as a result their breast cancer is receptor positive.

39. **(4)** Prostate cancer is usually found in men over age 50 and causes rapid onset of urinary obstructive symptoms. Palpation reveals asymmetric, discrete, hard nodule(s). Size of the prostate increases >4 mm.

40. **(4)** Rapid onset of obstructive symptoms of urine output would indicate a fast-growing tumor or obstruction of the urinary tract. All the other symptoms are indicative of BPH, tumor, or stricture of the urinary tract.

41. **(4)** Testicular cancer is primarily found in young men and presents as nonpainful nodules of the involved testicle. Trauma is not a causal factor.

42. **(2)** Acute bacterial prostatitis is caused by an infection in the urinary tract moving up the urethra into the prostate. The most common organisms are *Escherichia coli*, *Pseudomonas*, and *Streptococcus faecalis*. The condition tends to occur in men ages 30 to 50 but can be associated with BPH in older men. Chronic bacterial prostatitis is characterized by recurrent urinary tract infections. The usual antibiotic course is 12 weeks due to blockage of the antibiotics by fibrosis in prostatic tissue.

43. **(1)** Orchitis usually presents unilaterally with a tender, swollen testicle within 7–10 days of mumps (parotitis). Elevated serum amylase is associated with inflammation of the salivary glands (mumps).

44. **(2)** NGU is often asymptomatic and as such is difficult to diagnose. NGU typically has a clear discharge and usually is caused by chlamydiae. Gonococcal urethritis produces a yellow purulent discharge. If there is a discharge, NGU is difficult to differentiate from gonorrhea without a culture. Reiter's syndrome is also associated with untreated chlamydial infection of the urogenital tract.

45. **(1)** *Chlamydia trachomatis* is the most common organism in male clients with NGU.

46. **(3)** Cryptorchidism is the result of undescended testes, either bilateral or, more often, affecting the right testis. Normally, descent is in the seventh to eighth month of gestation.

47. **(1)** For rationale and discussion of AFP, PAP, and PSA, see Question 6 answer. ALP increases in osteosarcoma, hepatocellular carcinoma (metastatic to liver), and primary or secondary bone tumors.

48. **(3)** The mumps virus is responsible for causing orchitis. Arbovirus and echovirus are implicated in meningitis and encephalitis. Rubeola is associated with complications of otitis media, pneumonia, croup, and encephalitis.

49. **(3)** Obstructive symptoms are common in BPH. Dribbling, hesitancy, loss of normal urine stream, and recurrent urinary tract infections are present in chronic bacterial prostatitis. Dysuria, urgency, frequency, nocturia, and suprapubic heaviness are common symptoms of cystitis. Fever, chills, flank pain, headache, malaise, and costovertebral angle tenderness of acute onset with or without hematuria are indications of pyelonephritis.

50. **(3)** The symptoms described are consistent with testicular torsion. This is an emergent and surgical problem, and the client should be referred immediately.

51. **(2)** This is considered a urologic emergency because of the inability to void and because the circulation to the penis may be compromised. The client should be referred immediately to a physician.

52. **(4)** Dysuria is one of the most common complaints of young men with gonorrhea. No lesions, rash, or urinary dribbling accompanies the yellow discharge.

53. **(2)** The client's age, presentation, and uncircumcised state put him at risk for penile cancer. Balanitis does not present with a serosanguineous drainage.

54. **(2)** Diabetes is a common contributor to erectile dysfunction due to the impaired circulation.

Pharmacology

55. **(1)** Doxazosin is also used as an antihypertensive agent; the client may be experiencing orthostatic hypotension. The other options are directed toward evaluating his BPH, which has already been diagnosed.

56. **(3)** Antifungal agents such as topical nystatin (Mycostatin) and ciclopirox (Loprox) are the treatment of choice. Recalcitrant infection is treated with oral fluconazole (Diflucan) 150 mg/day or itraconazole (Sporanox) 100 mg/day. All the other treatments are inappropriate.

57. **(1)** The client is presenting with classic symptoms of acute bacterial prostatitis. The treatment of choice is TMP-SMX. It is important to treat the client for at least 30 days to prevent relapse. Treatment is started pending culture and sensitivity results.

58. **(2)** The client is presenting with classic symptoms of epididymitis. The treatment of choice is TMP-SMX. Nitrofurantoin is a urinary antiseptic, doxazosin is given for BPH, and oxbutynin is indicated for incontinence or enuresis. On differential diagnosis, the gradual onset of pain, voiding problems, urethral discharge, and swelling are more indicative of epididymitis than testicular torsion.

59. **(3)** It is important that women of childbearing age not be exposed to the sperm of a client taking finasteride. These women and pregnant women should avoid handling crushed tablets.

60. **(4)** The recommended treatment is for at least 30 days to prevent recurrence. Clients may require continued suppression therapy for an extended period.

61. **(2)** Vitamin E promotes softening of fibrous tissue, which forms the plaques in Peyronie's disease.

Women's Health

Physical Examination & Diagnostic Tests

1. When obtaining a cervical specimen for a Papanicolaou's (Pap) smear, the nurse practitioner:

   1. Lubricates the speculum with a water-soluble lubricant to assist in the insertion of the instrument.

   2. Uses a cotton-tipped applicator when obtaining the cervical cells from a prenatal client.

   3. Uses warm water to lubricate the speculum to assist in the insertion of the instrument. ✓

   4. Completes the bimanual portion of the examination first in order to determine the relative position of the cervix to assist in comfortable insertion of the speculum.

2. To promote client comfort before performing a pelvic examination, the nurse practitioner:

   1. Asks the client to bear down slightly as the speculum is inserted.

   2. Has the client empty her bladder. ✓

   3. Explains each step of the procedure in a calm manner.

   4. Carefully reassures the client that the exam will only take a few minutes.

3. What finding is considered a normal surface characteristic of the cervix?

   1. Small, yellow, raised round area on cervix. *Nabothis follicle*

   2. Red patches with occasional white spots.

   3. Friable, bleeding tissue at opening of cervical os.

   4. Irregular granular surface with red patches.

4. The primary role of a breast ultrasound is to:

   1. Screen for breast cancer. *misses 50% of lesions <2cm*

   2. Definitively diagnose breast cancer.

   3. Determine if a breast lesion is cystic or solid.

   4. Locate small lesions before surgery.

5. The screening bone mineral density (dexa) report ordered for a 60-year-old postmenopausal woman shows a result of −1.5 SD (standard deviation) at the hip. She gives a past history of myocardial infarction (MI) 1 year ago and wrist fracture at age 32. What option would **not** be considered for this client?

   1. Counsel on smoking cessation and alcohol consumption.

   2. Initiate therapy with continuous conjugated estrogen 0.625 mg and medroxyprogesterone acetate (MPA) 2.5 mg.

   3. Initiate therapy with raloxifene (Evista).

   4. Encourage weight-bearing exercises and increased calcium intake.

6. When is the optimal time to perform a hysterosalpingogram (HSG)?

   1. During menses.

   2. Immediately after ovulation.

   3. After menses, but before ovulation.

   4. 3–4 days before menses.

7. Which statement about mammography is **false**?

   1. Mammography detects all breast cancers.

   2. Mammography should be accompanied by breast exam.

   3. Negative mammography should not delay biopsy of a clinically suspicious mass.

   4. Mammography is a cost-effective method to screen for breast cancer.

8. The use of potassium hydroxide (KOH) when doing a wet mount assists in the diagnosis of:

   1. Bacterial vaginosis and candida vaginitis.

   2. *Trichomonas* and *Chlamydia*.

   3. Syphilis and gonorrhea.

   4. Herpes and condyloma.

9. The nurse practitioner is reviewing the laboratory results of an 18-year-old client seen recently for a Pap smear: Classification—high-grade squamous intraepithelial lesion; endocervical cells seen; adequate smear. The nurse practitioner phones the client and tells her which of the following?

   1. "Your Pap smear was normal. Follow up in 1 year, or sooner if problems arise."

   2. "Your Pap smear shows invasive cancer. I would like you to see a gynecologic oncologist for treatment."

   3. "Your Pap smear shows abnormal tissue that needs to be evaluated. Please schedule an appointment for a colposcopy."

   4. "Your Pap smear shows a minor abnormality. Sometimes this can signify a disease process just beginning. Please schedule another Pap smear in 4 months for follow-up."

10. A 27-year-old client reports the desire to become pregnant. She and her husband have had regular, unprotected intercourse for more than 1 year. The nurse practitioner completes a thorough history and gynecologic examination, which appear normal. What diagnostic test might be ordered early in the workup?

    1. Hysterosalpingogram.

    2. Tests for antisperm antibodies.

    3. Semen analysis.

    4. Endometrial biopsy.

11. For which of the following women does the National Osteoporosis Foundation (NOF) recommend a screening bone dexa scan?

    1. A 48-year-old Caucasian woman who smokes and has excessive alcohol intake.

    2. A 50-year-old woman having irregular menstrual cycles.

    3. A 51-year-old woman on long-term corticosteroid therapy for systemic lupus erythematosus.

    4. A 54-year-old woman receiving hormone replacement therapy (HRT).

12. When describing the findings from a normal breast examination, what would the nurse practitioner document on the client record?

    1. Left nipple everted, several coarse black hairs arising from areola, enlarged axillary lymph nodes palpated bilaterally, tender nodes in supraclavicular area.

2. No dimpling or retraction; 1-cm hard, fixed, stellate mass noted next to nipple with scant nipple discharge; no pain or tenderness on palpation.

3. Right breast slightly larger and denser than left with no nipple discharge, right areola dark pink in color and inverted, left areola dark brown in color and everted, breasts tender to palpation with no axillary nodes noted.

4. Pendulous breasts with no dimpling, retraction, nipple discharge, or areas of discoloration; numerous small nevi near areola with Montgomery's tubercles noted, no supraclavicular or axillary lymph nodes palpated. ✓

13. In an infertility workup, what is the best way to evaluate ovulation?

1. Hysterosalpingogram.
2. Postcoital test.
3. Endometrial biopsy.
4. Basal body temperature (BBT) chart. ✓

14. The nurse practitioner is reviewing the laboratory results of a 61-year-old client seen recently for a Pap smear: Atrophic changes, scant endocervical cells, adequate smear. She has been treated for breast cancer with mastectomy and tamoxifen (Nolvadex). She has never received hormone replacement therapy (HRT). What is appropriate for the nurse practitioner to tell the client when she phones her with her results?

1. "Your Pap smear is slightly abnormal. I would recommend the use of some estrogen vaginal cream nightly for 3 weeks, then return to the office to have the Pap smear repeated." N

2. "Your Pap smear is normal but shows a mild thinning of the tissue. This is to be expected in someone who is postmenapausal not on hormones and does not pose a threat to your health. Please return to the office in 1 year for your annual exam, or sooner if needed." \

3. "Your Pap smear shows that you don't have enough endocervical cells. Please make an appointment for endocervical curettage." N

4. "Your Pap smear is abnormal. This could signify a disease state of the cervix. Please schedule a colposcopy at your earliest convenience."

15. Which test is the "gold standard" for the diagnosis of chlamydial infection?

1. Use of KOH wet mount "whiff" test.
2. Presence of inflammatory cells in Pap smear.
3. Direct fluorescent antibody (DFA) test.
4. Culture with special media and collection technique. ✓

16. The nurse practitioner is discussing mammography with a group of women. What important information should the nurse practitioner include in the discussion?

1. A mammogram should be done annually for all women of childbearing age. N
2. All women age 40 years and older should have a mammogram annually. N 40-50?
3. A mammogram should be done annually after pregnancy, if the woman does not breast-feed. N
4. A mammogram should be done only if the woman has breast pain or nipple retraction. N

17. Which is the **most** accurate statement regarding a reactive serologic test for syphilis?

1. All reactive serologic tests require confirmation with a treponemal test.
2. Reactive serologic tests are highly suspicious for active syphilis.
3. A false-positive serologic test, although rare, can be unnecessarily traumatizing to a client.
4. A reactive serologic test most likely implies the need for re-treatment. —

18. In the workup for a client with secondary amenorrhea, the prolactin serum assay results show a level of 24 ng/ml. Appropriate management includes:

1. Administering MPA 10 mg bid × 5 days.
2. Referral to a physician.
3. Recording the results as WNL (within normal limits).
4. Assessment for nipple discharge.

prolactin >20ng - referral

19. In the evaluation of a young adult with amenorrhea and normal secondary sex characteristics, the purpose of the progesterone challenge is to determine the presence of:

    1. Endogenous estrogen. ✓

    2. Thyroxine.

    3. Prolactin.

    4. Adequate body fat.

20. A client comes to the office complaining of fatigue, breast tenderness, abdominal bloating, fluid retention, and irritability about a week before onset of her menses. This has been occurring for the past 4 months. What is the **most** important information for the nurse practitioner to obtain to assist in determining the diagnosis of premenstrual syndrome (PMS)?

    1. Point in menstrual cycle when symptoms occur.

    2. Severity of symptoms. –

    3. Number and frequency of symptoms over past 4 months.

    4. Presence or absence of anxiety or depression. ✓

    5x during luteal phase (p̄ ovulation)
    keep calendar x 3 months

21. A 65-year-old woman reports to the clinic stating she has been experiencing intermittent vaginal bleeding over the last 2 months. Her last menstrual period was more than 10 years ago. Her last Pap smear at the clinic 9 months ago was within normal limits (WNL). She is not taking any hormonal products. She is sexually active with occasional complaints of dyspareunia. What is the **most** appropriate response of the nurse practitioner at this time?

    1. Order CBC and TSH and repeat Pap smear.

    2. Schedule laparoscopy.

    3. Schedule endometrial biopsy. ✓

    4. Schedule pelvic/transvaginal ultrasonography.

Normal Gynecology

22. The endometrial cycle is often described in three phases. Select the correct phases:

    1. Follicular, menstrual, and luteal. ✓

    2. Proliferative, luteal, and menstrual.

    3. Follicular, secretory, and menstrual.

    4. Proliferative, secretory, and menstrual.

23. The nurse practitioner understands that PMS occurs with greatest frequency and severity in the:

    5-11 days ā menses

    1. Late luteal phase. *progesterone dominant*

    2. Follicular phase. *-estrogen dom.*

    3. Proliferative phase.

    4. Ovulatory phase.

24. Which hormone is **not** released from the anterior pituitary gland?

    1. Follicle-stimulating hormone (FSH).

    2. Luteinizing hormone (LH). ✓

    3. Oxytocin. *post. pit.*

    4. Prolactin.

25. What is the primary function of FSH?

    1. Stimulation of maturation of ovarian follicles. ✓

    2. Milk secretion. *(prolactin)*

    3. Triggering ovulation.

    4. Inhibiting release of LH from the pituitary gland.

26. How is the term *menopause* best defined?

    1. Cessation of ability for natural reproduction.

    2. Completion of 12 months of amenorrhea after last menstrual period. ✓

    3. FSH level of 30 and estradiol level of 30.

    4. Last menstrual period.

27. In the ovarian cycle, what phase begins with ovulation and ends with the onset of menses?

    1. Follicular phase. ✓

    2. Ovulation.

    3. Proliferative phase.

    4. Luteal phase.

28. Which is **not** a risk factor for heart disease in the postmenopausal female?

    1. Regular exercise. ✓

    2. Cigarette smoking.

3. Hormone replacement therapy.

4. Diabetes mellitus.

29. An adult client's last menstrual period (LMP) was 2 months ago. She has had a Paragard T 380 intrauterine device (IUD) in place for the last 4 months. She is complaining of nausea, fatigue, breast tenderness, and abdominal bloating. Physical examination reveals the following:

- Abdomen: WNL.
- Pelvic: Cervix—positive Chadwick's sign, IUD strings protruding from cervical os.
- Uterus: Enlarged and nontender.
- Adnexae: Nontender, without mass, no cervical motion tenderness.

What is the most likely diagnosis?

1. Uterine fibroid.

2. Ovarian cancer.

3. Dislodged IUD.

4. Pregnancy.

30. What function do the Bartholin's glands have in reproduction?

1. Prevent vaginitis by maintaining adequate pH.

2. Prepare the mucous plug that occurs during early pregnancy.

3. Produce an alkaline secretion that enhances sperm viability.

4. Produce small amounts of hormones necessary for ovulation.

31. Which is **not** a risk factor for osteoporosis?

1. Cigarette smoker.

2. Caucasian.

3. Alcohol consumption.

4. Obesity.

32. A young woman complains to the nurse practitioner that she is experiencing headaches, irritability, decreased appetite, and fatigue about 1 week before menses. Appropriate management includes which of the following?

1. Treat PMS with increased protein and salt in the diet.

2. Incorporate daily aerobic exercise and dietary changes into her lifestyle.

3. Order complete blood count (CBC), comprehensive metabolic panel, and urinalysis (UA).

4. Supplement her diet with an additional 1–2 gm of vitamin C.

33. A middle-aged female presents with abnormal uterine bleeding. A hormonal profile reveals increased FSH and LH levels. What is the most likely cause for these findings?

1. Hypothalmic disorder.

2. Onset of climacteric.

3. Premature ovarian failure.

4. Anterior pituitary disorder.

34. While assessing a 16-year-old girl, the nurse practitioner was asked about douching. What information would be used in the practitioner's teaching plan?

1. Douching during menstruation is safe.

2. Daily douching is important because the client has copious vaginal discharge.

3. Hypoallergenic douches include flavored or perfumed types.

4. Douching removes natural mucus and upsets normal vaginal flora.

35. A 29-year-old client presents to the family planning clinic for her annual examination. She had a tubal ligation postpartum 6 months ago. She has been feeling tired, is nauseated, and is slowly gaining weight. She had one menses postpartum, 4 months ago. The nurse practitioner notes the following on physical examination:

- Abdomen: Bowel sounds × 4, soft, no hepatosplenomegaly, palpable mass in lower abdomen measures 14 cm, no tenderness.
- Pelvic: Bartholin's/urethral/Skene's glands (BUS) normal; cervix—os closed, smooth pink mucosa.
- Bimanual: Uterus enlarged, nontender, smooth contours, no cervical motion tenderness.
- Adnexae: Not palpable.

What is the likely diagnosis?

1. Pregnancy. ✓
2. Uterine fibroid.
3. Premature menopause.
4. Colon cancer.

36. In the Western world, menopause occurs at a mean age of 51 years. Which of the following factors has been linked to influencing the age at which menopause occurs?

1. Use of oral contraceptives.
2. Socioeconomic status.
3. Age at menarche.
4. Smoking.

Gynecologic Disorders

37. During a yearly physical examination, a nurse practitioner asks a woman if she has any problems or questions about sexual function or activity. Initially the client hesitates, but with further questioning and discussion, she states that she is unsure if she has ever experienced an orgasm. The nurse practitioner suspects:

1. Vaginismus. *painful vaginal spasm*
2. Primary orgasmic dysfunction. *never achieved*
3. Secondary orgasmic dysfunction. *loss of later*
4. Dyspareunia.

38. The nurse practitioner is talking with a young women who has been diagnosed with herpes simplex type 2. In discussing her care, it would be important for the nurse practitioner to include what information?

1. The initial lesions are usually worse than lesions that occur with outbreaks at a later time.
2. Her sexual partner will not contract it if she does not have sex when the lesions are present.
3. This condition can be treated and cured if she takes all of the antibiotics for 2 weeks.
4. If she becomes pregnant in the future, she will need to have a cesarean delivery. ✓

vag OK if no lesions at time

39. The definition of bacterial vaginosis is:

1. A syndrome resulting from homeostatic disruption in the vagina.
2. Vaginitis caused by a flagellated protozoan.
3. A bacterial sexually transmitted disease (STD) that can be symptomatic or asymptomatic.
4. A virus characterized by recurrent outbreaks and remissions.

40. A 22-year-old married client complains of severe dysmenorrhea. Her gynecologic examination is normal. Which management protocol is preferred? *OCs ↓ prostaglandin production*

1. Assess for contraceptive interest and, if interested, suggest use of oral contraceptives (OCs). ✓
2. Suggest use of a prostaglandin synthetase inhibitor.
3. Suggest use of over-the-counter ibuprofen.
4. Assess exercise patterns and use of relaxation techniques.

41. Which is **not** a criterion for the diagnosis of bacterial vaginosis?

1. Positive amine test (whiff test). ✓
2. Presence of clue cells. ✓
3. Vaginal pH >4.5.
4. Presence of pseudohyphae.

42. A client with a history of dilatation and curettage (D&C) after a first-trimester spontaneous abortion and subsequent amenorrhea would lead the nurse practitioner to a working diagnosis of which of the following?

1. Polycystic ovarian syndrome.
2. Asherman's syndrome.
3. Hypogonadism.
4. Premature ovarian failure.

43. The LH/FSH ratio in polycystic ovarian syndrome (Stein-Leventhal syndrome) is:

1. 1.5:1
2. 3:1
3. 6:1
4. 1:3

44. What are common findings in a client with polycystic ovarian syndrome?

    1. Weight loss, dental caries, and amenorrhea.

    2. Hyperprolactinemia and galactorrhea

    3. Dysmenorrhea, nodules palpated on bimanual exam, and infertility.

    4. Chronic irregular menses, hirsutism, and increased abdominal girth.

45. What is the most common cause of dysfunctional uterine bleeding?

    1. Thyroid disorder.

    2. Blood dyscrasia.

    3. Anovulation.

    4. Uterine tumor.

46. A 30-year-old client presents with scant pubic hair, minimal breast development, absent cervix, and uterus with a 46,XY karyotype. Which diagnosis would the nurse practitioner suspect?

    1. Turner's syndrome.

    2. Müllerian agenesis.

    3. Testicular feminization.

    4. Gonadal dysgenesis.

47. The most common cause of a breast mass in clients ages 15–25 is:

    1. Fibroadenoma.

    2. Intraductal papilloma.

    3. Infiltrating lobular carcinoma.

    4. Fibrocystic breast syndrome.

    30-52 yrs old

48. An effective treatment for primary dysmenorrhea is:

    1. Nonsteroidal antiinflammatory drugs (NSAIDs).

    inhibit prostaglandin synthesis

    2. Tranquilizers.

    3. Progestins.

    4. Steroids.

49. What is a cause of secondary amenorrhea?

    1. Testicular feminization.

    0 menses? previously having

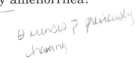

2. Hypogonadotropic hypogonadism.

3. Congenital absence of uterus.

4. Extreme exercise.

50. A young woman comes into the clinic for a well-woman checkup. She states that, about 3 weeks ago, she had a sore on her labia that went away. It was not particularly painful, did not itch, and apparently caused no residual problems. The nurse practitioner would treat this client by:

    syphilitic lesion

    1. Ordering the treponemal-specific test (FTA-ABS).

    2. Swabbing the area of the lesion for a viral culture.

    3. Advising her to notify her sexual contacts to determine if they have had any symptoms.

    4. Ordering nystatin (Mycostatin) cream to be applied to the area three or four times a day.

51. A high school athlete presents to the clinic with concerns regarding her menstrual periods. She states she has not had a period in the past 2 months. She has been in training and running about 3 miles a day for the past 3 months. She has lost approximately 15 lb. Her height is about 63 inches, and she currently weights 100 lb. What is the best response by the nurse practitioner?

    1. Determine the client's percentage of body fat and body mass.

    2. Obtain follicle-stimulating hormone (FSH) serum levels.

    3. Determine serum levels of human chorionic gonadotropin (hCG).

    4. Order thyroid function tests.

52. Which is **not** a risk factor for the development of cervical cancer?

    1. Human papillomavirus (HPV).

    2. Virginal status.

    3. Multiple sexual partners.

    4. Previous high-grade squamous intraepithelial lesion (HSIL).

53. A young woman is complaining of tenderness and burning of her vulva. On examination the vulva is edematous and excoriated. The nurse practitioner performs a wet mount prep of the vaginal secretions. It reveals pseudohyphae and spores. The diagnosis for this client is:

    1. Vulvovaginal candidiasis.
    2. Chlamydial infection.
    3. Bacterial vaginosis.
    4. Gonorrhea.

54. The leading cause of mortality in women with genital cancer, excluding breast, is:

    1. Ovarian cancer.
    2. Endometrial cancer.
    3. Cervical cancer.
    4. Vulvar/vaginal cancer.

55. A young woman presents with complaints of an irritation in the vaginal area. This is the first time it has occurred. On vaginal examination the cervix is inflamed and friable. Flagellated protozoa are seen on the wet prep. The most likely diagnosis is:

    1. Trichomoniasis.
    2. Cervicitis.
    3. Chlamydial infection.
    4. Bacterial vaginosis.

56. A 26-year-old female client presents to the emergency department complaining of gradual onset of abdominal pain. The pain started in the periumbilical region and is now in the right lower quadrant and is accompanied by nausea, anorexia, constipation, and low-grade fever. Physical examination confirms the diagnosis of acute appendicitis. What diagnostic studies are **least** useful in confirming this diagnosis?

    1. CBC with differential.
    2. Flat plate of abdomen, kidney-ureters-bladder (KUB).
    3. Pelvic ultrasound.
    4. Pregnancy test.

57. Which is **not** a risk factor for endometrial cancer?

    1. Obesity.

2. Oral contraceptive use.
3. Unopposed estrogen use.
4. Advancing age, >50 years.

58. Which statement is true regarding the diaphragm?

    1. May be inserted up to 24 hours before intercourse.
    2. May be inserted any time up to 6 hours before intercourse.
    3. Should be removed within 1 hour after intercourse.
    4. May only be left in place up to 12 hours.

    insert 2 hrs before
    leave for at least 6 up to 12

59. A contraceptive method associated with an increase in urinary tract infection (UTI) is the:

    1. Intrauterine device.
    2. Diaphragm.
    3. Norplant.
    4. Oral contraception.

60. Which is **not** a risk factor for ovarian cancer?

    1. Family history of ovarian cancer.
    2. Advancing age, >50 years.
    3. Oral contraceptive use.
    4. Positive BRCA-2 gene.

61. What is the most common female genital malignancy, excluding the breast?

    1. Ovary.
    2. Endometrium.
    3. Cervix.
    4. Vulva/vagina.

62. A 20-year-old college student presents to urgent care with new onset of painful sores in the vulva. These erupted yesterday and are associated with exquisite pain, fever, and flu-like symptoms of headache, general body aches, and mild dysuria. She has a new sexual partner and thinks she saw a sore on his external genitalia after coitus. The examination reveals vesicular lesions covering the labia, extreme tenderness of external genitalia to palpation, normal BUS, normal vaginal

inspection with mild leukorrhea, normal cervical mucosa, and slightly tender, minimally enlarged inguinal lymph nodes bilaterally. What is the likely diagnosis?

1. Gonorrhea.

2. Chlamydial infection.

3. Herpes simplex virus.

4. Lymphogranuloma venereum.

63. A 21-year-old client is seen for her annual gynecologic examination. She is sexually active, rarely uses condoms for STD prevention, and has multiple sexual partners. She smokes one pack of cigarettes per day, admits to a sedentary lifestyle, and eats two meals per day, most often at fast-food restaurants. Her exam is negative for any abnormality. Her family history and personal medical history are negative for major disease. She has no menstrual abnormalities; her LMP was 1 week ago. The nurse practitioner has done her Pap smear. Which would **not** be appropriate for this client?

1. Cultures for gonorrhea and *Chlamydia*.

2. Laboratory testing of glucose, cardiac risk profile, and TSH.

3. Human immunodeficiency (HIV) titer and rapid plasma reagin (RPR).

4. Counseling on safe sex practice and contraceptive information.

64. Which is **not** considered to be a risk factor in the development of breast cancer?

1. Early menopause.

2. High-fat diet.

3. Advancing age.

4. Early menarche.

65. A 32-year-old female client, G2 T1 P1 A0 L2, is seen in the clinic by the nurse practitioner for her annual examinaion and is requesting information on preconception counseling. She has been taking oral contraceptives (OCs) for 3 years without complications. During the past year she has started an exercise program at a health club 5 days a week and is eating three nutritionally sound meals daily. She has lost 33 lb and is now at her ideal body weight. She quit her job as a postal worker and now stays home with her children. As part of her preconception care, what should the nurse practitioner recommend?

1. Start prenatal vitamins with folic acid.

2. Discontinue exercise.

3. Update measles-mumps-rubella (MMR) vaccine.

4. Start genetic counseling due to advanced maternal age.

66. The initial workup for abnormal uterine bleeding should include:

1. Referral for diagnostic D&C.

2. Referral for endometrial biopsy to rule out cancer.

3. CBC, pregnancy test, and endocrine studies.

4. Coagulation studies and STD cultures.

67. Which is **not** a risk factor for breast cancer?

1. History of maternal breast cancer, premenopausal onset.

2. First pregnancy after age 35.

3. Late menopause, after age 54.

4. Fibrocystic breast disease.

68. A 20-year-old female client presents for her first well-woman examinaion; she never has been sexually active. Her family history and past medical history are negative for any gynecologic diseases. Her menses occur every 28 days, lasting 5 days, with a relatively moderate flow and no significant abdominal cramps. Her physical exam/visit today should include which tests?

1. Pap smear. — Not New

2. Cultures for gonorrhea and *Chlamydia*.

3. Stool Hemoccult.

4. Baseline mammogram.

69. What is the leading cause of death for women in the United States?

1. Breast cancer.

2. Colon cancer.

3. Heart disease.

4. Stroke.

70. During a gynecologic examination at the family planning clinic, an underweight 17-year-old presents with bruising around her upper torso and genitalia. She is minimally interactive and avoids eye contact as much as possible. Priority intervention should focus on:

    1. Lab work to rule out bleeding disorder.
    2. Nutritional assessment to determine possible anemia.
    3. Determination of possible physical abuse.
    4. Finding out if she has a support system.

71. Reactive cellular changes noted on a Pap smear are most often associated with:

    1. Inflammation.
    2. Use of estrogen vaginal cream.
    3. Drying artifact.
    4. Use of OCs.

72. Risk factors for cervical cancer include:

    1. Pregnancy after age 35.
    2. Viral exposure.
    3. Low parity.
    4. Prolonged contraceptive use.

73. What is the most common cancer in women in the United States?

    1. Breast cancer.
    2. Colon cancer.
    3. Malignant melanoma.
    4. Lung cancer.

74. A 48-year-old client presents to the clinic complaining of hot flashes, no menses for 14 months, insomnia, crying spells, irritability, decreased libido, and fatigue. At the end of her history and physical examination, she begins to cry and tells the nurse practitioner that she "thinks she's going crazy." She then begs the nurse practitioner to tell her what is wrong. Which action is **inappropriate** for the nurse practitioner to do at this point?

    1. Obtain laboratory tests, including FSH and LH.

2. Discuss HRT, including risks and benefits and short-term and long-term treatment strategies.

3. Provide antidepressant therapy and a referral for counseling sessions for depression.

4. Provide written information regarding menopause and options for treatment of symptoms.

75. Care for a client with chancroid should include:

    1. Screening for HIV as well as syphilis.
    2. Mandatory notification and treatment of all sexual partners.
    3. Screening for lymphogranuloma venereum.
    4. Culture for gonorrhea.

76. During her annual examination a 39-year-old client complains of recent breast changes. She states that her breasts are painful and frequently feel "lumpy." Because of this, she has stopped doing monthly breast self-examination (BSE), believing BSE is a "waste of time." What would be the most appropriate advice for the nurse practitioner to give to this client?

    1. Stress the importance of continuing monthly BSE to detect unusual lumps because the client knows the "feel" of her breasts.
    2. Suggest she at least do BSE every 2 months.
    3. Suggest she start having mammograms to establish some baseline data about her breasts.
    4. Determine when her breasts are nontender and least "lumpy," and change her BSE schedule.

77. During a breast examination on a young woman, palpation reveals a painless, 2-cm lobular mass in the right breast that is firm and freely mobile. Appropriate management includes:

    1. Continued observation and rechecking in 3 months.
    2. Referral for a mammogram.
    3. Referral for probable surgical excision.

4. Detailed family history to determine breast cancer risk.

78. A woman with bilateral breast implants asks if it is really necessary to do monthly BSE because she "does not know what to feel for." The most appropriate response would be:

   1. Suggest she involve her sexual partner in assessing her breasts on a regular basis.
   2. Review the steps in BSE until she feels comfortable with the process.
   3. Acknowledge the difficulty of doing BSE after implant surgery. ✓
   4. Explain the usefulness of regular mammograms for implant clients.

79. An adult client comes to the clinic complaining of abnormal vaginal discharge (dark watery brown) along with postcoital bleeding. The nurse practitioner suspects the possibility of cancer of the cervix. During the vaginal examination, suspicious physical results would be:

   1. Soft, sill-shaped cervix.
   2. Very firm cervix with an ulcer. —
   3. Vague lower abdominal discomfort.
   4. Tender, enlarged lymph nodes.

80. A postmenopausal client is worried about pain in the upper outer quadrant of her left breast. The nurse practitioner should:

   1. Do a breast exam and order a mammogram. ✓
   2. Explain that the pain is related to hormone fluctuations, and order laboratory studies.
   3. Reassure the client that pain is not a presenting symptom of breast cancer, and check for proper fit of the brassiere.
   4. Teach the client BSE.

81. A 22-year-old female client comes to the nurse practitioner's office with a complaint of 1 day of fever of 102°F, a diffuse macular rash, vomiting, headache, and decreased urine output. The history obtained by the nurse practitioner must include: *toxic shock syndrome*

   1. Whether the client's immunizations are up to date. ✓
   2. If the client is currently menstruating.

3. If the client has a history of tuberculosis.
4. What type of contraception the client uses.

82. A young female client presents to the nurse practitioner's office with a complaint of abdominal pain. In the United States, which of the following diagnoses results in about 1 death per 1000 and therefore must be considered early in the decision process?

   1. Irritable bowel syndrome.
   2. Appendicitis.
   3. Pyelonephritis.
   4. Ectopic pregnancy. ✓

83. A young adult client presents with a history of vaginal itching and heavy white discharge. The client gives a history of no sexual activity. On examination the nurse practitioner finds a red, edematous vulva and white patches on the vaginal walls. The discharge has no odor. The nurse practitioner expects which factors in the client's history?

   1. Vegetarian diet.
   2. Recent diarrhea.
   3. Early menopause.
   4. Recent antibiotic use. ✓

84. A young client comes to the office complaining of vaginal bleeding. The client states that she has used five tampons in the past 3 hours. She admits to sexual activity and takes OCs. On further questioning, the client states that she started her last pack of OCs "about 2 weeks late." The nurse practitioner should:

   1. Perform a STAT urine pregnancy test. ✓
   2. Perform a STAT CBC.
   3. Discuss proper use of OCs.
   4. Send the client for a pelvic sonogram.

85. The nurse practitioner knows that the majority of breast cancers occur in which area of the breast?

   1. Upper inner quadrant.
   2. Upper outer quadrant.
   3. Beneath the nipple and areola.
   4. Lower outer quadrant.

86. The client presents with abnormal uterine bleeding and has been found to have endometrial cancer. She returned to the nurse practitioner because she does not understand how this is possible when the Pap smear 6 months ago was negative. What is the nurse practitioner's best response?

    1. "Uterine cancer develops quickly."

    2. "Pap smears are difficult to read, and mistakes can happen."

    3. "Pap smears are not useful in detecting uterine cancers in most cases."

    4. "The previous Pap smear did not have an adequate sample."

87. A postmenopausal woman is seen in the office with complaints of frequent urination, stress incontinence, vaginal dryness, and dyspareunia. Her last menstrual cycle was 6 years ago, and she elected not to take HRT. She has increased her intake of soy products. What is the most common cause of her symptoms?

    1. Urinary tract infection.

    2. Cystocele

    3. Bacterial vaginitis.

    4. Atrophic vaginitis.

Pharmacology

88. A 42-year-old female client presents to the office with complaints of dysuria, urinary frequency, and urgency. These symptoms began early this morning. She leaves a clean-catch midstream urine specimen, which shows white blood cells (WBCs) too numerous to count (TNTC)/high-power field (HPF), 4–5 red blood cells (RBCs)/HPF, and positive nitrites. A urine culture will be ready in 3 days. Which is **not** a correct treatment for an uncomplicated lower urinary tract infection (UTI)?

    1. Phenazopyridine (Pyridium) 200 mg 1 tab PO tid × 2 days.

    2. Trimethoprim-sulfamethoxazole (TMP-SMX; Septra DS) 1 tab PO bid × 5 days.

    3. Ceftriaxone (Rocephin) 1 gm IM.

    4. Nitrofurantoin (Macrobid) 1 tab PO bid × 5 days.

89. The results of the Women's Health Initiative (WHI) provided evidence-based data that have led to new guidelines in assessing the risk/benefit ratio for initiation of HRT in postmenopausal women. Which statement is **not** correct?

    1. HRT is indicated for the treatment of menopausal symptoms, such as vasomotor and urogenital symptoms.

    2. HRT should be continued for primary prevention of coronary heart disease.

    3. HRT can be continued for the prevention of postmenopausal fractures due to osteoporosis.

    4. HRT should be limited to the shortest duration consistent with treatment goals and benefits in consideration with risks in the individual woman.

90. A 46-year-old female client is being seen in the clinic by the nurse practitioner. She was last seen 2 weeks ago for an upper respiratory tract infection and was treated with amoxicillin (Amoxil) 250 mg PO tid × 10 days. She completed her medication last week but now is aware of vaginal itching and a cottage cheese–like vaginal discharge. She states that she has never experienced such intense itching. She is in a mutually monogamous relationship. Her LMP was 2 weeks ago. Her partner had a vasectomy 2 years ago. Wet mount with KOH shows negative whiff test, rare clue cells, positive lactobacilli, positive hyphae and spores, few WBCs, and no trichomonads. She is leaving tomorrow for a week-long cruise. She is not taking any medications and has no known drug allergies. The nurse practitioner knows that the best treatment for this problem is:

    1. Metronidazole (Flagyl) 500 mg PO bid × 7 days.

    2. Clindamycin (Cleocin) vaginal cream one applicator full vaginally hs × 7 days.

3. Fluconazole (Diflucan) 150 mg 1 tab PO one time. ✓

4. Hydrocortisone (Cortaid) 1% cream sparingly bid × 7 days.

91. A 25-year-old client presents with complaints of a malodorous vaginal discharge described as white and watery. She douches with vinegar and water every 2 weeks. She uses a diaphragm for contraception. She and her boyfriend have been sexually active for 2 years, using condoms for STD prevention with every act of coitus. She denies any dyspareunia. Her LMP was 1 week ago, and there are no noted changes in her normal menstrual pattern. Her wet mount with KOH results show a positive whiff test, TNTC clue cells/HPF, no lactobacilli, no hyphae or spores, no trichomonads, and few WBCs. What is the diagnosis and treatment for this client?

1. *Chlamydia*; doxycycline (Vibratabs) 100 mg PO bid × 10 days.

2. *Candida albicans*; terconazole (Terazol 7) vaginal cream 1 applicator hs × 7 days.

3. Herpes simplex type 2; acyclovir (Zovirax) 200 mg PO q4h × 5 days.

4. Bacterial vaginosis; metronidazole (Metrogel) vaginal gel 1 applicator hs × 5 days.

92. A 55-year-old client, G2 T2 P0 A0 L2, is being seen in the clinic for her annual examination. She went through a natural menopause 5 years ago and has never been interested in HRT. She smokes one pack per day and does no formal exercise. Her family history is positive for osteoporosis in her mother, positive for myocardial infarction (MI) in her father, and negative for cancer. She has a normal physical exam today and had a negative mammogram yesterday. She is now interested in HRT but wants to know her alternatives. Which choice has **not** been clinically proven for prevention of osteoporosis?

1. Estradiol (Estrace) 0.5 mg 1 tab PO qd and micronized progesterone (Prometrium) 100mg 1 tablet PO qd.

2. Weight-bearing exercise three times weekly.

3. Discontinue cigarette smoking.

4. Wild Mexican yam cream applied to skin tid.

93. A young woman is seen in the STD clinic. She noticed some itchy bumps in the vulvar area and is concerned that they could be cancer. On careful inspection the nurse practitioner notes five cauliflower-like, warty, pinkish lesions in the lower introitus. Two smaller lesions nestled anterior to hymeneal ring of vagina and cervix fail to reveal any abnormalities. Wet mount with KOH is negative. Culture for gonorrhea and *Chlamydia* was obtained, Pap smear done, and HIV titer and RPR drawn. Which is **not** an appropriate treatment for this client?

1. Podophyllin (Podoben) application; wash off in 6 hours with soap and water.

2. Trichloroacetic acid application; do not wash off.

3. Cryotherapy with liquid nitrogen to lesions.

4. Benzathine penicillin 2.4 million units IM weekly × 3 weeks.

94. A young adult complaining of vaginal itching, thick yellow mucous discharge, and urinary discomfort is seen in the urgent care unit by the nurse practitioner. She is sexually active and uses condoms with only one of her two partners. On physical examination the abdomen is negative; pelvic exam reveals the Bartholin, urethra, and Skene's (BUS) WNL, cervix with mucopurulent discharge from the os, and mucosa friable to palpation; bimanual exam is negative. Cultures were taken but are not yet available. Wet mount with KOH reveals a negative whiff test, few clue cells, TNTC WBCs/HPF, no yeast, and no trichomonads. What is the likely diagnosis and appropriate treatment?

1. *Chlamydia*; azithromycin (Zithromax) 1 gm PO single dose.

2. *Chlamydia*; ceftriaxone (Rocephin) 125 mg IM.

3. Herpes simplex virus; acyclovir (Zovirax) 200 mg 1 cap PO q4h × 5 days.

4. Trichomoniasis; metronidazole (Flagyl) 2 gm PO single dose.

95. A 52-year-old woman presents for her annual gynecologic examination from her primary care provider. She received a hysterectomy with ovarian conservation at age 40 for uterine fibroids and dysfunctional uterine bleeding. She has been taking oral estrogen (conjugated equine estrogen 0.625 mg) replacement therapy (ERT) for 1 year. Although ERT has definitely reduced the discomfort of hot flashes, vaginal dryness, and mood swings from insomnia, she still experiences flushes and some night sweats. Her diagnostic lipid panel shows total cholesterol 180, LDL 112, HDL 52, and triglycerides 325. What, if any, change might be considered in her medication regimen?

    1. No change should be considered at this time.

    2. Decrease estrogen dosage to 0.3 mg daily.

    3. Recommend stopping estrogen therapy.

    4. Suggest changing route of administration to transdermal.

96. An adult female client is seen in the family planning clinic for a consultation on contraception. She is using OCs but forgets to take them because her work schedule changes every week; she is looking for an effective method that will be easy to remember. She has been married for 14 years, is G2 T2 P0 A0 L2, and is a nonsmoker. She has a negative past history for major diseases and a negative gynecologic history for abnormalities. She has never been treated for an STD and is in a mutually monogamous relationship. She is needle phobic and faints when she has to have blood drawn. What contraceptive method would be a good choice for the client?

    1. Depo-Provera injection every 3 months.

    2. Norplant implantation system for 5 years.

    3. Intrauterine device (IUD).

    4. Diaphragm.

97. A young woman is seen at the family planning clinic by the nurse practitioner. The client wants birth control pills but has heard that OCs are "dangerous to one's health." When asked for clarification, she lists weight gain, ovarian cancer, heavy or irregular periods, and infertility. After saying, "I can see that you are concerned about your health," would be appropriate for the nurse practitioner to tell this client?

    1. "There are a lot of fallacies about birth control pills. They actually are thought to reduce the risk of ovarian cancers and to help regulate the bleeding, and they are not associated with causing infertility. There can be a minor increase in body weight of 3 to 5 pounds."

    2. "Perhaps you would be better off trying the Norplant system or Depo-Provera."

    3. "What you have heard is true. They can be dangerous to your health, and many women experience these problems."

    4. "There are a lot of fallacies about birth control pills. Ovarian cancer and infertility are risks when taking the pills, but they do not cause weight gain or bleeding changes during periods. Pap smears done every year will detect such problems as ovarian cancer."

98. A 41-year-old female client is seen in the family planning clinic. She is seeking information about contraceptive methods because her Norplant system is due for removal next month. She is in a new sexual relationship and plans to use condoms for STD prevention. She is in excellent health, is a nonsmoker, and is nulliparous. Her menses are every 28 days, with light flow. Which is **inappropriate** for the nurse practitioner to recommend for this client?

    1. OCs.

    2. IUD.

    3. Norplant system.

    4. Depo-Provera injections.

99. An adult female client is taking OCs. She calls into the clinic with complaints of bleeding through the first 2 weeks of every package of pills. She has been taking this pill for 4 months at the same time every day. Her present OC is a low-dose monophasic pill. She is not taking any other medications and denies any adverse effects from the OCs. She would prefer to keep taking the OCs if possible. The nurse practitioner's advice should include:

    1. Discontinue the pills and do not restart them. Use an alternative contraceptive method.

    2. Change to a higher dosage, higher progestational agent.

3. Try taking the pills early in the morning on an empty stomach to improve their metabolism.

4. There is no cause for concern; breakthrough bleeding is a normal side effect of OCs.

100. An adult female client is seen by the nurse practitioner at the family planning clinic. The client notes heavy, irregular menses and an increase in facial acne and facial/abdominal hair growth over the past few years. She is G1 T1 P0 A0 L1 and is not planning future pregnancies. After a normal pelvic examination, she decides she wants OCs. What is a good choice for this client?

1. Loestrin 1/20.

2. Triphasil.

3. Demulen 1/35.

4. OCs are inappropriate for this client.

101. A 41-year-old client is seen for her 6-week postpartum examination by the nurse practitioner. She is breast-feeding without difficulty and plans to continue for a year. She wants to begin using a contraceptive and plans no further pregnancies. Which of the following is an **inappropriate** choice for this client?

1. Depo-Provera 150 mg IM every 3 months.

2. Intrauterine device.

3. Progestin-only OC.

4. Combination OC.

102. A 38-year-old client is seen for her 6-week postpartum examination by the nurse practitioner. The client was breast-feeding for a short time but discontinued 4 weeks ago. Her menses have resumed. She is contemplating another pregnancy in about a year, but if she became pregnant before then, she "wouldn't mind." She is seeking contraception. She smokes one pack per day. Her exam is normal, with the uterus well involuted. Which of the following is **contraindicated** in this client?

1. Progestacert IUD.

2. Oral contraception.

3. Depo-Provera injection.

4. Condoms and spermicide.

103. A 25-year-old female client is seen by the nurse practitioner for her annual examination. The client is interested in contraceptive choices. She just quit smoking and is well motivated to remain a nonsmoker. She is taking phenobarbital and phenytoin (Dilantin) for seizure control. She is G3 T2 P0 A1 L1 and may be planning future pregnancies but is unsure at this time. She is in good health other than the seizure disorder, and the exam is normal. Which contraceptive method is **contraindicated** in this client?

1. Diaphragm.

2. Depo-Provera injection.

3. IUD.

4. Norplant system.

104. A 22-year-old female client presents to the urgent care department and is seen by the nurse practitioner. She is complaining of abdominal pain, low-grade fever, and mucopurulent vaginal discharge. Her symptoms began 3 days ago and are worsening. She has a new sexual partner and has not yet used condoms with him. Her menses just ended; she is taking OCs. She denies nausea, vomiting, or anorexia. Her exam reveals findings consistent with pelvic inflammatory disease (PID). Cultures are taken for gonorrhea and *Chlamydia*. Which of the following represents an **inappropriate** treatment plan for the nurse practitioner to follow?

1. Ceftriaxone (Rocephin) 250 mg IM.

2. Doxycycline (Vibratabs) 100 mg PO bid × 10 days.

3. CBC, erythrocyte sedimentation rate (ESR).

4. Hospitalization.

105. What is the primary role of progestins in prescribing postmenopausal HRT?

1. Reduce side effects of estrogen-related breast tenderness.

2. Provide endometrial protection against hyperplasia.

3. Stabilize mood swings and reduce hot flashes.

4. Reduce occurrence of breakthrough bleeding.

106. An older female client is seen by the nurse practitioner for her annual examination. She has been on HRT for 6 months, having started herself on the pills left over by her deceased mother. She brings the pills, which she wants to keep taking, and requests a prescription for Estrace 1 mg daily. She has an intact uterus, is in excellent health, and denies any complaints. She does not have any contraindications to the use of HRT. Her exam is normal. Which represents an **incorrect** and potentially dangerous plan for the nurse practitioner to follow?

    1. Endometrial biopsy.

    2. Prescription for Estrace 1 mg daily plus medroxyprogesterone acetate (Provera) 2.5 mg daily.

    3. Prescription for Estrace 1 mg daily. _unopposed estrogen_

    4. Instruct client on the risks and benefits of HRT.

107. An older adult client is seen for follow-up to discuss her HRT that she began 3 months ago. She needs a refill on her HRT but is not sure "if it is working right." She continues to feel hot flashes, moodiness, and decreased libido and has many sleep disturbances. She is taking Premarin 0.625 mg daily and Provera 2.5 mg daily. She denies any vaginal bleeding. Which is **not** an acceptable choice for the client?

    1. Premarin 0.9 mg 1 tab PO qd and Provera 5 mg 1 tab PO qd days 1–12.

    2. Premarin 0.9 mg 1 tab PO qd and Provera 5 mg 1 tab PO qd days 16–25.

    3. Premarin 0.3 mg 1 tab PO qd and Provera 2.5 mg 1 tab PO qd.

    4. Premarin 1.25 mg 1 tab PO qd and Provera 10 mg 1 tab PO qd days 1–12.

108. Which is **not** a contraindication to the use of HRT in the postmenopausal woman?

    1. Recent deep vein thrombosis.

    2. Chronic active hepatitis.

    3. Controlled hypertension.

    4. Undiagnosed abnormal genital bleeding.

109. A young adult client presents to the clinic with complaints of a malodorous, yellowish vaginal discharge and vulvovaginal itching. She has never had a gynecologic examination and is extremely apprehensive. She is sexually active and has had a new sexual partner for 2 months. She states that they use condoms "most of the time" and are not interested in alternate forms of contraception at this time. Her LMP was 1 week ago. Her wet mount with KOH shows few clue cells, moderate lactobacilli, few WBCs, no yeast, and TNTC mobile trichomonads. Appropriate treatment for this client would include:

    1. Metronidazole (Flagyl) 2 gm PO single dose.

    2. Metronidazole (Metrogel) vaginal cream 1 applicator hs × 5 days.

    3. Fluconazole (Diflucan) 150 mg PO single dose.

    4. Terconazole (Terazol) vaginal cream 1 applicator hs × 7 days.

110. Which dose of conjugated equine estrogen (Premarin) is the minimal effective dose to prevent osteoporosis?

    1. 0.3 mg.

    2. 0.625 mg.

    3. 0.9 mg.

    4. Premarin is inappropriate.

111. A single woman presents for contraceptive counseling expressing preference for a diaphragm. Which factor in her history would make a diaphragm a poor choice?

    1. Three urinary tract infections (UTIs) in the past year.

    2. Strong desire to avoid pregnancy.

    3. Last two Pap smears showing atypical cells.

    4. Nulliparous cervix.

112. Combination OCs prevent pregnancy primarily by:

    1. Decreasing fallopian tube motility.

    2. Thinning of cervical mucus.

    3. Suppressing ovulation.

    4. Causing inflammation of the endometrium.

113. A young adult client is hesitant to be fitted for an IUD because of strong antiabortion views

and asks your opinion. Which explanation **least accurately** describes an IUD's probable action?

1. Slows transport of ovum through the fallopian tube, causing it to age and die in transit.

2. Prevents effective implantation of a fertilized ovum.

3. Action no different than that of a spermicide.

4. Slows transport of sperm.

114. What is a unique advantage of a Progesterone T IUD?

1. Lowest failure rate of IUDs.

2. May be left in place for up to 10 years.

3. Decreases menstrual blood loss and dysmenorrhea.

4. Must be replaced annually.

115. An older female client is seen by the nurse practitioner for her annual examination and needs a refill on her HRT. She is feeling well and has not voiced concerns. The client had a total abdominal hysterectomy and bilateral salpingo-oophorectomy 2 years ago for benign fibroids. Her exam is normal. She takes conjugated estrogen (Premarin) 0.625 mg days 1–25 and medroxyprogesterone acetate (Provera) 10 mg from days 16–25. What changes would be appropriate for the nurse practitioner to make in the HRT regimen?

1. No changes needed; the client is doing well on the present regimen.

2. Premarin 0.625 mg daily and discontinue the Provera.

3. Premarin 0.625 mg daily and Provera 2.5 mg daily.

4. Premarin 0.625 mg days 1–25 and Provera 5 mg days 16–25.

116. Which statement about progestin-only pills is true?

1. Women who are breast-feeding should not use progestin-only pills.

2. Ovulation suppression is as effective with progestin-only pills as with combination OCs.

3. There is an increased incidence of functional ovarian cysts.

4. The risk of ectopic pregnancy is lower for women using progestin-only pills.

117. Before prescribing HRT, which clinical approach should have the highest priority?

1. The decision about use should rest primarily with the client after providing appropriate education and counseling.

2. For most women the benefits of HRT far outweigh any possible side effects, so HRT should be actively encouraged.

3. Involving the sexual partner in the counseling session is likely to lead to a higher compliance rate for HRT.

4. Education regarding HRT should include a thorough review of risk factors and possible side effects to avoid liability issues.

118. The most common side effect associated with depomedroxyprogesterone (DMPA; Depo-Provera) is:

1. Nausea.

2. Acne.

3. Menstrual cycle changes.

4. Increased menstrual cramps.

119. What information should the nurse practitioner include when teaching a client about taking alendronate (Fosamax)?

1. Take it midmorning.

2. Take with food.

3. Take with a full glass of orange juice.

4. Remain upright after taking medication.

120. The addition of a progesterone to an estrogen regimen in a postmenopausal woman with a uterus reduces the risk of:

1. Endometrial cancer.

2. Cervical cancer.

3. Gallbladder disease.

4. Breast cancer.

121. The single-dose treatment of choice for trichomoniasis is:

    1. Azithromycin (Zithromax) 1 gm PO.

    2. Ofloxacin (Floxin) 500 mg PO.

    3. Metronidazole (Flagyl) 2 gm PO. ✓

    4. Clindamycin (Cleocin) 300 mg PO.

122. A 25-year-old woman comes into the office with complaints of profuse malodorous discharge. The nurse practitioner makes a diagnosis of bacterial vaginosis and then would:

    1. Advise the client to notify her sexual contacts regarding the diagnosis.

    2. Treat the problem with metronidazole (Flagyl) 2 gm for one dose.

    3. Initiate treatment with doxycycline (Vibramycin) 100 mg PO bid × 7 days.

    4. Determine the presence of pregnancy before initiating a course of treatment.

123. A young woman who is taking a low-dose OC calls the clinic in a panic stating that she forgot her pill 2 days ago. She is taking phenytoin (Dilantin) for seizure activity and has been seizure free for over a year. She asks, "What should I do about my pills?" What would be the nurse practitioner's most appropriate response?

    1. "Take the forgotten dose today along with the regular dose." ✓

    2. "See your physician for advice about the Dilantin."

    3. "Continue pills, but use another contraceptive through the rest of this cycle."

    4. "Come to the clinic for a 'morning-after' pill."

124. A vaginal culture has confirmed the presence of chancroid in a homeless woman who presented with a painful genital ulcer. The treatment regimen of choice should be:

    1. Ceftrixone (Rocephin) 250 mg IM single dose.

    2. Erythromycin (E-Mycin) 500 mg PO qid × 7 days.

    3. Metronidazole (Flagyl) 2 mg PO single dose.

    4. Clindamycin (Cleocin) 2% vaginal cream 1 applicator × 5 days.

125. You are counseling a 49 year-old woman who had her LMP 10 months ago. She is experiencing some hot flashes and night sweats and is not sleeping well. These symptoms are affecting her ability to work effectively because she finds herself tired and "cranky." She does not want HRT. Which of the following evidence-based alternative measures is most accurately described?

    1. Venlafaxine (Effexor SR) has been effective in reducing hot flashes in randomized controlled trials.

    2. Raloxifene (Evista) has demonstrated a significant reduction in hot flashes compared with placebo in clinical trials.

    3. Black cohosh (Cimicifuga racemosa) has been reported as efficacious in treating menopausal symptoms in many large, controlled trials. ✓

    4. Isoflavones, specifically soy, have been shown in studies to be significantly more effective than placebo in reducing hot flashes.

126. A young woman presents to the office for evaluation of abdominal pain. The client admits to recent sexual activity and states that she does not have her partner use condoms. On examination the nurse practitioner finds vaginal discharge and cervical motion tenderness. Besides sending cultures to the laboratory, the practitioner's treatment plan for this client would also include:

    1. Penicillin G 2.4 million units IM.

    2. Metronidazole (Flagyl) 500 mg PO bid × 7 days.

    3. Ceftriaxone (Rocephin) 125 mg IM and azithromycin (Zithromax) 1 gm PO. ✓

    4. Acyclovir (Zovirax) 400 mg PO bid × 7 days.

127. Which information about HRT should the NP understand when discussing HRT with clients?

    1. Estrogen replacement delays the onset of menopause.

    2. Estrogen and progesterone cause vasomotor symptoms.

    3. Estrogen decreases the risk of osteoporosis. ✓

    4. Estrogen replacement with progesterone increases risk of ovarian cancer.

Answers & Rationales

Physical Examination & Diagnostic Tests

1. **(3)** Lubricants, other than water, should not be used if a cervical specimen is being obtained for Pap smear analysis; some can alter the appearance of the cells and affect cytologic accuracy. The endocervical cell retrieval is diminished with use of a cotton-tipped applicator and is not recommended in any female client regardless of pregnancy status. The bimanual exam is performed after the internal vaginal exam.

2. **(2)** To aid in the examination, an empty bladder provides comfort for client and assists the nurse practitioner in making a more accurate assessment during the bimanual portion of the exam. Options #1 and #3 help reduce the client's anxiety, which ultimately may help achieve comfort.

3. **(1)** A nabothian cyst (Naboth's follicle) is a small, white or yellow, raised, round area on the cervix and is considered to be a normal variant. The surface of the cervix should be smooth and may have a symmetric, reddened circle around the os (squamocolumnar epithelium, or ectropion). The other options are all unexpected, abnormal findings.

4. **(3)** A breast ultrasound is used to determine if a lesion is solid or cystic. Ultrasound misses 50% of lesions <2 cm. The test is not sensitive enough to be used for routine screening and cannot replace mammography. The definitive diagnosis of breast cancer is the breast biopsy.

5. **(2)** The World Health Organization defines osteoporosis as a bone mineral density T-score below −2.5 SD and osteopenia as a T-score

between −1 and −2.5. This woman has early signs of osteopenia. She is not a candidate for HRT (estrogen + MPA) because of her past cardiovascular history. Raloxifene has been shown to prevent the progression of osteoporosis and, as a selective estrogen-receptor modulator (SERM), may be a good alternative to HRT. The other two lifestyle modifications are important counseling issues to reduce the risk of developing osteoporosis.

6. **(3)** The HSG is used to document the presence of a normal uterine cavity and the patency of the fallopian tubes. A contrast dye is injected into the uterus, and radiographs are taken to assess anatomy. The best time to do this test is 2–5 days after menses but before ovulation.

7. **(1)** Approximately 10% of breast cancers are not seen mammographically.

8. **(1)** KOH lyses epithelial and white blood cells, making it easier to visualize *Candida* (yeast). *Candida* cells are resistant and remain intact. KOH also assists with diagnosing bacterial vaginosis by alkalinizing vaginal discharge, causing a distinct fishy odor. This is a positive amine or whiff test.

9. **(3)** The Pap smear is a screening test for cervical cancer and precancerous states. The diagnostic test needed to confirm the diagnosis of a high-grade lesion is the colposcopy with guided biopsies. The results of this test are clearly abnormal and must be addressed. Waiting a year could be deleterious to the client's health. This is not a Pap smear report that one would choose to redo in

4 months; the client needs a diagnostic test, not another screening test. Because this is not a diagnosis of cervical cancer on this Pap smear, referral to a gynecologic oncologist is premature at this time.

10. **(3)** All the tests listed may be included in the workup for infertility. Because male factors account for 35%–40% of infertility, a semen analysis should be done early in the workup. HSG and endometrial biopsy require scheduling at specific times of the menstrual cycle. Tests for antisperm antibodies would be done if the postcoital test revealed abnormalities.

11. **(3)** The NOF has conducted cost analyses on the value of screening bone dexas for evaluation of bone mineral density (BMD). The NOF reports that BMD testing is cost-effective for postmenopausal women ages 50–60 who have other risk factors for development of osteoporosis, including lifestyle factors of minimal exercise, smoking, excessive alcohol intake, and low calcium intake. Other risk factors include genetic history of disease, slender physical frame, premature menopause, hyperthyroidism, multiple myeloma, rheumatoid arthritis, chronic renal disease, corticosteroid use, and long-term anticonvulsant therapy. The woman with the history given in Option #3 would meet the NOF criteria.

12. **(4)** Longstanding nevi and Montgomery's tubercles are normal findings; pendulous breast is only a description of size, which is important to note. Enlarged lymph nodes and tender supraclavicular nodes are potential cause for concern. A fixed stellate mass with nipple discharge is not normal, and although asymmetry might be normal, the different colors of the areolae and unilateral nipple inversion could represent a problem.

13. **(4)** The BBT chart is an easy and inexpensive tool to evaluate for ovulation. Clients should be instructed on the first visit how to use a BBT thermometer and record the findings on a BBT chart. The remaining answers are usually included in an infertility workup but do not evaluate the presence of ovulation.

14. **(2)** Atrophic changes on the cervix of a postmenopausal woman are to be expected, as is the paucity of endocervical cells. Because of her past medical history of breast cancer, she is not a candidate for the use of estrogen vaginal cream, and the Pap smear interpretation is not abnormal. Endocervical curettage is used as a biopsy technique for sampling tissue from the endocervical canal; however, it is not appropriate to recommend this invasive procedure for someone with scant endocervical cells, but rather for one with abnormal endocervical cells. Since this Pap smear report really is not classified as abnormal, there is no need to recommend a diagnostic procedure for the client.

15. **(4)** Culture is the only certain or definitive method of diagnosis. It is a collected cervical specimen, and the results take about 2–6 days to obtain. The DFA is fast and has good sensitivity and specificity.

16. **(2)** Mammography is recommended annually by the American Cancer Society for all women 40 years of age and older. There is no place for annual mammographic testing for all women of childbearing age. Breast-feeding does not preclude the use of mammography, and screening is not done only for breast symptoms.

17. **(1)** Serologic tests are good screening tests, but positive results require follow-up with a treponemal test to detect specific antibodies.

18. **(2)** Serum prolactin assay levels >20 ng/ml indicate the need for medical referral, usually to an endocrinologist. The most common cause of hyperprolactinemia and galactorrhea (milky breast discharge) is a pituitary tumor or lesion of the hypothalamus. Other causes include hypothyroidism, medications (narcotics, tranquilizers, antihypertensives), and oral contraceptives.

19. **(1)** A positive withdrawal bleed after a progesterone challenge indicates adequate levels of endogenous estrogen. A serum prolactin level should be obtained as part of the amenorrhea workup in addition to a serum pregnancy test. A diagnosis of anovulation can be made on the basis of the successful withdrawal bleed and normal prolactin levels. Low body fat and abnormal thyroxine levels can also lead to amenorrhea but do not affect the progesterone challenge test.

20. **(1)** The occurrence of the symptoms during the luteal phase of the cycle (following ovulation) will assist the nurse practitioner in making the diagnosis of PMS. Having the

client keep a calendar to track her symptoms for three cycles is helpful in making the diagnosis and measuring successful treatment. Severity of symptoms, although important, is not the most important information.

21. **(3)** If bleeding resumes after 1 year of amenorrhea in a postmenopausal woman or persists longer than 6 months after HRT initiation, further evaluation is necessary. The most common cause of this abnormal finding is endometrial atrophy, but more serious pathology must be definitively ruled out. An endometrial biopsy should be scheduled to further evaluate the cause of bleeding.

Normal Gynecology

22. **(4)** The uterine lining first proliferates and then prepares for implantation. During the secretory phase, glandular epithelium develops, further enhancing the lining. If no fertilized egg arrives for implantation, the lining sloughs off; this is the menstrual phase.

23. **(1)** PMS occurs approximately 5–11 days before onset of menses (late luteal phase) and subsides within 1–2 days of menses onset. This phase is progesterone dominant. The follicular phase is estrogen dominant.

24. **(3)** Oxytocin is released from the posterior pituitary. FSH, LH, and prolactin are all released from the anterior pituitary gland. The other hormones released from the anterior pituitary are thyroid-stimulating hormone (TSH), adrenocorticotropic hormone (ACTH), and growth hormone.

25. **(1)** FSH stimulates the maturation of ovarian follicles, resulting in a dominant follicle. Milk secretion depends on prolactin. The production and release of LH is regulated by estrogen. LH is responsible for ovulation.

26. **(2)** In 2001 the Stages of Reproductive Aging Workshop (STRAW) developed standardized definitions for menopause events. The phrases "in menopause" or "going through menopause" are misnomers and actually refer to the period preceding menopause, appropriately termed "menopause transition," or perimenopause. Menopause is one point in time and is defined after 12 months of amenorrhea following the final menstrual period. In postmenopause, FSH levels rise 10-fold to 15-fold with marked reductions in estradiol, but other menstrual irregularities can create a variation in these levels. Therefore these levels are not considered the best definition for menopause.

27. **(4)** The ovarian cycle is divided into three phases. The follicular phase begins on the first day of menses and continues until day 14, when ovulation usually occurs. Immediately after ovulation, the empty follicle begins to enlarge and develops into a corpus luteum, which releases increasing amounts of progesterone. If implantation does not occur, the corpus luteum regresses, causing the onset of menses. This phase, from ovulation to menses, is the luteal phase.

28. **(1)** As many as 30% of all coronary events are associated with tobacco use. HRT increases the risk of cardiovascular disease. Diabetes increases the mortality from cardiovascular disease two to four times compared with nondiabetic patients.

29. **(4)** Pregnancy is the most likely diagnosis in this client, given the list of symptoms and physical findings. She could have a uterine fibroid, but it is not contributing to the symptoms listed. Ovarian cancer could present with nausea, fatigue, and abdominal bloating but would not cause the enlarged uterus or the positive Chadwick's sign. A dislodged IUD will usually change the position of the IUD, decreasing visibility of the strings or causing the IUD itself to be expelled into the vagina or endocervical canal.

30. **(3)** Maintaining an alkaline pH is important to promote viability of sperm that are deposited into the vaginal vault.

31. **(4)** Obesity is not a risk factor for osteoporosis. Cigarette use, Caucasian race, and alcohol consumption, among others, are considered risk factors for osteoporosis.

32. **(2)** Conservative management for PMS includes daily exercise, stress reduction, dietary changes, and reassurance that her symptoms are valid should help the client gain more control. A low-salt diet is encouraged; when necessary, a diuretic may be used for fluid retention. The use of

vitamins B$_6$, A, and E may be helpful as well. Laboratory studies are not indicated here but might be helpful if the symptoms were sustained throughout the menstrual cycle.

33. **(2)** As the function of the ovaries declines and the amount of circulating estrogen begins to fall, the middle-aged woman may begin to experience the symptoms typically associated with menopause. The body's feedback system will attempt to stimulate the ovaries and increase estrogen level. FSH and LH levels rise in response to these efforts.

34. **(4)** Douching is never necessary. It changes the normal pH and upsets the normal vaginal flora. Douching during menstruation could cause "retrograde menstruation," a potential precursor to endometriosis. Copious vaginal discharge can be a symptom of infection and warrants workup.

35. **(1)** Pregnancy is the most likely diagnosis, requiring a pregnancy test and pelvic ultrasound to confirm it. Even though the client has had a tubal ligation, failure rates of 1 in 300 have been reported. This client could have uterine fibroids, but these do not generally present with this symptom complex and are not associated with amenorrhea, although they do cause uterine enlargement. Premature menopause could cause all these symptoms, including amenorrhea, but not the enlarged uterus. Colon cancer can present with these symptoms and could be responsible for an abdominal mass, but not for uterine enlargement or amenorrhea.

36. **(4)** The age of menopause has fluctuated little over the past several centuries, even though life expectancy has increased. Of the options, only smoking has been found to cause an earlier menopause (average 1.5 years). Research shows a direct correlation among number of cigarettes smoked, number of years of smoking, and age at menopause. Nulliparity and epilepsy have also been associated with an earlier age at menopause.

Gynecologic Disorders

37. **(2)** Dyspareunia is painful intercourse, and vaginismus is painful vaginal spasms on penetration. Primary orgasmic disorder is

when an individual has never achieved orgasm, usually a lifelong problem. Secondary orgasmic dysfunction refers to an acquired problem of loss of orgasmic function after an individual has experienced orgasm.

38. **(1)** The initial outbreak is usually the worst. It can be transmitted even when there is no lesion present, and it cannot be cured. Vaginal delivery is allowed if there are no genital lesions at the time of labor.

39. **(1)** Bacterial vaginosis results when the normal environment in the vagina is disrupted. The normal vaginal lactobacilli are decreased or absent, and there is an overgrowth of many different types of anaerobic bacteria. Trichomoniasis is caused by a flagellated protozoan, and gonorrhea is caused by a bacteria and may be asymptomatic. The virus that causes recurrent outbreaks of genital lesions is herpes simplex type 2 (HSV-2).

40. **(1)** OCs will reduce prostaglandin production, which is thought to be the primary cause of dysmenorrhea.

41. **(4)** The criteria for the diagnosis of bacterial vaginosis are characteristic milky homogeneous discharge, pH >4.5, amine odor (positive whiff test) with addition of KOH, and presence of epithelial cells studded with coccibacilli that obscure the borders (clue cells). Pseudohyphae are present in candidiasis.

42. **(2)** In Asherman's syndrome a normally functioning uterus has been damaged and scarred secondary to instrumentation, usually a D&C. Ovulation may be occurring normally, but no endometrium is built up and therefore no endometrium is shed (menstruation does not occur). Pregnancy should be ruled out in this client, as well as the other diseases listed.

43. **(2)** The LH/FSH ratio in polycystic ovarian syndrome is 3:1. The normal LH/FSH ratio is 1.5:1.

44. **(4)** The criteria for the diagnosis of polycystic ovarian syndrome include menstrual irregularity, increased body weight, hirsuitism, androgen excess evidenced by lab studies and physical findings, chronic anovulation, and multiple bilateral ovarian cysts. Option #1 would be more common in

anorexia nervosa/bulimia, Option #2 a prolactin-secreting pituitary tumor, and Option #3 endometriosis.

45. **(3)** Anovulation causes 90% of dysfunctional uterine bleeding. The lack of progesterone allows asynchronous, excessive proliferation of the endometrium. This tissue is fragile, and the normal hemostatic mechanism is altered. Thyroid disease, blood dyscrasias, and uterine tumors can mimic dysfunctional uterine bleeding and must be excluded.

46. **(3)** A female-appearing person with a 46,XY karyotype has androgen insensitivity syndrome, or testicular feminization. This maternal X-linked recessive disorder accounts for approximately 10% of all cases of amenorrhea, and these persons appear normal until puberty. These clients present with amenorrhea, scant or absent pubic hair, and abnormal or no breast development. Persons with müllerian abnormalities have a normal XX karyotype with abnormalities of fallopian tubes, uterus, and upper vagina occurring in fetal development. In Turner's syndrome, congenital absence of ovaries results from loss of one X chromosome.

47. **(1)** The most common breast mass in young women <30 years old is the fibroadenoma. This benign breast mass is the third most common breast mass after fibrocystic changes and carcinoma. Fibrocystic breast changes are seen most commonly in women 30–50 years old. Intraductal papilloma is a wartlike growth located in the mammary duct and occurs in women 40–50 years old. Malignant breast neoplasms occur most frequently in women over 40 and are rarely seen in women 15–25 years old.

48. **(1)** NSAIDs inhibit prostaglandin synthesis and are effective agents in primary dysmenorrhea. The other agents listed have not demonstrated effectiveness in primary dysmenorrhea. Other measures to decrease discomfort are exercise, relaxation techniques, heat application, and low-dose OCs.

49. **(4)** Secondary amenorrhea is defined as no menses for three cycle lengths or 6 months in a woman with previously established menses. Exercise can cause an increase in estrogen and endorphin levels, which influences the release of gonadotropin-releasing hormone (GnRH). Without appropriate GnRH release,

FSH and LH are not released adequately, resulting in anovulation, which may lead to amenorrhea. The other conditions listed are causes of primary amenorrhea.

50. **(1)** This has the characteristics of a syphilitic lesion and needs to be evaluated. Only after determining the presence or type of STD can it be treated effectively. The herpes viral culture should be done while the lesion is present and the fluid from the vesicles can be obtained.

51. **(3)** Pregnancy is the most common cause of amenorrhea in young women. It is important to rule out pregnancy in a female client with a problem of amenorrhea, even if she is very athletic. Interviewing the client regarding her sexual practices is unreliable. The presence or absence of pregnancy should be determined before other diagnostic studies.

52. **(2)** A person who has never engaged in coital activity is not considered at risk for cervical cancer because exposure to HPV is unlikely. In addition to other factors not listed, the presence of HPV, multiple sexual partners, and previous HSIL are considered to be risk factors in the development of cervical cancer.

53. **(1)** The pseudohyphae and spores on the wet mount with KOH are diagnostic for candidal infection. *Chlamydia trachomatis* is diagnosed by direct immunofluorescent assay or by chlamydial culture. Gonorrhea is diagnosed by cervical culture, and bacterial vaginosis has microscopic findings of clue cells and positive amine odor.

54. **(1)** Cancer of the ovary is the leading cause of death from female genital cancer, excluding the breast, in the United States.

55. **(1)** Flagellated protozoan confirms the diagnosis of trichomoniasis. Chlamydial infection is best diagnosed by direct immunofluorescent assay or culture. Bacterial vaginosis is diagnosed by wet mount revealing clue cells and positive amine test. Inflammatory cervicitis is generally asymptomatic and will not cause vaginal irritation.

56. **(3)** The pelvic ultrasound is not a useful test for appendicitis because it does not allow for adequate examination of the appendix. The CBC with differential is useful because of the

expected rise in WBCs seen in this inflammatory state. The flat plate of the abdomen and KUB are helpful to determine the extent of the problem and to rule out other diagnoses. Since pregnancy can cause these symptoms if complicated by an ectopic state, the practitioner should consider it as part of the differential diagnosis.

57. **(2)** OCs have been shown to reduce the risk of endometrial cancer. Obesity, unopposed estrogen use, and advanced age, in addition to others not listed here, are considered to be risk factors for developing endometrial cancer.

58. **(4)** The diaphragm may be inserted up to 2 hours before intercourse and should be removed no sooner than 6 hours after intercourse has ended. It should not be left in place longer than 24 hours.

59. **(2)** Urethral discomfort and recurrent UTIs are associated with diaphragm use and are the most common reasons for discontinuing use and changing birth control methods.

60. **(3)** OC use has been shown to reduce the risk of ovarian cancer. Family history of ovarian cancer, advancing age, and positive BRCA-2 gene are considered risk factors for developing ovarian cancer.

61. **(2)** Endometrial cancer is the most common female genital cancer.

62. **(3)** Herpes simplex virus type 2 (HSV-2) typically presents dramatically in the newly infected primary outbreak. Gonorrhea generally is associated with a mucopurulent vaginal discharge and is not accompanied by vesicular lesions. Chlamydial infection may be associated with dysuria and, unless accompanied by PID, is not generally accompanied by fever or body aches and is not associated with vesicular lesions. Lymphogranuloma venereum is a rare disease classically accompanied by pustular enlargement of the lymph nodes, particularly the inguinal nodes. It is associated not with vesicles, but bubos.

63. **(2)** Screening blood studies for glucose, cardiac risk profile, and TSH in this age group without any stated risk factors is not cost-effective and is of little value. The client can be better served with a discussion regarding diet and exercise. Since this client

is at risk for STDs, counseling and testing for these is a reasonable approach. Contraceptive information educates the client and allows her to make wiser choices in her family planning.

64. **(1)** Early menopause has not been associated with the development of breast cancer. High-fat diet, advancing age, and early menarche have been identified as risk factors in the development of breast cancer.

65. **(1)** The use of prenatal vitamins with folic acid before conception has been found to reduce the risk of neural tube defects in the fetus. It is important for the client to continue her exercise program, although some discussion about the type of exercise and any limitations are important once pregnancy is achieved. Because the client has had two previous pregnancies, it is likely that her rubella immune status has been determined; if she is found to not be immune to rubella, an MMR should be recommended. This client is not of advanced maternal age and therefore does not require genetic counseling for this reason. (See Chapter 17, Question 15, for gravida/para and TPAL acronym.)

66. **(3)** Baseline laboratory work should be obtained to determine the presence of anemia, possible pregnancy, and endocrine dysfunction.

67. **(4)** Fibrocystic breast disease is not a risk factor for breast cancer. In addition to others, those listed in Options #1, #2, and #3 are considered to be risk factors for breast cancer.

68. **(1)** The recommended age for a female to begin screening Pap smears is at the onset of sexual activity or at 18 years of age. Because this client is 20 years old and has not yet had her first Pap smear, this would be the most appropriate test to perform. It is not necessary to perform STD screening on clients who have not been sexually active. Stool guaiac (Hemoccult) testing and mammography are not recommended as screening procedures in the young adult.

69. **(3)** Heart disease remains the leading cause of death for women in the United States.

70. **(3)** The presence of bruising, particularly on genitalia, should raise suspicion of abuse. Combined with her nonverbal behavior, the

bruising should prompt the nurse practitioner to explore the possibility of abuse.

71. **(1)** Reactive cellular changes are most often associated with inflammation, including typical repair. Other causes include atrophy with inflammation (atrophic vaginitis), IUD use, radiation, and diethylstilbestrol exposure in utero. OCs do not cause reactive changes, and estrogen vaginal cream may be used to improve atrophy.

72. **(2)** Cervical cancer has been directly linked with high-risk types of human papillomavirus (HPV). Pregnancy after 35, low parity, and prolonged contraceptive use are not risk factors for cervical cancer.

73. **(1)** Breast cancer is the most common cancer in women in the United States. Lung cancer mortality is higher than that for breast cancer.

74. **(3)** These symptoms are classic for menopausal syndrome, although some depressive symptoms are listed. Antidepressant therapy and counseling for depression at this stage of treatment is not appropriate. Testing, teaching, and treatment in this case should be aimed at the menopause. The depressive symptoms will undoubtedly improve with greater understanding and treatment of the menopausal symptoms.

75. **(1)** Chancroid is well established as a cofactor for HIV transmission.

76. **(4)** Monthly BSE is an important preventive practice to identify early breast changes.

77. **(2)** Symptoms are most likely indicative of benign fibroadenoma. Mammography is indicated. Surgical excision is unlikely for a young woman.

78. **(2)** This client needs to become more knowledgeable about the normal feel of implants as well as her own breast tissue. Mammography is not a substitute for BSE.

79. **(2)** A very firm cervix along with a cervical lesion/ulcer is suspicious for cancer of the cervix, which can be confirmed with a Pap smear.

80. **(1)** This complaint is an indication for clinical breast examination and mammography.

Although uncommon, breast pain can be a presenting symptom for breast cancer. Teaching BSE is important, but not the most important action at this point. Hormonal fluctuations can explain breast pain, as can excessive caffeine intake, but should be a diagnosis of exclusion after ruling out malignancy.

81. **(2)** Toxic shock syndrome occurs primarily in menstruating women ages 12–24 who use tampons. The diagnosis is made with the presence of fever over 102°F, macular rash, hypotension, and involvement of three or more organ systems.

82. **(4)** More than 16% of ectopic pregnancies present as surgical emergencies. In the United States, blood loss causes one death in 1000 ectopic pregnancies.

83. **(4)** Almost half of all vaginal infections are caused by candidiasis. The majority of women who develop the disease have recently taken antibiotics. It is not an STD.

84. **(1)** It is important to evaluate the client for threatened abortion as soon as possible. It is most likely too soon for the CBC to reflect blood loss. A pelvic sonogram takes longer than a urine pregnancy test, and the client must be immediately referred for a D&C if her pregnancy test is positive.

85. **(2)** The most common site for breast cancer occurrence is the upper outer quadrant, followed by the area beneath the nipple.

86. **(3)** Pap smears are crucial for the detection of cervical cancer but do not diagnose uterine cancer. In the early stages, uterine cancer can be asymptomatic and would not be detectable even on bimanual examination.

87. **(4)** Vulvovaginal changes such as atrophic vaginitis often become apparent and bothersome several years after the LMP in women not receiving estrogen therapy. Insufficient data are available to demonstrate that isoflavones have a positive effect on vaginal symptoms. Vaginal lubricants are therapeutic in relieving symptoms of vaginal dryness. If nonprescription remedies do not provide relief and no contraindications exist, estrogen (often topical) is the treatment of choice.

Pharmacology

88. **(3)** Ceftriaxone is an effective drug for complicated UTI but is unnecessary in uncomplicated lower UTI. TMP-SMX and nitrofurantoin are both effective against UTI. Phenazopyridine helps to make the client more comfortable until the antibiotic reaches effective levels for treatment.

89. **(2)** The WHI study was stopped early because after 5.2 years, in the opinion of the Safety/Data Monitoring Board, the health risks for the women on the study (mean age 63) taking estrogen plus progestin exceeded the benefits. Women taking estrogen/progestin were at higher risk for developing MIs, strokes, and thromboemboli as well as developing breast cancer than women taking placebo. However, women taking HRT were less likely to have a fracture caused by osteoporosis and less likely to develop colorectal cancer. The study did not address the shorter term use of HRT for treatment of menopausal symptoms, the primary indication for initiating the therapy. This landmark study stresses the need for providers to discuss the risks/benefits of initiating or continuing HRT with postmenopausal women.

90. **(3)** Fluconazole is now approved for single-dose oral treatment of uncomplicated vulvovaginal candidiasis. It is most convenient approach for this client, who is unlikely to be compliant with vaginal creams given the upcoming travel. She does not have contraindications to its use. Metronidazole and clindamycin are for bacterial vaginosis, not *Candida* infections. Hydrocortisone is a topical steroid used for inflammatory dermatologic conditions, and although it may help the itching, it would not treat the candidiasis.

91. **(4)** Metronidazole vaginal gel is the treatment of choice for bacterial vaginosis in the nonpregnant female. The presence of clue cells and the associated malodorous discharge and the absence of lactobacilli are markers for the diagnosis of bacterial vaginosis.

92. **(4)** Although some authors may recommend herbal treatments for menopausal symptoms, no controlled studies have been done on disease prevention. Traditional allopathic Western medicine supports the use of HRT for the prevention of osteoporosis. Weight-bearing exercise and increased calcium intake have been shown to help maintain bone health. Cigarette smoking increases the risk for bone loss. This client can reduce her risk by quitting smoking.

93. **(4)** Benzathine penicillin 2.4 million units IM is the treatment of choice for syphilis, but this client has condyloma acuminatum, not condyloma latum. Topical use of podophyllin, trichloroacetic acid, and cryotherapy are all accepted treatment modalities for condyloma acuminatum.

94. **(1)** *Chlamydia* often presents this way (dysuria, mucopurulent discharge, cervical friability). The treatment of choice in ambulatory care settings is single-dose azithromycin 1 gm PO. The treatment listed in Option #2 is for gonorrhea, not chlamydial infection. Herpes simplex virus will present with painful vesicles in the vulvovaginal region and is treated with acyclovir 200 mg 1 cap PO q4h × 5 days for recurrences. Trichomoniasis can present this way, but trichomonads on the wet mount are absent. Therapy for trichomoniasis is single-dose metronidazole 2 gm PO.

95. **(4)** A hepatic effect due to the first-pass metabolism in the liver occurs with oral estrogen products. A 25% increase in triglycerides has been associated with this route of administration. Because transdermal estrogen is not dependent on gastrointestinal absorption or affected by the first-pass metabolic effect, this option should be considered. A discussion regarding risks/benefits of continuing ERT is appropriate from the primary provider. Because the client is only 52 years old and is still experiencing menopausal symptoms, reducing the most common dosage or stopping the medication unless significant risks are apparent is probably not the most therapeutic option.

96. **(3)** The IUD would be a good choice for this client because it is extremely effective (>99%). Maintenance is minimal, and no injections are involved for insertion or removal. The Depo-Provera injections, although extremely effective as well (>99%), require an injection every 3 months, which could lead to decreased client compliance. The Norplant system of

implants is also very effective (>99%) but also requires injections for insertion and removal, which this client is trying to avoid. The diaphragm is a noninvasive contraceptive that is effective (88%) but requires her to be more active in its use. None of these methods is contraindicated for this client, but an attempt should be made to help her choose one with which she is likely to be comfortable.

97. **(1)** The nurse practitioner should try to determine what the client has heard and dispel the fallacies if possible. Recent research supports the protective benefit of OCs against ovarian cancer as well as endometrial cancer. Amount of menstrual bleeding usually is decreased and the cycle regulated. Minimal weight fluctuations are reported. Infertility is not associated with OC use. To suggest either Norplant or Depo-Provera injections to someone who voices concerns about irregular menses or weight gain is sure to lead to an unhappy client, because these are common side effects of both methods. Options #3 and #4 are incorrect and misleading; Pap smears do not screen for ovarian cancer.

98. **(2)** The IUD is not recommended for nulliparous women or those not in a stable, mutually monogamous relationship due to the increased risk of complications. OC use in a 41-year-old nonsmoker in good health is acceptable without concern. The client is already familiar with Norplant and may not be aware that she could have a new set of implants inserted when she has the others removed. Depo-Provera would be equally appropriate for this client.

99. **(2)** Changing to a pill with a stronger progestational agent or changing to a different progestational agent often will resolve the problem of bleeding irregularities with OCs. Many choices are available regarding dosage or strength of an OC, and her problem likely can be resolved with a different pill. Taking the pills at a different time of day or on an empty stomach will do nothing to resolve the stated problem, which is not breakthrough bleeding but rather prolonged bleeding probably secondary to poor endometrial support. If a change is not made in the pills, the client will continue to bleed and may eventually develop anemia.

100. **(3)** An OC such as Demulen 1/35 is a good choice for women with more androgenic characteristics due to its strong estrogenic effect with moderate progestational effect. Loestrin 1/20 is a poor choice; the weaker dose of estrogen and progestin may not adequately support her endometrium and will not have a positive effect on this client's androgenic characteristics. Triphasil is a triphasic pill and does have a positive progestational effect that should support the endometrium, but the progestin in this OC tends to be slightly more androgenic, which is undesirable in this client.

101. **(4)** Combination OCs are not recommended for breast-feeding mothers due to the potential effect on decreasing milk quantity and quality. Progestin-only OCs are approved for nursing mothers because no deleterious effect on milk quantity or quality have been shown. Depo-Provera and the IUD are also accepted contraceptive methods for lactating females.

102. **(2)** OCs are contraindicated in a cigarette smoker age 35 years or older. No contraindication exists to the use of Depo-Provera injection in the cigarette smoker. The Progestacert IUD would probably be a good IUD choice for this client because it is only approved for 1 year's use and is safe in a cigarette smoker. The only contraindication to condoms and spermicide is allergy to either substance.

103. **(4)** The Norplant implantation system is contraindicated in the client with seizure disorder taking phenobarbital or phenytoin because of the potential for reduced anticonvulsant or reduced contraceptive effect. This does not occur with Depo-Provera, allowing the client to use this method freely without concern. The IUD is not contraindicated with anticonvulsants, and the client is a good candidate. The diaphragm is not contraindicated with anticonvulsant therapy.

104. **(4)** It is not necessary to hospitalize the client with acute PID who is not vomiting or pregnant. If she does not respond well to outpatient treatment, hospitalization may be recommended. The medications listed are the accepted treatment of choice for outpatient management of PID and should be started before lab results are available, based on the client's clinical presentation. The CBC and ESR are helpful to track the WBC count and inflammatory response of the body.

105. **(2)** Unopposed estrogen in a woman with an intact uterus increases her risk of endometrial hyperplasia and progression to endometrial cancer. Women who have taken unopposed estrogen for more than 3 years have a fivefold increased risk of endometrial cancer compared with women not on this regimen. The addition of progesterone to the regimen provides uterine protection. However, the progestin component of HRT is responsible for the breakthrough bleeding, a chief complaint at the initiation of therapy that may lead to discontinuance of the drug. Some women also are intolerant of progestins, which have been linked to irritability.

106. **(3)** The use of unopposed estrogen in the client with an intact uterus could put her at risk for endometrial hyperplasia or cancer. The addition of a progestin protects the endometrium adequately. The client is an excellent candidate for endometrial biopsy to document the status of the endometrium. This client also needs to be educated on the risks and benefits of HRT.

107. **(3)** Lowering the dosage of the estrogen would not help this client's symptoms. The other dosage regimens listed are all acceptable choices for this client, proving that there are many effective ways to utilize HRT, allowing for individualization of the regimen to the client.

108. **(3)** Well-controlled hypertension is not a contraindication to the use of HRT.

109. **(1)** Metronidazole 2 gm PO in a single dose is the treatment of choice for trichomoniasis. Metronidazole vaginal cream does not effectively treat vaginal trichomoniasis. Fluconazole and terconazole are treatments for vaginal candidiasis.

110. **(4)** A dose of 0.625 mg of conjugated equine estrogen (Premarin) is the minimal effective dose to prevent osteoporosis. HRT helps to maintain bones, but this effect only lasts as long as HRT is taken. Because of the risks for cardiovascular disease from using HRT, it is no longer recommended for osteoporosis prevention. Other methods of osteoporosis prevention include regular exercise, smoking cessation, and sufficient calcium (1200–1500 mg elemental calcium) and vitamin D (400–800 IU) daily.

111. **(1)** The diaphragm predisposes many women to UTIs. Some women are sensitive to the contraceptive cream or jelly. The diaphragm has been associated with toxic shock syndrome, so its use should be avoided during menses, and it should not be left in place longer than 24 hours.

112. **(3)** The primary mechanism of action of OCs is suppression of ovulation. Ovulation is suppressed in 95%–98% of clients. Should ovulation occur, the other mechanisms of action likely to prevent conception are thickening of cervical mucus, causing the endometrium to become atrophic, and making the uterine environment unfavorable for implantation.

113. **(3)** Although still unproven conclusively, mechanisms of action for IUDs include prevention of blastocyst implantation by inducing low-grade endometritis, the copper's effects on enzymes, progesterone's actions on the endometrium, and inhibition of sperm/ovum migration.

114. **(3)** A progesterone-releasing IUD acts to decrease blood loss and cramping.

115. **(2)** The client no longer requires Provera to protect the endometrium from the potential effects of estrogen; therefore the progestin can be discontinued and the client given continuous estrogen therapy without concern. The other dosage regimens listed are appropriate for an HRT client with an intact uterus.

116. **(3)** The progestin-only pill does not consistently suppress ovulation. This suppression only occurs in 40%–60% of cycles, which makes the progestin-only pill less effective than combination OCs. Mechanisms of action that contribute to the progestin-only pill's effectiveness include creating an atrophic endometrium and possibly altering tubal physiology by decreasing ovum transport. Progestin-only pills contain no estrogen and are a good choice for the breast-feeding woman. There is an increased incidence of functional ovarian cyst.

117. **(1)** Informed consent is essential. The pros and cons of HRT should be explained, but the choice is up to the client.

118. **(3)** Depo-Provera is frequently associated with menstrual cycle changes. In fact, this

irregular bleeding is the most frequently cited reason for discontinuation. These menstrual changes range from heavy, irregular bleeding to spotting and even amenorrhea. Nausea and acne are usually effects of estrogen and are not seen with Depo-Provera.

119. **(4)** Clients taking alendronate are instructed to take the medication on arising, 30 minutes before eating, and with a full glass of water. Clients should be instructed to remain upright to prevent esophageal irritation. Taking medication with food (reduces bioavailability by 40%), coffee, or orange juice (decreases bioavailability by 60%) or after eating significantly reduces absorption.

120. **(1)** Women with a uterus taking unopposed exogenous estrogen have an increased risk of endometrial cancer. The addition of progesterone decreases this risk. The addition of progesterone may prompt bleeding, which many women view unfavorably. Progesterone does not affect cervical cancer, breast cancer, or gallbladder disease.

121. **(3)** Metronidazole in a single 2-gm dose is the treatment of choice for trichomoniasis. An alternative is giving the 2 gm in divided doses the same day to reduce nausea and improve compliance.

122. **(4)** Metronidazole is the treatment of choice for bacterial vaginosis. However, pregnancy should be ruled out before beginning treatment because metronidazole should not be used if the woman may be pregnant. The sexual partners do not require treatment, and doxycycline is not the drug of choice.

123. **(3)** This client requires added protection through this cycle because of the low-dose OC. Phenytoin may also decrease effectiveness of OCs, especially low-dose forms.

124. **(1)** Because of homeless status, the nurse practitioner needs to use a single-dose treatment. Erythromycin, although a correct medication, is a poor dosing choice for this client.

125. **(1)** The most accurate answer is venlafaxine. This combination serotonin and norepinephrine reuptake inhibitor has been found to reduce hot flashes at doses of 25–150 mg/day in several clinical trials. Although many individuals consider the "natural" over-the-counter products to be safer than prescription drugs, these products can have pharmacologic effects and side effects. Use of these drugs by clients should be questioned at the time of the exam. Critics argue that the trials studying black cohosh (*C. racemosa*) have been too small, uncontrolled, and not randomized to provide evidence-based information on the herb's efficacy and safety. Soy has been found to be moderately effective in reducing hot flashes, but comparable results have been seen in the placebo groups as well. A side effect of raloxifene, used to prevent postmenopausal osteoporosis, is hot flashes.

126. **(3)** The most common cause of PID in sexually active women is gonococcal infections. These infections are often accompanied by *Chlamydia*, and usually both are treated.

127. **(3)** HRT may be considered for short-term use (3–4 years) to alleviate menopausal symptoms and the risk of osteoporosis in high-risk clients. The ovarian cancer risk may increase for women using estrogen alone for 10 years or longer. Current data are insufficient to know if combination HRT has the same risk. HRT reduces the colorectal cancer risk.

Perinatal & Newborn

Physiology of Pregnancy

1. Normal cardiovascular physiologic responses to pregnancy include:

   1. Increased heart rate, increased cardiac output, decreased blood volume, and systolic murmur.

   2. Increased heart rate, decreased cardiac output, increased blood volume, and systolic murmur.

   3. Increased heart rate, increased cardiac output, increased blood volume, and systolic murmur.

   4. Decreased heart rate, increased cardiac output, increased blood volume, and diastolic murmur.

2. How does progesterone effect the gastrointestinal (GI) system during pregnancy?

   1. Causes nausea and vomiting early in pregnancy.

   2. Causes hypertrophy and bleeding of gums.

   3. Delays gastric emptying time and decreases intestinal peristalsis.

   4. Causes diarrhea due to increased intestinal peristalsis.

3. A pregnant client has a hemoglobin value of 11.7 gm/dl. Which factor explains this finding?

   1. Presence of iron deficiency anemia.

   2. The trimester of pregnancy.

   3. Physiologic anemia of pregnancy.

   4. Anemia of chronic disease.

4. Several physiologic changes in pregnancy may mimic heart disease. Which of the following is an **abnormal** finding in pregnancy?

   1. Third heart sound.

   2. Leg edema.

   3. Systolic murmur.

   4. Diastolic murmur.

5. Which of the following is **not** a common urinary system finding during pregnancy?

    1. Physiologic hydronephrosis.
    2. Increased glomerular filtration rate.
    3. Increased urinary frequency.
    4. Proteinuria.

6. Which laboratory finding remains unchanged during pregnancy?

    1. White blood cell (WBC) count.
    2. Red blood cell (RBC) volume.
    3. Fibrinogen level.
    4. Prothrombin level.

7. During pregnancy, estrogen is responsible for:

    1. Hyperpigmentation.
    2. Facilitating implantation.
    3. Reducing smooth muscle tone.
    4. Decreased uterine contractility.

8. Which is **not** a placental hormone?

    1. Human chorionic gonadotropin (hCG).
    2. Estrogen.
    3. Relaxin.
    4. Cortisol.

9. What is the function of the placental hormone relaxin?

    1. Causes changes in endometrium and relaxes smooth muscle.
    2. Stimulates development of the ductal system of the breasts and causes hypertrophy and hyperplasia of the uterus.
    3. Aids in softening smooth muscle and connective tissue.
    4. Involved with metabolizing certain nutrients and aids in the growth of breasts and other maternal tissues.

10. The nurse practitioner understands that at 12 weeks of fetal development:

    1. Quickening is felt.

    2. Fetal heart tones should be heard with Doppler ultrasound.
    3. Fetal heart tones are heard with the stethoscope.
    4. Respiratory movements occur.

11. A positive sign of pregnancy is:

    1. Softening of the cervix.
    2. Fetal heartbeat.
    3. Enlargement of uterus and abdomen.
    4. Mother's perception of fetal movement.

12. The bluish discoloration of the cervix and vagina is known as:

    1. Goodell's sign.
    2. Chadwick's sign.
    3. Hegar's sign.
    4. Braxton Hicks sign.

13. What is MacDonald's method of abdominal measurement in the pregnant woman?

    1. With woman on her back and knees slightly flexed, top of fundus is palpated, and measuring tape is stretched from top of symphysis pubis over the abdomen to top of fundus.
    2. Midline of abdomen is determined, and measuring tape is placed around abdomen and measured at the point where fundus is determined to be at midline.
    3. Distance from xiphoid process to symphysis pubis is measured, and dimensions of abdominal curve or fundus is calculated.
    4. With woman on her back and knees flexed, bony pelvis is determined, ischial tuberosities are identified, and distance from tuberosities to top of fundus is measured.

14. During the regular prenatal visits, what assessment data other than vital signs and weight are determined with each visit?

    1. Fundal height, fetal heart rate, presence of venous congestion, posture, and gait.
    2. Urinalysis, glucose screen, fundal height, and fetal heart rate.

3. Presence of/changes in Chadwick's sign, complete blood count, and blood glucose screening.

4. Pelvic measurements, fundal height, urinalysis, and complete blood count.

Perinatal Care & Newborn

15. A client is pregnant for the fifth time. She had two spontaneous abortions in the first trimester. She has a son and daughter, both full-term pregnancies. What is her calculation of gravida and para using the TPAL acronym?

1. Gravida 2, para 5, T1, P1, A2, L4.

2. Gravida 5, para 2, T2, P0, A2, L2.

3. Gravida 2, para 4, T0, P2, A0, L2.

4. Gravida 5, para 2, T0, P2, A2, L2.

16. A client comes in for her first prenatal visit. Her last menstrual period (LMP) was on June 15, 2003. Using Nagele's rule, the nurse practitioner computes estimated date of delivery (EDD) as:

1. March 22, 2004.

2. April 20, 2004.

3. February 15, 2004.

4. April 3, 2004.

17. Dietary changes to reduce nausea and vomiting in pregnancy include:

1. Consuming small, frequent, low-fat meals and avoiding spicy foods.

2. Avoiding carbonated beverages.

3. Avoiding eating first thing in the morning.

4. Increasing iron and prenatal vitamins to twice daily.

18. The pregnant woman requires an average of how many extra calories per day?

1. 100.

2. 300.

3. 500.

4. 800.

19. A pregnant client at 22 weeks' gestation is planning a prolonged car trip. The nurse practitioner's recommendations would **not** include:

1. Support stockings.

2. Frequent (every 1–2 hours) walking.

3. Wearing a seat belt.

4. Knee-high stockings.

20. The recommended office visit interval for a low-risk client at 28 weeks of pregnancy is every:

1. 4 weeks.

2. Week.

3. 2 weeks.

4. 6 weeks.

21. At 20 weeks' gestation, the nurse practitioner would expect to palpate the fundus at:

1. The symphysis pubis.

2. The umbilicus.

3. Halfway between symphysis pubis and umbilicus.

4. The xiphoid.

22. Which is **not** an expected complication of the pregnant client 35 years or older?

1. Spontaneous abortion (SAB).

2. Pregnancy-induced hypertension (PIH).

3. Gestational diabetes mellitus (GDM).

4. Anemia.

23. At an initial prenatal visit occurring in the first trimester, which blood test is **not** recommended?

1. Antibody screen.

2. Rubella.

3. Maternal serum alpha-fetoprotein (MSAFP).

4. Hepatitis B surface antigen.

24. The most common indication for genetic counseling is:

1. Maternal age.

2. Drug exposure during the first trimester.

3. Increased maternal alpha-fetoprotein.

4. History of previous stillbirth.

25. Clients at highest risk for having a child with Tay-Sachs disease are:

    1. Black.

    2. Jewish.

    3. Oriental.

    4. 35 years or older at conception.

26. The nurse practitioner teaches a prenatal client that a significant source of toxoplasmosis is:

    1. Rare hamburger.

    2. Fresh fruits.

    3. Raw oysters.

    4. Raw vegetables.

27. A pregnant diabetic client is in the clinic for a prenatal visit; she is at 34 weeks' gestation. She was last seen in the clinic 1 month earlier and her dose of insulin had not changed from the previous month. This month her blood sugar remains in control with the same amount of insulin. How would the nurse practitioner interpret this information?

    1. This is normal and indicates the woman has been on her diet, and her insulin needs are stable.

    2. The infant is developing well, and his pancreas is assisting to control the increased blood sugar from the mother.

    3. With the developing fetus, there should be an increase in the serum glucose for increased nourishment.

    4. The mother may be developing problems with placental insufficiency and should be thoroughly evaluated.

28. Which finding would the nurse practitioner assess in a client with a ruptured tubal pregnancy?

    1. Sharp, stabbing pain localizing to left lower quadrant with blood pressure (BP) of 90/58.

    2. Boardlike rigidity of the uterus with abdominal distention.

    3. Dilatation of the cervix and rapidly falling BP and pulse.

    4. Serosanguineous vaginal fluid with grape-like vesicles.

29. A pregnant client at 20 weeks' gestation comes into the clinic with complaints of vaginal bleeding for the past 6 hours as well as abdominal cramping before the bleeding started. Vaginal examination reveals a decrease in the uterine size, loss of pregnancy symptoms, and a closed, firm cervix. The most likely diagnosis for this client is:

    1. Threatened abortion.

    2. Braxton Hicks contractions.

    3. Placenta abruptio.

    4. Missed abortion.

30. The nurse practitioner schedules a 38-year-old primigravida for an amniocentesis at 16 weeks' gestation. The nurse practitioner would explain that the purpose of this procedure is to:

    1. Assess for the possibility of twins.

    2. Determine the bilirubin level.

    3. Perform genetic studies.

    4. Assess lecithin/sphingomyelin (L/S) ratio.

31. Management of a client after an amniocentesis includes assessing for:

    1. Increased fetal activity.

    2. Elevated temperature.

    3. Spontaneous rupture of the membranes.

    4. Abnormal lung sounds.

32. What would be appropriate management for a primigravida at term who experiences rupture of the membranes?

    1. Begin timing contractions.

    2. Begin pushing.

    3. Take a warm bath.

    4. Immediately go to the emergency department (ED).

33. The nurse practitioner would note which finding as a possible sign of pregnancy-induced hypertension (PIH)?

    1. Urgency to urinate at night.

    2. Edema in extremities and puffy face.

    3. Stomach cramps.

    4. Clear fluid discharge from nipple.

34. The nurse practitioner is discussing the monitoring of the growth of twins during the pregnancy with a client in the first trimester. Which test would the practitioner explain to the client?

    1. Nonstress test (NST).

    2. Sonogram.

    3. L/S ratio.

    4. Amniocentesis.

35. A woman who has missed her period for 5 weeks states that she has been having nausea with some vomiting in the morning hours. The woman also states that she may have a urinary tract infection due to frequency and fatigue. The nurse practitioner would recognize these symptoms to be:

    1. A possible systemic infection.

    2. Positive signs of pregnancy.

    3. Presumptive signs of pregnancy.

    4. Probable signs of pregnancy.

36. The nurse practitioner managing a pregnant client with sickle cell trait would include which information in the plan?

    1. Complete blood count (CBC) each trimester.

    2. Weekly nonstress test.

    3. Urine cultures each trimester.

    4. Frequent ultrasounds for growth.

37. Screening for gestational diabetes mellitus (GDM) during pregnancy includes:

    1. 1-hour postprandial 100-gm glucose screen for all women at 24–28 weeks' gestation.

    2. 3-hour 100-gm glucose tolerance test (GTT) at initial visit for all women with GDM history.

    3. 1-hour postprandial 50-gm glucose screen at initial visit for women at risk.

    4. Glycosylated hemoglobin A_{1c} (HgbA$_{1c}$) for all women at 24–28 weeks' gestation.

38. A 23-year-old G3 P0 has a 1-hour postprandial 50-gm glucose screen result of 210 mg/dl. What is the next appropriate step for the nurse practitioner to take?

    1. Order 3-hour 100-gm GTT.

    2. Order fasting blood sugar (FBS).

    3. Order HgbA$_{1c}$.

    4. Refer immediately for diabetic treatment.

39. A teenager returns to the clinic for contraceptive follow-up after being on a low-dose oral contraceptive (OC) for 3 months. She complains of amenorrhea for 2 months, urinary frequency, and leukorrhea. Vaginal examination reveals uterus about 6 cm and presence of Chadwick's sign. The first diagnostic test indicated should be:

    1. Pregnancy test.

    2. Complete blood count.

    3. Microscopic urinalysis.

    4. Culture for gonorrhea and *Chlamydia*.

40. An adult client presents with her spouse for a prenatal visit. During the examination the nurse practitioner notices bruises on her abdomen and back. The spouse does most of talking during the history. What is the best approach for the nurse practitioner to take in this situation?

    1. Ask the spouse to leave the room so the nurse can do a pelvic exam.

    2. Ask the woman to accompany the nurse to the lab for blood work, and ask about bruises.

    3. Ask the woman about the bruises during the exam.

    4. Do nothing; domestic violence is beyond the scope of the nurse's practice.

41. A pregnant employee who works at a day care center is concerned about a recent outbreak of "fifth disease." The nurse practitioner understands that:

    1. Most parvovirus B19 infections in utero are associated with an increased number of congenital anomalies.

    2. There are no isoimmunization-associated problems for the mother exposed to a young child with fifth disease.

    3. Parvovirus B19 has caused hydrops fetalis and death in some fetuses infected in utero.

    4. Mortality risk for a fetus is extremely high, especially if the mother has never had fifth disease.

42. Which is an **abnormal** complaint in the second trimester of pregnancy?

    1. Frequent uterine contractions.
    2. Frequent fetal movement.
    3. Calf cramps.
    4. Heartburn.

43. Which statement is true about smoking during pregnancy?

    1. The rate of spontaneous abortion among smokers is the same as in nonsmokers.
    2. Risks of complications increase with the number of cigarettes smoked.
    3. Discontinuation of smoking during pregnancy has no effect on pregnancy outcome.
    4. No relationship exists between smoking and sudden infant death syndrome (SIDS).

44. Chlamydial infections during pregnancy may be associated with:

    1. Transplacental transmission to fetus.
    2. Congenital anomalies of the eyes.
    3. Premature rupture of membranes.
    4. Fetal hydrops.

45. Cocaine use during pregnancy is associated with:

    1. Abruptio placentae.
    2. Postdate pregnancy.
    3. Macrosomatia infant.
    4. Maternal hypotension.

46. Which is **not** a normal cervical finding in the second trimester?

    1. Cervix firm.
    2. Cervical dilatation.
    3. Cervix 2 cm long.
    4. Cervix posterior.

47. During pregnancy, sexual relations are contraindicated:

    1. During the first trimester when client has a history of spontaneous abortion.
    2. After 36 weeks' gestation.
    3. With the diagnosis of placenta previa.
    4. With excessive maternal weight gain.

48. Which is an **abnormal** complaint in the first trimester of pregnancy?

    1. Nausea and vomiting.
    2. Fatigue.
    3. Vaginal bleeding.
    4. Low backache.

49. The recommended screening test for gestational diabetes mellitus (GDM) is:

    1. 3-hour glucose tolerance test (GTT).
    2. 1-hour blood sugar measurement after 50 gm of glucose.
    3. 2-hour postprandial blood sugar measurement.
    4. Random blood sugar measurement.

50. Which is an **abnormal** complaint of the third trimester of pregnancy?

    1. Leukorrhea.
    2. Headache with blurred vision.
    3. Urinary frequency.
    4. Uterine contractions.

51. Which would be **incorrect** for the treatment of mild PIH?

    1. Modified bed rest.
    2. Monitor BP, weight, and urinary protein.
    3. Methyldopa (Aldomet) 250 mg PO tid.
    4. Daily urine dipstick for protein.

52. What would be **incorrect** advice to a nonlaboring pregnant client with a second-trimester diagnosis of marginal placenta previa?

    1. Pelvic rest.
    2. Report any bright-red bleeding.
    3. Planned cesarean section.
    4. Follow-up ultrasound at 32 weeks' gestation.

53. A pregnant client requests further information regarding exercise guidelines. She runs on the treadmill 4 mph for 30 minutes daily, then does 30 additional minutes of free weight and lower leg exercises at the gym. General guidelines should include all **except**:

    1. Keep the heart rate <140 beats/min.

    2. Limit free weight for upper body to <10 lb each.

    3. Limit exercise time to 30 minutes total.

    4. Avoid breathlessness and excessive heat.

54. Testing for GDM should be done in which of the following clients?

    1. Client with previous macrosomatia infant.

    2. Obese clients.

    3. All pregnant clients.

    4. Client with glycosuria.

55. Which is **not** a predisposing factor of PIH?

    1. Primigravida.

    2. Age >35.

    3. Multiple gestation.

    4. Hyperthyroidism.

56. For a pregnant client at 32 weeks' gestation with a BP of 140/92, weight gain the past 2 weeks of 4 lb, trace protein on urine dip, 1+ pitting edema in the feet, and 2+ reflexes, the probable diagnosis would be:

    1. Mild PIH.

    2. Severe PIH.

    3. Eclampsia.

    4. Hemolysis, elevated liver enzymes, low platelets (HELLP) syndrome.

57. The nurse practitioner is assessing a client who has a positive pregnancy test. Laboratory data indicate that the mother's blood group is O positive and the father's AB negative. What risk is associated with this pregnancy?

    1. The mother may build up antibodies to the infant's blood if the infant is type B positive, which will be significant in future pregnancies.

    2. The mother is Rh positive; if the infant is Rh negative, there is an increased incidence of the infant building up Rh antibodies.

    3. Since the mother is O and the father is AB, there is an increased risk for the development of an ABO incompatibility.

    4. Type O blood is the dominant characteristic; the infant's blood will be in the O group, with no complications.

58. A young adult client, G2 P1 A0 L1, 10 weeks' gestation with intrauterine pregnancy (IUP), is seen for her first obstetric intake history and physical examination. She knows when she conceived and denies any vaginal bleeding or abdominal pain. The client has a soft, nontender fundus that measures 14 cm; adnexal exam negative for mass or tenderness; no fetal heart tones (FHTs) audible with doptone. What is the most likely diagnosis seen on ultrasound?

    1. Multiple gestation.

    2. Fibroid uterus.

    3. Ectopic pregnancy.

    4. 14-week viable IUP.

59. A healthy client is at 36 weeks' gestation. On her regular clinical visit, the fundus is measured at the level of the xiphoid process. At the 40-week gestational visit, the fundus is measured at just below the xiphoid process. What is the most likely interpretation of this observation?

    1. Fetus has stopped growing.

    2. Fetal head has descended into pelvic cavity.

    3. Labor will probably begin within 24 hours.

    4. Amount of aminotic fluid is decreased.

60. On her first prenatal visit, a client's blood work indicates that she is Rh negative. This is her first pregnancy, and she has no history of abortions. What will the nurse practitioner explain to the client regarding this information?

    1. To prevent complications of future pregnancies, the client will receive an injection of RhoGAM at about 28 weeks' gestation and after the birth of an Rh-positive infant.

    2. Her husband needs to be tested to determine if his blood type is Rh positive and if there is a problem.

    3. The client needs to receive RhoGAM at about 20 weeks' gestation and after the birth of the first child to prevent hemolytic disease.

    4. There could be a problem with the mother's blood sensitizing the infant's blood to the Rh factor, the mother will receive RhoGAM after the birth of each child.

61. During a postpartum assessment, the nurse practitioner notes a cluster of external hemorrhoids. Which statement made by the client indicates a need for additional teaching?

    1. "I can give myself an enema every other day to reduce constipation."

    2. "I can take sitz baths for pain."

    3. "I can decrease the swelling by using a topical hydrocortisone cream."

    4. "I can take a stool softener to decrease the pain of a BM."

62. A 28-year-old female client is seen by the nurse practitioner for an office visit. Her LMP was 8 weeks ago; she is complaining of left lower quadrant (LLQ) abdominal pain, spotting, and fatigue. Her pelvic exam reveals cervical os closed, minimal blood in vaginal vault, uterus minimally enlarged, mild cervical motion tenderness (CMT), left adnexal fullness and tenderness, and right adnexa within normal limits (WNL). Vital signs are stable. The serum pregnancy test is positive. What is the most cost-effective and useful test for the nurse practitioner to order?

    1. Abdominopelvic computed tomography (CT) scan.

    2. Barium enema.

    3. Pelvic ultrasound.

    4. Flat plate of abdomen.

63. Ten days after delivery a client is diagnosed with mastitis. Which of the following would the nurse practitioner expect to find on physical examination?

    1. Tender, hard, and reddened breast with increased temperature over the affected area.

    2. Dimpled skin on breasts and firm nodules around areola.

    3. Decreased milk production, inverted nipple, and firm, inflamed breast tissue.

    4. Soft, tender palpable masses with cracked, bleeding nipples.

64. In discussing the timing of contractions with a client, the nurse practitioner explains "frequency" as the interval from the:

    1. Beginning of one contraction to the beginning of the next.

    2. Beginning of one contraction to the end of that contraction.

    3. End of one contraction to the start of the next.

    4. End of one contraction to the end of the next.

65. Which is **not** an expected complication of the pregnant adolescent age 17 or younger?

    1. Premature labor and birth.

    2. Anemia.

    3. Gestational diabetes mellitus (GDM).

    4. Pregnancy-induced hypertension (PIH).

66. The biophysical profile includes which of the following parameters?

    1. Fetal breathing movements, fetal muscle tone, and amniotic fluid volume.

    2. Ultrasonography, alpha-fetoprotein screening, and fetal heart reactivity.

    3. Amniocentesis, amniotic fluid volume, and nonstress test.

    4. Contraction stress test, nonstress test, and gross fetal movement.

67. The most common reason for a nonreactive nonstress test (NST) is:

    1. Fetal hypoxia.

    2. Maternal drug use.

3. Fetal inactivity or sleep.

4. Congenital heart defect.

68. Which is **least** likely to be found in a client presenting with an ectopic pregnancy?

1. Pain.

2. Missed menses.

3. Vaginal bleeding.

4. Abdominal mass.

69. Which is **not** true about an ectopic pregnancy?

1. 90% occur in the fallopian tube.

2. Ectopic pregnancies account for approximately 10% of maternal deaths.

3. Prior history of pelvic inflammatory disease (PID) is reported in 50% of these clients.

4. Previous ectopic pregnancy does not increase risk of another ectopic pregnancy.

70. A client presents to the clinic with a diagnosis of threatened abortion. The nurse practitioner describes this as:

1. Vaginal bleeding with or without cramping and no cervical change.

2. Vaginal bleeding with cramping and cervical change.

3. Loss of pregnancy symptoms, decrease in uterine size, and cervix closed and firm.

4. Cramping, bleeding, and incomplete expulsion of products of conception.

71. A predisposing factor in preterm labor is:

1. Obesity.

2. Previous spontaneous abortions.

3. Prior preterm delivery.

4. White race.

72. The ability of amniotic fluid to produce a ferning pattern when dried may be altered by:

1. Meconium.

2. Changes in vaginal pH.

3. Presence of cervical mucus.

4. Heavy contamination with blood.

73. Ten weeks into her pregnancy, a client begins to experience light vaginal bleeding. Her human chorionic gonadotropin (hCG) levels remain elevated. The nurse practitioner would instruct the client to report which of the following symptoms?

1. Nausea and vomiting.

2. Abdominal pain or severe cramping.

3. Urinary frequency.

4. Fatigue.

74. Which statement is true regarding the course of pruritic urticaria papules and plaques of pregnancy (PUPPP)?

1. Perinatal mortality is increased.

2. Pruritus is increased postpartum.

3. Lesions first appear on abdomen.

4. Onset is usually in the first trimester.

75. Why does an infant have increased loss of scalp hair 2–4 months after delivery?

1. Increased number of hairs in telogen.

2. Hyperthyroidism.

3. Fatigue.

4. Sudden postpartum cardiovascular changes.

76. In a breast-feeding client having difficulty with milk production, the nurse practitioner understands that milk production will be increased by:

1. More frequent suckling of infant.

2. Longer duration of suckling.

3. Cessation of suckling for 24 hours.

4. Cold compresses to the breast.

77. During a breast examination on a lactating woman, which finding is cause for concern?

1. Leaking of "watery" fluid from left breast.

2. Cracked nipples that are tender to touch.

3. Warm breasts that are distended.

4. Inverted left nipple and flat right nipple.

78. A new first-time mother is being evaluated for a complaint of breast pain. Her infant is 3 weeks old, and she is breast-feeding. The infant is gaining weight and seems satisfied after feeding. On examinaion the nurse practitioner finds a red, irritated nipple on one breast but no masses or tenderness to the breast itself. What is an important part of the nurse practitioner's evaluation?

    1. Mammogram of the breast.

    2. Examination of the infant's mouth.

    3. STAT complete blood count (CBC).

    4. Analysis of the milk.

79. A client delivers a healthy newborn with a cleft lip and cleft palate. Which action by the nurse practitioner would promote maternal-infant bonding?

    1. Point out the newborn's normal characteristics.

    2. Explain to the mother how the problem is not significant.

    3. Have the mother begin taking care of the newborn immediately after delivery.

    4. Explain to the mother that orofacial surgery will completely correct the defect.

80. The nurse practitioner is measuring a newborn's frontal-occipital circumference (FOC). Correct technique involves:

    1. Placing the tape measure at the maximal occipital prominence, just above the eyebrows.

    2. Placing the cloth tape measure at a level 2 inches above the ears.

    3. Using a cloth tape to prevent inaccuracy due to stretchable materials.

    4. Having another person hold the tape in the center of the forehead and repeating the measurement.

81. Which newborn screening tests are mandatory state requirements?

    1. CBC and urinalyisis.

    2. Thyroid function test and phenylketonuria (PKU).

    3. PKU and alpha-fetoprotein.

    4. Glucose and thyroid function tests.

82. The nurse practitioner notes an undescended testicle on a newborn. She understands that testicular function and the ability to produce healthy sperm as an adult may be impaired if the repair is not made by age:

    1. 6 years.

    2. 2 years.

    3. 1 year.

    4. 6 months.

83. The nurse practitioner is examining a full-term infant who developed physiologic jaundice and is being treated with phototherapy. What is the mechanism of action of phototherapy in the treatment of this infant?

    1. The light is absorbed by bilirubin and promotes the conversion of a toxic bilirubin to an unconjugated product that can be excreted in the bile.

    2. It increases hemolysis of the excessive red blood cells that are received by the full-term infant during labor and delivery.

    3. The ultraviolet light decreases sensitivity to the destruction of red blood cells secondary to the Rh incompatibility.

    4. It increases enzymatic activity in breaking down the unconjugated bilirubin to a nontoxic form to be eliminated by the kidney.

84. A 4-day-old infant who is being breast-fed begins to develop jaundice. What is a common theory regarding the precipitating cause of this jaundice?

    1. Decreased intake in the first few days and the subsequent weight loss.

    2. Decreased tolerance and digestion of the breast milk.

    3. Increased destruction of red blood cells with release of bilirubin.

    4. Antigen-antibody reaction that increases destruction of fetal red blood cells.

85. Which infant is at an increased risk for development of "bronze baby syndrome?"

    1. Premature infant with ABO incompatibility.

    2. Oriental infant who is bottle-fed.

3. Caucasian infant who is breast-fed.

4. Presence of obstructive liver disease.

86. A mother brings her 6-week-old infant to the office with concern over the child's "constant crying." She states she did not have this problem with her other two children. She is bottle-feeding the infant, and there is no problem with feeding. The infant has a bowel movement every day, and the stools are soft. The infant is afebrile with no evidence of ear, throat, lung, or abdominal problems. What is the best diagnosis for this infant?

1. Infantile colic.

2. Spastic colon.

3. Infant stress syndrome.

4. Lactose intolerance.

87. The nurse practitioner suspects infantile colic in a 2-month-old infant. A complete physical examination reveals no abnormalities. What further study might the nurse practitioner order?

1. Chest radiograph.

2. CBC and differential.

3. Blood culture.

4. None of the above.

88. The nurse practitioner is discussing with the parents the care of their 1-month-old infant, who has been diagnosed with infantile colic. What is important to explain to the parents?

1. The problem may be decreased by not feeding the infant more often than every 3 hours.

2. No specific medication is indicated to treat the problem.

3. The problem is often related to increased stress in the home; family therapy may be indicated.

4. The formula should be changed from a milk-based to a soy-based formula.

89. The nurse practitioner is assessing an infant who was delivered by cesarean section. What is a complication frequently associated with cesarean delivery?

1. Increased levels of serum bilirubin.

2. Respiratory distress.

3. Meconium aspiration.

4. Hypoglycemia.

90. The nurse practitioner is assessing an infant's respiratory status immediately after birth. Breath sounds are normal, no retractions present, acrocyanosis present, respirations 70 and irregular with 5-second periods of apnea, pulse regular at 160, and first and second heart sounds normal with no murmurs. What is the initial interpretation of these findings?

1. Normal newborn findings for immediately after birth.

2. Symptoms suggestive of respiratory distress syndrome.

3. Increased probability of neonatal asphyxia.

4. Presence of choanal atresia.

91. The nurse practitioner is performing a newborn assessment on a full-term infant approximately 6 hours after birth. When evaluating the infant's head, the practitioner identifies an edematous area that crosses the cranial suture lines, is soft, and varies with size. The cranial suture lines have minimal space between them. What is the practitioner's interpretation of these findings?

1. A cephalhematoma is present.

2. The cranial suture lines indicate premature closing.

3. Molding of the infant's head is present.

4. A caput succedaneum is present

92. The nurse is evaluating an infant 8 hours after delivery. The infant was full term, weighed 10 lb at birth, and is being breast-fed. The mother has a history of gestational diabetes during the pregnancy. What findings indicate the need for further evaluation?

1. Blood glucose 50 mg/dl with glucose screening strips.

2. Respirations 70, tremors, and jitteriness.

3. Bilirubin level 3 mg/dl.

4. No passage of meconium stool.

93. The nurse practitioner is assessing a postpartum client about 12 hours after delivery. On assessment of the uterus, at what position would the practitioner expect to palpate the uterus?

    1. At the level of the umbilicus.

    2. Two fingerbreadths below the umbilicus.

    3. About 2 cm above the umbilicus.

    4. Three fingerbreadths above the symphysis pubis.

94. When do most non-nursing mothers resume menstruation after childbirth?

    1. 30 days.

    2. 7–9 weeks.

    3. 45 days.

    4. 2–4 weeks.

95. What risk factor is often associated with puerperal infection?

    1. Rupture of membranes 36 hours before delivery.

    2. Excessive weight gain during pregnancy.

    3. 10 hours in the labor process.

    4. Premature labor and delivery.

Pharmacology

96. Which immunization is contraindicated in pregnancy?

    1. Polio vaccine.

    2. Hepatitis B vaccine.

    3. Measles-mumps-rubella (MMR).

    4. Tetanus.

97. If studies in animals or pregnant women demonstrate evidence of fetal abnormality or risk, or if the potential for fetal risk clearly outweighs the possible benefit of a drug, the U.S. Food and Drug Administration (FDA) category for this drug is:

    1. B.

    2. C.

    3. D.

    4. X.

98. The nurse practitioner is aware that fetal exposure to tetracycline causes:

    1. Blindness.

    2. Hearing loss.

    3. Tooth discoloration.

    4. Limb deformities.

99. Which of the following may reduce the risk of neural tube defects when taken before conception?

    1. Vitamin A.

    2. Pyroxidine.

    3. Folic acid.

    4. Vitamin C.

100. The current recommendation for antepartum treatment of Rh-negative pregnant women with $Rh_o(D)$ immune globulin (RhoGAM) includes:

    1. Administration of 300 μg at 28 and 36 weeks' gestation.

    2. Administration of 300 μg at 28 weeks' gestation.

    3. Administration of 300 μg in each trimester.

    4. No administration is needed until postpartum.

101. The client comes in for her first prenatal visit. She is healthy and has no history that would contribute to complications during the pregnancy. She asks the nurse practitioner what she can take for her occasional headaches caused by eyestrain and allergies. Which of the following would the nurse practitioner recommend for this client?

    1. Ibuprofen (Advil) 200 mg q4–6h, not to exceed 600 mg over 24 hours.

    2. Naproxen (Aleve) 220 mg q8–12h.

    3. Aspirin (ASA) 60mg q6h, not to exceed 300 mg over 24 hours.

    4. Acetaminophen (Tylenol) 650 mg q4–6h, not to exceed 650 mg over 24 hours.

102. Which medication would be considered safe to use in all trimesters of pregnancy?

    1. Metronidazole (Flagyl).

    2. Tetracycline (Achromycin).

    3. Isotretinoin (Accutane).

    4. Angiotensin-converting enzyme (ACE) inhibitors.

103. For the client who wants to breast-feed and take oral contraceptives, the pill of choice is:

    1. 1/35 preparation.

    2. Triphasic preparation.

    3. Progestin-only preparation.

    4. 1/50 preparation.

104. A pregnant client in the last trimester complains of a constant backache aggravated by walking, moving, and bending. The pain does not radiate to either leg. In addition to rest,

massage, and physiotherapy, which of the following medications is appropriate?

    1. Acetaminophen.

    2. Codeine.

    3. Naproxen.

    4. Aspirin.

105. The nurse practitioner has diagnosed mastitis in a 6-week postpartum client. The client has no known drug allergies. Which medication is appropriate for treatment?

    1. Doxycycline (Vibramycin) 100 mg PO bid × 10 days.

    2. Dicloxacillin (Dynapen) 250 mg PO qid × 10 days.

    3. Metronidazole (Flagyl) 500 mg PO bid × 10 days.

    4. Ciprofloxacin (Cipro) 500 mg PO bid × 7 days.

Answers & Rationales

Physiology of Pregnancy

1. **(3)** During pregnancy, a hyperdynamic state is caused by an increase in blood volume, which results in a slightly increased heart rate and increased cardiac output. Systolic ejection murmurs are common and caused by increased flow across the pulmonic and aortic valves. Diastolic murmurs are abnormal and require referral.

2. **(3)** Progesterone affects the GI system by decreasing smooth muscle tone, delaying gastric emptying, and decreasing intestinal peristalsis. Human CG is associated with nausea and vomiting early in pregnancy. Estrogen causes the gums to become hyperemic, soft, and swollen with a tendency to bleed.

3. **(3)** The increase in plasma volume combined with a slower rise in RBC production produces a dilutional anemia. Hemoglobin and hematocrit decrease in relation to plasma volume. True anemia occurs with hemoglobin <11 gm/dl and hematocrit <35%.

4. **(4)** Leg edema is caused by increased venous pressure in the legs. Both components of the first heart sound become louder, with exaggerated splitting, and a third heart sound gallop is common after midpregnancy . Systolic ejection murmurs are common and result from the increased flow across the aortic and pulmonic valves. Diastolic murmurs are an abnormal finding.

5. **(4)** Changes in renal structure are influenced by estrogen, progesterone, increased blood volume, and uterine pressure. Changes in the collection system, such as dilatation of the renal pelvis and ureters, cause a physiologic hydronephrosis. The glomerular filtration rate does increase during pregnancy. Increased urinary frequency is related to increasing size of uterus and its pressure on the bladder. Proteinuria is abnormal except in very concentrated urine or in the first voided specimen on arising. Proteinuria is a warning of impaired kidney function or PIH.

6. **(4)** RBC volume increases approximately 30%, and WBCs increase 5000–12,000/mm³. Fibrin, fibrinogen, and plasma levels of factors VII, IX, and X are also increased. Prothrombin levels remain unchanged.

7. **(1)** During pregnancy, estrogen is responsible for stimulation of melanin-stimulating hormone, resulting in hyperpigmentation. Progesterone from the corpus luteum and later the placenta is responsible for facilitating implantation, decreasing uterine contractility, and reducing smooth muscle tone.

8. **(4)** There are five placental hormones: hCG, estrogen, progesterone, human placental lactogen, and relaxin. Cortisol is not a placental hormone.

9. **(3)** Relaxin helps to soften smooth muscle and connective tissue in preparation for labor and delivery. Progesterone relaxes smooth muscle and causes changes in the endometrium. Estrogen stimulates the development of the ductal system of the breasts and causes hypertrophy and hyperplasia of the uterus. Human placental lactogen is involved with metabolism of glucose, fatty acids, and amino

acids. It also aids in the growth of the breasts and other maternal tissues.

10. **(2)** Fetal heart tones should be heard by 12 weeks' gestation and may be heard as early as 10 weeks. Quickening is felt at 16–20 weeks. Fetal heart tones can be heard by stethoscope at 20 weeks. Respiratory movements occur later in fetal development, at about 24 weeks.

11. **(2)** Positive evidence of pregnancy includes fetal heartbeat, palpation of fetal movement by examiner, and visualization of fetus by ultrasonography. Amenorrhea, nausea, emesis, urinary frequency, fatigue, skin changes, and mother's perception of fetal movement are presumptive evidence of pregnancy. Probable evidence of pregnancy includes softening of cervix, softening of lower uterine segment, cyanosis of cervix and vagina, Braxton Hicks contractions, ballottement, palpation of fetal outline by examiner, and pregnancy tests.

12. **(2)** Chadwick's sign occurs at 6–8 weeks' gestation and is the bluish discoloration of the cervix and vagina. Goodell's sign is the softening of the cervix that is seen as early as 4 weeks' gestation. Hegar's sign is the softening of the lower uterine segment. Braxton Hicks sign consists of contractions of the uterus that can occur as early as 16 weeks' gestation.

13. **(1)** MacDonald's measurement is taken at each prenatal visit to determine abdominal contour and size. Fundal height is measure with a tape that is stretched from the top of the fundus to the symphysis pubis. If the fundal height is less than expected based on the gestational age, the estimated date of delivery (EDD) should be reevaluated and confirmed. Further fetal assessment may be necessary.

14. **(1)** Fundal height, fetal heart rate, presence of venous congestion, posture, and gait are common assessments to be determined with each prenatal visit. Urinalysis and CBC are done as part of initial exam and are repeated as necessary. Chadwick's sign is an early indication of pregnancy, and pelvic measurements are done to determine adequacy of the pelvic outlet for delivery.

Perinatal Care & Newborn

15. **(2)** *Gravida* is the number of pregnancies, including the present pregnancy, gravida 5 for this client. *Para* is the number of pregnancies that have progressed past 20 weeks, para 2. *T* is the number of pregnancies that have progressed to term, T2. *P* is the number of pregnancies with delivery preterm, P0. *A* is abortions, A2. *L* is living children, L2.

16. **(1)** The nurse practitioner counts back 3 months to March 15, and adds 7 days. This brings the date to March 22 of the next year.

17. **(1)** Clients should eat frequent small meals to keep some food in the stomach at all times and to avoid stomach distention. Sipping on carbonated beverages may be helpful. Having crackers at the bedside to take before rising in the morning may be a successful preventive measure.

18. **(2)** The pregnant woman requires about 15% more calories per day than the nonpregnant woman. This is approximately 300 calories per day and depends on the client's weight and activity level.

19. **(4)** Venous stasis occurs with prolonged sitting and may be a risk factor for thrombophlebitis. Support stockings and frequent walking should be encouraged. Knee-high stockings have elastic around the calf that may act as a tourniquet. They should be avoided during pregnancy. Seat belts are recommended.

20. **(3)** The American College of Obstetricians and Gynecologists (ACOG) recommends visits every 2 weeks starting at 28 weeks until 36 weeks. At 36 weeks, visits are weekly until delivery.

21. **(2)** The expected fundal height at 20 weeks' gestation is at the umbilicus. At 12 weeks the fundus can be palpated just above the symphysis pubis, and at 16 weeks between the symphysis and umbilicus. The fundus is palpated at the xiphoid process at approximately 36 weeks.

22. **(4)** The risk for anemia in pregnancy does not increase with age. The risks for SAB, PIH, and GDM do increase with maternal age.

23. **(3)** Routine prenatal laboratory studies include CBC, blood type and Rh, antibody screen, hepatitis B surface antigen, syphilis screen, and rubella immune status. The MSAFP is done between 15 and 20 weeks. Before this time the fetus produces little alpha-fetoprotein, and results would be inaccurate.

24. **(1)** The largest group of women who potentially benefit from genetic counseling are those 35 and older. The number of births to women between 35 and 40 years old has increased by approximately 35% in the 1990s. The primary cause of congenital abnormalities in women older than 35 years is chromosomal abnormalities. The other answers are all reasons for genetic counseling, but to a much lesser degree.

25. **(2)** The incidence of the Tay-Sachs gene in the Jewish population is 1 in 30, compared with 1 in 300 for the non-Jewish population.

26. **(1)** Undercooked red meat is a major source of toxoplasmosis. Pregnant women should be cautioned against eating undercooked meats. Cats are also shown to be hosts. Toxoplasmosis is spread through cat feces. Pregnant women should be warned about cleaning the litter box and about contaminated soil.

27. **(4)** In the last two trimesters of pregnancy, the insulin needs should steadily increase due to the insulin antagonism from the placenta, as well as from the fetus. By not increasing her need for insulin, she could be showing signs of placental insufficiency.

28. **(1)** The ruptured fallopian tube causes a sharp, sudden, stabbing pain. Symptoms of shock (decreased BP, increased pulse, increased respiration) occur, and the client quickly becomes a surgical emergency. Boardlike abdominal rigidity is often noted with abruptio placentae. Grapelike vesicles are associated with hydatidiform mole, a gestational trophoblastic disease.

29. **(4)** A missed abortion is characterized by vaginal bleeding and a closed cervix. A threatened abortion has vaginal bleeding and cramping, but the symptoms of pregnancy are still present. Placenta abruptio is bleeding without pain, and symptoms of pregnancy are present.

30. **(3)** The woman's age places her at risk for a Down syndrome baby. The L/S ratio is tested in the third trimester for fetal lung maturity.

31. **(3)** Damage to the membranes is a possibility and a high-priority situation. Fever would not be an immediate problem. Fetal heart rate is monitored, not activity.

32. **(1)** This client should begin to count the contractions to determine the progress of beginning labor. Because she is a primagravida, delivery probably is not imminent, so going to the ED is not appropriate. She should not try to "push" this early in labor. Without the protective barrier of the amniotic membrane, the mother and fetus are susceptible to infection. Bathing would be a hazard due to the possibility of contracting an infection from the bath water. The client should count the contractions and call the physician.

33. **(2)** Classic signs of PIH are generalized edema of the extremities and around the face, proteinuria, and hypertension. Stomach cramps could be an indication of early labor or GI upset. Clear nipple fluid would be an early sign of colostrum.

34. **(2)** The ultrasound test (sonogram) is used to assess growth of the fetus and position of the placenta and fetus. The NST is used to observe the response of the fetal heart rate to the stress of activity. The L/S ratio determines if there is sufficient surfactant. An amniocentesis is performed to obtain amniotic fluid for analysis later in the pregnancy, if indicated.

35. **(3)** Missed menstrual periods, nausea, vomiting, frequency, and fatigue are presumptive signs (subjective) of pregnancy. Probable signs of pregnancy are objective, such as Chadwick's sign, ballottement, and positive pregnancy test. Positive signs of pregnancy are fetal heart rate and sonographic evidence.

36. **(3)** Sickle cell trait occurs in 8% of American blacks. These women are asymptomatic, not anemic, and usually have no problems except under conditions of hypoxia. There is no difference in perinatal outcome, and these women do not require frequent ultrasounds or nonstress testing. They are at increased risk for asymptomatic bacteriuria and require a urine culture each trimester.

37. **(3)** This is standard screening for women at risk of GDM. This glucose screen should also be done for all other pregnant women between 24 and 28 weeks of gestation.

38. **(2)** This is a standard diagnostic decision tree for a screen >200 mg. If FBS >130 mg, the nurse practitioner would refer the client to or consult with the physician about the treatment plan.

39. **(1)** This clinical picture is highly indicative of pregnancy.

40. **(2)** Although Option #1 may work, it may also arouse the spouse's suspicion and create a situation. Option #2 is best because it gives a legitimate reason to move the woman quickly from the room, offers privacy to inquire about the bruises, and provides an opportunity to move the woman to a safe place, if needed, without creating confrontation.

41. **(3)** Most fetuses are not affected; however, some undergo isoimmunization, which leads to hydrops fetalis and death. The mortality risk is actually low, and there are usually no associated congenital anomalies.

42. **(1)** Contractions could represent early premature labor and should be monitored to rule out early cervical change. Not all contractions are "Braxton Hicks," and contractions require serious consideration. The other symptoms listed are important to discuss and to rule out other associated symptomatology.

43. **(2)** The risk of complications and perinatal loss increases with the number of cigarettes smoked. Discontinuation of or decrease in the amount of cigarettes smoked during pregnancy can reduce the risk of complications, especially for high-risk women.

44. **(3)** Premature rupture of membranes may be associated with chlamydial infections. Intrauterine transmission of *Chlamydia trachomatis* to the fetus has not been demonstrated. There is no evidence of fetal eye anomalies; without prophylaxis, however, conjunctivitis will develop in 30%–50% of infants 7 days after birth.

45. **(1)** Use of cocaine during pregnancy is associated with placental abruption, spontaneous abortion, and preterm labor.

Maternal blood pressure and heart rate are increased. The fetus is at risk for intrauterine growth retardation, fetal distress, seizures, and death.

46. **(2)** It is not considered normal or expected for a woman to have a dilated cervix at any time in the second trimester of pregnancy. The cervix will typically be firm, 2 cm long, and posterior, as well as closed.

47. **(3)** In placenta previa the placenta is improperly positioned in the lower uterine segment, covering all or part of the cervical os. There is an increased risk of bleeding. Management includes bed rest, no intercourse, no vaginal exams, instruction on managing bleeding, and close fetal surveillance.

48. **(3)** Vaginal bleeding could represent a potential problem in the pregnancy during the first trimester. The other symptoms listed are important as well and warrant further discussion to rule out a problem.

49. **(2)** The recommended screening test for gestational diabetes is a blood sugar measurement 1 hour after 50 gm of glucose at 24–28 weeks' gestation. If the result of this test is 140 or above, a 3-hour GTT is done.

50. **(2)** Headache associated with blurred vision could represent early symptoms of mild preeclampsia or PIH and warrants further workup to rule out a problem. The other symptoms are not of concern if not associated with other symptoms.

51. **(3)** The use of medication is no longer thought to be useful in the treatment of mild PIH and could be hazardous. The client is best treated conservatively with modified bed rest on the left side and dietary counseling, along with close monitoring of BP, weight, and urinary protein. Close follow-up with examination for edema or symptomatic change and monitoring of the fetus are also performed.

52. **(3)** There is no reason to plan a cesarean section on diagnosis of the placenta previa at this stage of the pregnancy, since the lower segment of the uterus goes through its final maturation between 28 and 32 weeks of gestation. The placenta could likely migrate by the third trimester, thus allowing for vaginal birth, barring any other unforeseen factors.

53. **(3)** No reason exists to limit the amount of time for exercise, provided the client is feeling well. Keeping the heart rate below 140 beats/min reduces the risk of internal overheating and exhaustion. The ACOG suggests limiting free weights to <10 lb to avoid undue stress and strain on muscles and ligaments. Avoidance of breathlessness and excessive heat allows for better circulation to the fetus.

54. **(3)** More than one half of pregnant women who exhibit GDM lack the classic risk factors of family history of diabetes, unexpected stillbirth, prior macrosomatia infant, obesity, advanced maternal age, and glycosuria. The best answer is that all women should be screened for gestational diabetes.

55. **(4)** Predisposing factors in PIH include primigravida, <20 years or >35 years, women with vascular diseases (hypertension, systemic lupus erythematosus, diabetes mellitus, renal disease), family history, previous history of preeclampsia, and multiple gestation. Hyperthyroidism does not predispose to PIH.

56. **(1)** Mild PIH (preeclampsia) is consistent with systolic BP >140 mm Hg or systolic rise >30 mm Hg, diastolic >90 or diastolic rise >15 mm Hg, weight gain >2 lb/wk, and nondependent edema >1+ with normal reflexes. Severe preeclampsia symptoms include BP >160/100, weight gain >2 lb/wk, generalized edema, proteinuria >3+, decreased urine output, and hyperreflexia. Eclampsia includes the above plus seizures. The HELLP syndrome includes signs and symptoms of severe preeclampsia, an enlarged and firm liver, epigastric or right upper quadrant pain, and frequently jaundice.

57. **(3)** There is an increased incidence of ABO incompatibility if the mother is blood group O and the infant is either blood group A or B. Rh incompatibility occurs only when the mother is Rh negative and is carrying an Rh-positive infant. In the most common cases of ABO incompatibility, there is production of maternal antibodies against the A or B cells.

58. **(1)** Multiple gestation will cause the uterus to enlarge faster than normal. FHTs may be inaudible with the doptone at 10 weeks' gestation. A fibroid could cause the uterus to enlarge, but it is generally accompanied by firmness to palpation of the uterus. Ectopic pregnancy could be the cause of inaudible FHTs but is usually accompanied by adnexal tenderness, a mass, or vaginal bleeding. A 14-week viable IUP should have an audible FHT with the doptone.

59. **(2)** "Lightening" often occurs at about 40 weeks' gestation when the infant's head descends into the pelvic cavity and becomes "engaged." At any other time during pregnancy, a decrease in fundal height would cause concern for the infant's growth. There has been no decrease in amniotic fluid, and it does not indicate that labor is imminent.

60. **(1)** The unsensensitized Rh-negative pregnant woman is given RhoGAM at 28 weeks' gestation as a preventive measure. It effectively prevents the formation of active antibodies if there is accidental transport of fetal Rh-positive blood cells into the circulation during the remainder of the pregnancy. At delivery the infant's blood type is determined. If the infant is Rh positive, the mother will receive another dose of RhoGAM within 72 hours of delivery. If the infant is Rh negative, there is no antibody formation and RhoGAM is unnecessary.

61. **(1)** An enema every other day to reduce constipation would negatively affect the normal bowel movement pattern and deplete the client's natural intestinal flora. Sitz baths, antiinflammatory and analgesic topical ointments and sprays, stool softeners, and increased bulk in the diet would be indicated in the management of the external hemorrhoids.

62. **(3)** This easy, inexpensive, and relatively noninvasive test assists the nurse practitioner with confirming the diagnosis of ectopic pregnancy. It can be obtained quickly and is often available rapidly. Abdominopelvic CT will also show an ectopic pregnancy but is neither cost-effective nor noninvasive. Barium enema and flat plate of the abdomen are not useful in this client.

63. **(1)** A tender, hard, and reddened breast with increased temperature over the affected area is typically found with mastitis. Dimpled skin (peau d'orange, or orange peel appearance) is a potential sign of breast cancer. Decreased milk production, inverted nipple, and firm breast tissue may be complications of engorgement. Cracked nipples may result from improper

positioning or oversuckling. Soft, tender breast masses may be engorged milk ducts.

64. **(1)** Frequency of contractions should be timed from the beginning of one contraction to the beginning of the next contraction.

65. **(3)** The pregnant adolescent is at increased risk for premature labor, anemia, and PIH. There is no documentation that the pregnant teen is at greater risk of gestational diabetes.

66. **(4)** The biophysical profile includes observation of fetal respiratory movement, fetal tone, gross fetal movement, measurement of amniotic fluid volume, and fetal heart reactivity. Each parameter is given a score of 0 to 2; and normal is 8 to 10. Ultrasonography, alpha-fetoprotein screening, nonstress testing, and stress test are not part of this profile.

67. **(3)** The most common reason for a nonreactive NST is fetal sleep or inactivity. The fetal sleep-wake cycle ranges from 20–40 minutes. If reactivity is not demonstrated in 20 minutes, continuing to 40 minutes usually accommodates the sleep-wake cycles. Fetal hypoxia and maternal smoking and drug use certainly affect fetal heart rate but are not the most common causes. Infants with a congenital heart defect do not exhibit a significant incidence of nonreactive NSTs.

68. **(4)** Greater than 90% of clients presenting with ectopic pregnancies will complain of pain and report a missed period. Approximately 80% will describe vaginal bleeding. Only 50% will have a palpable abdominal mass.

69. **(4)** It is true that 90% of ectopic pregnancies are found in the fallopian tubes. Clients with PID have a sevenfold increase in the rate of ectopic pregnancy. A previous ectopic pregnancy is a risk factor and does increase the risk of a subsequent ectopic pregnancy.

70. **(1)** A threatened abortion progresses to complete spontaneous abortion in 50% of cases. Clinical findings are vaginal bleeding with or without cramping and no cervical change. Vaginal bleeding with cramping and cervical change is an inevitable abortion. An incomplete abortion is demonstrated by vaginal bleeding, cramping, and incomplete expulsion of the products of conception. A missed abortion is diagnosed when products

of conception are retained after fetal death. There is a decrease in uterine size, loss of pregnancy symptoms, and often a closed and firm cervix.

71. **(3)** History of preterm birth is associated with a 20%–40% recurrence risk. Low prepregnancy weight and inadequate weight gain, not obesity, are associated with preterm labor. Maternal smoking, drug use (especially cocaine), low socioeconomic status, maternal age <17 and >35, and nonwhite race are all predisposing factors for preterm labor. Previous spontaneous and elective abortions are not risk factors.

72. **(4)** When air-dried, amniotic fluid produces a fern pattern. This microscopic arborization is accurate in confirming rupture of membranes in 90%–95% of cases. Samples heavily contaminated with blood may not fern.

73. **(2)** Contractions, cramping, or abdominal pain along with continued bleeding could signify a spontaneous abortion. The other symptoms are common during the first trimester.

74. **(3)** Lesions typically start on the abdomen and spread to the thighs and possibly the buttocks. Onset of lesions is usually in the third trimester and usually resolves postpartum. There is no associated adverse perinatal outcome.

75. **(1)** Normally, 15%–20% of hairs are in telogen (resting phase of hair cycle). In late pregnancy this is reduced to <10%. After delivery the percentage increases, and by 2 months postpartum, 20% of hairs are in telogen. Therefore a marked increase occurs in hair loss at 2–4 months after delivery.

76. **(1)** More frequent suckling will increase production of milk more effectively than increasing the duration of suckling. Stopping or decreasing breast-feeding or applying cold compresses to the breasts will decrease milk production.

77. **(2)** Cracked nipples are a sign of irritation and may eventually cause skin breakdown with severe pain.

78. **(2)** Breast irritation in nursing mothers is often caused by *Candida albicans*. The source of infection is most likely the infant's mouth (thrush).

79. **(1)** Initially after delivery, the mother needs an opportunity to accept that her newborn has a congenital defect. Pointing out normal characteristics of the newborn will allow her to put the problem in perspective. Often the mother will focus on the defect. Orofacial surgery will provide closure of the defect but will not completely correct it, since scarring will undoubtedly occur.

80. **(1)** Using a paper or a plastic tape, rather than cloth, prevents error due to the stretching of the fabric. Measurements should be repeated to confirm accuracy. The tape should not lie over the ears.

81. **(2)** Neonatal screening for PKU and congenital hypothyroidism is done in all states. Other tests are up to the primary care provider. Alpha-fetoprotein is usually a maternal blood test done during the prenatal period to screen for genetic defects, primarily neural tube anomalies.

82. **(2)** Normal morphology and testes tissue development will be impaired if the testes are not descended by age 2 years. These children are at higher risk for development of testicular cancer in the young adult male (20–30 years old).

83. **(1)** Phototherapy is effective secondary to the absorption of the light by bilirubin across the infant's skin. The light energy is absorbed by bilirubin and promotes the conversion of bilirubin to a nontoxic form that can be excreted in the bile without the need for conjugation. The increase in hemolysis will increase the bilirubin level, and this is physiologic jaundice that is *not* associated with an Rh incompatibility problem.

84. **(1)** Neonatal jaundice is more common in breast-fed infants and is thought to result from the decreased intake in the first few days. It usually begins between 4 and 7 days after birth, and the bilirubin levels range from 10 to 30 mg/dl. Increasing the infant's intake of water does not improve the condition. Breast-feeding may be temporarily interrupted, but phototherapy is usually unnecessary.

85. **(4)** Bronze baby syndrome describes a grayish brown pigmentation that occurs in neonates. It may occur in infants undergoing phototherapy but is usually associated with infants who have obstructive liver problems. The pigmentation is not permanent but may last for several months.

86. **(1)** Infantile colic is unexplained crying and restlessness that lasts longer than 3 hours per day, 3 days a week. Most often it stops spontaneously at about 3 months. Other causes, particularly infections, should be ruled out. Spastic colon and lactose intolerance are unlikely and would include problems with diarrhea and constipation. Infant stress syndrome is not a valid problem.

87. **(4)** With a normal physical exam, in the absence of fever or sepsis, the listed lab tests are not necessary to diagnose colic. If there were positive findings or fever, the complete laboratory workup should be obtained, with the addition of urinalysis and lumbar puncture.

88. **(2)** After the infant has been carefully evaluated and there is no evidence of other problems, it is important to explain to the parents that no medication is available to treat the condition. The condition is not resolved by changing the feeding schedule of the infant, it is not related to stress within the home, and a change to soy formula will not solve the problem. The parents must be informed that the colic most often resolves with no residual problems by age 3 months.

89. **(2)** The physiology of normal vaginal delivery causes pressure against the infant's thorax and helps to remove amniotic fluid. If the cesarean section was done as an emergency prior to term, the infant may have inadequate surfactant for good pulmonary function. Increased levels of bilirubin, meconium aspiration, and hypoglycemia are not associated with an increase in cesarean delivery.

90. **(1)** These are normal newborn findings. The respiratory rate is increased but is usually increased immediately after birth (transient tachypnea) and during the second period of reactivity. Continued tachypnea is abnormal. The respiratory rate should be counted for a full minute due to the irregularity of the infant's breathing. Periodic pauses may occur for up to 10 seconds, but apnea lasting longer

than 20 seconds is abnormal. Acrocyanosis is normal immediately after birth. Choanal atresia occurs when one or both of the nasal passages are blocked by an abnormality of the septum. In respiratory distress syndrome the infant exhibits other symptoms that are consistent with hypoxia.

91. **(4)** Caput succedaneum results from pressure against the mother's cervix during labor. The edematous area crosses the suture lines and will resolve within hours to days after birth. There is normally a space between the cranial suture lines; if there is no space or an overriding suture line, it may be caused by molding. Widening of the suture line may indicate increased intracranial pressure. Cephalhematoma is characterized by bleeding between the bone and the periosteum, and it does not cross the suture line.

92. **(2)** Early signs of hypoglycemia are jitteriness, poor muscle tone, tremors, and symptoms of respiratory difficulty. The blood sugar of 50 mg/dl is within normal limits at this time (40–60 mg/dl the first 24 hours). If blood sugar levels are less that 45 mg/dl on the screening strip, a follow-up serum glucose should be done. The meconium stool should be passed within the first 24 hours, and the bilirubin level is normal.

93. **(1)** Within a few hours after birth, the fundus rises to the level of the umbilicus and remains there for about 24 hours. After 24 hours the fundus begins to descend by about 1 cm or one fingerbreadth per day. It often is not palpable by day 10.

94. **(2)** Most non-nursing mothers will resume menstruation 7–9 weeks after birth. About one half of them will ovulate during the first cycle. Most lactating women will resume menstruation in 12 weeks, although some do not menstruate during the entire lactation period.

95. **(1)** Prolonged rupture of the membranes is defined as membrane rupture >24 hours before delivery. The rupture provides an increased opportunity for bacterial growth. Excessive weight gain and premature delivery are not associated with postpartum infection. Ten hours in labor is well within the normal time for labor.

Pharmacology

96. **(3)** The MMR is a live virus and is contraindicated in pregnancy. Polio, tetanus, and hepatitis B vaccine are inactivated bacterial or DNA-based vaccines and are safe when indicated.

97. **(4)** The FDA has five pregnancy risk categories for drugs. Category X indicates that fetal risk outweighs any benefit, and use in pregnancy is contraindicated. Category B drugs show no evidence of fetal abnormalities, and risk to the fetus is relatively unlikely. Category C drugs have potential for animal fetal abnormalities and/or no adequate well-controlled studies in pregnant women, but benefits of drugs are thought to justify risks to the fetus. Drugs classified as Category D demonstrate positive evidence of human fetal risk and should be used only in serious disease or life-threatening situations when safer drugs are ineffective.

98. **(3)** Tetracycline binds with developing enamel and discolors the deciduous teeth between 26 weeks of gestation and 6 months of infancy.

99. **(3)** Recent studies have confirmed that folic acid taken before conception can reduce the risk of neural tube defect.

100. **(2)** Current recommendations for RhoGAM is administration of 300 μg to all Rh-negative women at 28 weeks of pregnancy. This is considered protective for the remainder of the pregnancy.

101. **(4)** Acetaminophen is a risk category B drug, but problems have not been documented; it should be used with caution. Aspirin is risk category D and may cause bleeding disorders. Nonsteroidal antiinflammatory drugs (NSAIDs; ibuprofen, naproxen) are risk category B but have been associated with prolonging pregnancy and labor due to antiprostaglandin effects.

102. **(1)** Metronidazole is safe to use in all trimesters of pregnancy. The other medications are known teratogens and therefore contraindicated in pregnancy.

103. **(3)** Estrogen inhibits milk production. Progestin-only preparations are ideal for the breast-feeding client because they do not contain estrogen and therefore do not inhibit milk production. The other OCs listed contain estrogen in varying amounts.

104. **(1)** Acetaminophen can be safely prescribed to the pregnant client. Aspirin and NSAIDs are contraindicated in the third trimester.

The use of narcotics for this client is inappropriate.

105. **(2)** Dicloxacillin will treat *Staphylococcus aureus,* which is the most common organism associated with mastitis. None of the other medications is appropriate for treatment of mastitis, and both doxycycline and ciprofloxacin are contraindicated when breast-feeding.

18

Mental Health

Psychosocial Examination & Diagnostic Tests

1. The mental status examination enables the nurse practitioner to identify:

   1. Intelligence quotient and reasoning.

   2. Abstract thinking and memory functioning.

   3. Reasoning and psychomotor skills.

   4. Memory functioning and intelligence quotient.

2. A client with a history of psychiatric problems arrives at the clinic shouting that he is a messenger of God and knows the meaning of the prophecies in Revelations. This behavior is assessed as:

   1. A delusion.

   2. A hallucination.

   3. Magical thinking.

   4. An illusion.

3. An assessment of a client experiencing auditory hallucinations would most likely reveal:

   1. Client mumbling to self, tilted head, eyes darting back and forth.

   2. Performance of obsessive-compulsive rituals of turning off and on a radio, talking to self.

   3. Hyperactivity, expansive mood, easy distractibility.

   4. Cool, aloof, unapproachable, avoiding enclosed areas.

4. The MAST and the CAGE are screening instruments for which disease process?

   1. Glaucoma.

   2. Depression.

   3. Alcoholism.

   4. Diabetes.

5. When receiving records from another agency, the nurse practitioner notes on the summary sheet that the client has a dual diagnosis. This means the client has:

   1. Both manic and depressive symptoms of bipolar affective disorder.

   2. Two closely related psychiatric disorders (e.g., panic disorder and bulimia nervosa).

   3. Coexistence of both a psychiatric disorder (e.g., depression) and a substance abuse disorder (e.g., alcohol dependence).

   4. Coexistence of a personality disorder (e.g., borderline personality) and a psychiatric disorder (e.g., panic disorder).

6. A child is being evaluated for attention deficit hyperactivity disorder (ADHD). Which test is helpful in evaluating the difference between ADHD and a learning disability?

   1. Standardized IQ achievement test.

   2. Denver Developmental Screening Test.

   3. Audiologic and visual testing.

   4. Complete neurologic examination.

7. While completing the history on an older adult, the nurse practitioner understands that when a client "makes up stories or answers" to the questions, this is known as:

   1. Perseveration.

   2. Confabulation.

   3. Echolalia.

   4. Alcoholic encephalopathy.

8. In taking a history from a client with depression, which is the most important question for the nurse practitioner to ask?

   1. Have you ever experienced hallucinations, delusions, or illusions?

   2. Have you ever been hospitalized in a psychiatric facility?

   3. Do you regularly take antidepressants or other medications?

   4. Have you thought about or attempted suicide?

9. While taking a history, the nurse practitioner is aware that the following drug is most commonly first used by an adolescent:

   1. Nicotine.

   2. Alcohol.

   3. Marijuana.

   4. Crystal methamphetamine.

10. A common laboratory finding associated with bulimia nervosa is:

    1. Hyperkalemia.

    2. Hypochloremia.

    3. Elevated liver enzymes.

    4. Platelet abnormalities.

11. The nurse practitioner knows habituation is suggested when a client gives a history of:

    1. The same dose of the drug has reduced effects.

    2. Less of the medication produces the desired effects.

    3. No withdrawal symptoms when the drug is stopped.

    4. Increasing side effects with an increase in the dosage of drug.

12. Which statement is correct about mental health in the older adult and supports research findings in the literature?

    1. Self-esteem does not decline as a person ages.

    2. Older adults are consistently concerned about their physical appearance.

    3. Older adults have a negative self-image in comparison with younger adults.

    4. Learning ability is not maintained due to loss of short-term memory.

13. When doing a mental status examination, which questions would be helpful to assess the ability of the client for abstract thinking?

    1. Can you repeat the following numbers: 1, 3, 5, 7, 9?

    2. What is today's date?

3. How are a carpet and a hardwood floor alike?

4. Can you tell me the name of three past U.S. presidents?

Psychiatric Disorders

14. An elderly client is experiencing a recent onset of confusion. The nurse practitioner is trying to determine whether the confusion is related to depression or dementia. In evaluating this client, what specific assessment finding would be helpful in making this distinction?

1. Determining whether confusion worsens in the evening.

2. Assessing early morning agitation, hyperactivity, and insomnia.

3. Noting signs of anger, hostility, and loss of control.

4. Assessing reality distortions and preoccupation with family matters.

15. A client calls the clinic and asks to speak to the nurse practitioner. When she answers the telephone, the client states that he is going to commit suicide. The priority goal is to:

1. Refer the client to an appropriate treatment facility.

2. Encourage ventilation of angry and depressed feelings.

3. Assess the lethality of the suicide plan.

4. Establish rapport with the client.

16. During an intake interview with a 26-year-old man diagnosed with generalized anxiety disorder, the nurse practitioner might observe what type of behaviors?

1. An inflated sense of self.

2. Constant relation to future events.

3. Inability to concentrate and irritability when questioned.

4. Nervousness and fear of the nurse practitioner during the interview.

17. An elderly woman answers the nurse practitioner's questions by mumbling in low tones with answers that seem inappropriate. What would be initial findings associated with a diagnosis of dementia?

1. Sees people floating across the ceiling of her room.

2. Has problems with cognition and confusion.

3. Hears voices at night telling her to change her clothes.

4. Shows fear when the nurse makes any movements toward her.

18. An older client comes to the office with the complaint of confusion. The daughter is concerned that her mother is developing Alzheimer's disease. Which of these assessments would indicate this client is experiencing delirium versus dementia?

1. The confusion has been slowly developing.

2. The confusion started after the client started taking cimetidine (Tagamet).

3. The client's attention span has not been affected.

4. The client's memory has been impaired.

19. When the nurse practitioner talks with a client about his chemical dependency, the client states, "I wish I would have never used cocaine. It has ruined my life!" What would be the most appropriate response by the nurse practitioner?

1. "You should think before you do something."

2. "Things will work out, don't worry."

3. "It sounds like you've thought a lot about your cocaine use."

4. "You shouldn't be so hard on yourself. You can change."

20. The nurse would expect which symptoms in a client with a diagnosis of schizophrenia?

1. High energy with varying sleep patterns and nonstop conversation.

2. Extreme and frequent mood swings with hyperactivity and difficulty concentrating.

3. Paranoia, delusions, hallucinations, and diminished self-care.

4. Antisocial behavior, manipulativeness, charisma, and ability to lie convincingly.

21. Dementia can be distinguished from delirium by:

    1. Dementia lasts days to weeks compared to delirium, which lasts months to years.

    2. Dementia is often associated with medications or systemic illness.

    3. Dementia exhibits a disturbance in attention that is not present in delirium.

    4. Dementia does not include altered perception, including hallucinations and illusions.

22. An elderly client is brought to the nurse practitioner by his family for evaluation of increasing confusion over the past few days. The client has a history of dementia; however, the family states that this is a definite change. What course of action would the nurse practitioner consider?

    1. Help the family look for a nursing home.

    2. Order an immediate magnetic resonance imaging (MRI) scan.

    3. Perform a comprehensive medication review.

    4. Order a urine analysis (UA).

23. A middle-aged, upper-middle class, married woman presents to your clinic for the third time in 2 months with a complaint of headache, gastrointestinal upset with abdominal pain, and difficulty sleeping. Past exams have been essentially negative. You suspect the client suffers from depression, but she has been reluctant to complete even the briefest of screenings for this. Today, the client requests "something for sleep," again stating she "doesn't have time to take a bunch of tests." Which tentative diagnosis seems most likely?

    1. Hypochondriasis.

    2. Domestic violence.

    3. Addiction.

    4. Irritable bowel syndrome.

24. An elderly client was taken to the clinic in a confused state that began suddenly 24 hours ago. She fails to be oriented to person, time, or place. She was incontinent of urine due to her confusion. She looks apathetic and is drowsy. The nurse practitioner would suspect:

    1. Delirium.

    2. Dementia.

3. Depression.

4. A psychotic disorder.

25. Which of the following groups of clients fall under mandatory reporting laws for abuse and neglect in a majority of states in the United States?

    1. Children, adult women, dependent elderly.

    2. Children, disabled individuals, adult women.

    3. Disabled individuals, adult women, dependent elderly.

    4. Children, disabled individuals, dependent elderly.

26. A mother brings her young child to the clinic, stating she fell off the porch swing. What assessment finding would cause the nurse practitioner to consider the possibility of child abuse?

    1. Mother is very upset and stroking her daughter's hair.

    2. Child is crying and says her head and arm hurt.

    3. Child has red, blue, and green colored bruised areas on her trunk.

    4. Child has a bruised, edematous area on forehead and shoulder.

27. In evaluating a 16-year-old female client, which symptom would indicate anorexia nervosa?

    1. Refuses to discuss questions pertaining to food.

    2. Reflects a positive body image.

    3. States she is eating very well but has episodes of vomiting.

    4. The family states she refuses to stop her severe dieting.

28. A mother is concerned about her child having nightmares. The nurse practitioner understands the difference between nightmares and night terrors is:

    1. Nightmares are vivid, frightening dreams recalled by the child.

    2. Nightmares rarely occur in children before age 4.

    3. Nightmares are accompanied by gross motor movements, labored breathing, and enuresis.

    4. Nightmares and night terrors are essentially the same and are unrelated to stressful events.

29. A 16-year-old adolescent boy is 54 inches in height. The nurse practitioner identifies the following as a positive effective coping behavior:

    1. Acts as the class clown.

    2. Has a rehearsed reply to teasing comments.

    3. Spends most of his free time watching television.

    4. Has predominantly friends that are short statured.

30. The nurse practitioner is examining an older adolescent who has been a long-term intravenous cocaine user. What other findings would alert the nurse practitioner to a frequent complication?

    1. Epistaxis and chronic rhinorrhea.

    2. Cardiac arrhythmias and hypertension.

    3. Chest congestion and wheezing.

    4. Hepatitis and cellulitis.

31. The nurse practitioner is comparing the typical signs of depression in the adolescent with the adult client. The depressed adolescent would present with:

    1. Lonely feelings.

    2. Sad, flat affect.

    3. Anger and acting-out behavior.

    4. Feelings of powerlessness and anxiety.

32. The effects of prenatal cocaine exposure on newborns includes:

    1. Increased incidence of prematurity.

    2. Large-for-gestational-age.

    3. Caput succedaneum.

    4. Hypotonia and lethargy.

33. While interviewing a teenager to determine her level of health, the nurse practitioner recognizes symptoms of anorexia nervosa. Which characteristics of anorexia nervosa would be noted in the admission assessment interview?

    1. Below to average intelligence.

    2. Increased libido.

    3. Vigorous daily exercise.

    4. Tachycardia.

34. The nurse practitioner expects a preschool child with ADHD to have:

    1. Delayed growth and development, especially language skills.

    2. Negativism, overactivity, and active curiosity.

    3. Diminished fine motor skills and frequent mood swings.

    4. Easy distractibility, impulsiveness, and fidgeting.

35. The nurse practitioner is completing a history and physical exam on a child who she suspects may be autistic. Findings associated with autism include:

    1. Delay in language development.

    2. Delay in physical growth.

    3. Overprotective parents who provide minimal social interaction for the child.

    4. Warm, cuddling child with excessive need for interaction.

36. The mother of a preschooler is concerned because her child has begun to stutter. The nurse practitioner should:

    1. Refer the child to a speech pathologist.

    2. Encourage the mother to correct the child when she stutters.

    3. Give the child verbal exercises to perform at home.

    4. Reassure the mother that stuttering is normal in a preschooler.

37. A teenaged female client is brought to the nurse practitioner for evaluation by her grandmother with whom she lives. The teenager has been vomiting and her grandmother believes that she is becoming confused. The grandmother relates that the client has been upset lately over a breakup with her boyfriend. What will the nurse practitioner investigate as a possible cause for this teenager's symptoms?

    1. Appendicitis.

    2. Ectopic pregnancy.

    3. Drug overdose.

    4. Sexually transmitted disease.

38. An adult client has a history of irritability, loss of appetite, inability to concentrate, and feelings of depression and "burn out" at work. Recently, he relates missing several days at work. He is doing and taking everything he can to relax. What would be an appropriate question to ask this client?

    1. "Do you drink alcohol or take drugs?"

    2. "Have you ever felt this way before?"

    3. "When you feel depressed, do you talk to your wife?"

    4. "Have you lost your job?"

39. A teenager comes to the office of the nurse practitioner and states that she was raped several hours ago by her boyfriend. The immediate action taken by the nurse practitioner is:

    1. Perform a pelvic examination to determine injuries to the client.

    2. Accompany her to the emergency department for an exam.

    3. Send her immediately for counseling to help her deal with this situation.

    4. Call the client's parents so they can be with her.

40. Physical findings of cocaine abuse include:

    1. Bradycardia, miosis, hypertension.

    2. Hypertension, tachycardia, tremor.

    3. Hypotension, bradycardia, abdominal cramps.

    4. Decreased level of consciousness, tachycardia, excessive salivation.

41. While interviewing an adolescent female presenting with her mother for birth control counseling and examination, you detect signs of family tension. During the physical exam, while the mother is out of the room, the daughter admits to frequent marijuana use and occasional drinking. What assessment information would most confirm the presence of active or potential violence in the home?

    1. Signs of general neglect.

    2. Injuries at different stages of healing.

    3. Client's response to a direct question.

    4. Admitted fear of mother's boyfriend.

42. The parents of a 7-year-old boy ask advice regarding sugar intake stating the teacher has said not to allow the child to have any sugar products such as cookies at lunch due to behavior problems. Advice would include:

    1. The child needs further assessment for ADHD.

    2. Moderate sugar consumption rarely produces inappropriate behavior.

    3. Increase the protein and fat in his diet to decrease nerve overstimulation.

    4. Research has shown increased sugar intake directly affects cognitive performance.

43. Which neurotransmitters are associated with the etiology of acute mania in bipolar affective disorder?

    1. Epinephrine and norepinephrine.

    2. Serotonin and dopamine.

    3. Dopamine and norepinephrine.

    4. Gamma-aminobutyric acid (GABA) and renin-angiotensin.

44. All of the following behaviors meet the criteria for substance abuse in the *Diagnostic and Statistical Manual of Mental Disorders, Fourth Edition (DSM-IV)* **except**:

    1. Repeated arrests for drunk driving.

    2. Multiple absences from work due to substance use.

    3. Chronic anxiety attacks.

    4. Recurrent arguments with spouse about his/her drinking behavior.

45. An elderly client's wife is concerned about her husband's increasing confusion and agitation. Not only has he exhibited symptoms of increased confusion, but he also is unable to care for his physical needs. He has been incontinent of urine and feces and sometimes is totally unaware of other people. What would be an assessment priority for this client?

    1. Evaluate changes in social habits.

    2. Assess for hallucinations and impaired reality testing.

    3. Evaluate his orientation to person, place, and time.

    4. Determine if he is experiencing a problem with impaired judgement.

46. A client is transferred to the alcohol treatment unit from the emergency room. What is important to include in the therapeutic milieu during detoxification?

    1. Keep the environment adequately lit to diminish illusions.
    2. Keep a radio or television on in the room to assist to maintain orientation.
    3. Speak quietly when in the room to avoid overstimulation.
    4. Keep the suction equipment available in case of seizures.

47. What condition of a child would the nurse practitioner identify as most likely to be the result of abuse?

    1. Concussion in a 4-year-old.
    2. Fractured wrist in a 6-year-old.
    3. Femur fracture in a 6-month-old.
    4. Scald burn on the arm of a 1-year-old.

Pharmacology

48. A client has been receiving fluphenazine (Prolixin) for the past 3 weeks. The nurse practitioner's assessment notes the following: temperature elevated (41°C), marked muscle rigidity, agitation, and confusion. The nurse practitioner understands these findings are often associated with the diagnosis of:

    1. Acute dystonia.
    2. Tardive dyskinesia.
    3. Neuroleptic malignant syndrome.
    4. Extrapyramidal disorder.

49. The preferred antidepressant for an elderly client is:

    1. Amitriptyline (Elavil).
    2. Citalopram (Celexa).
    3. Trazodone (Desyrel).
    4. Haloperidol (Haldol).

50. A client has been referred to the nurse practitioner. The client's medical history reveals long-term use of antianxiety agents that the client considers harmless. The nurse practitioner understands that antianxiety agents can:

    1. Cause drug dependency.
    2. Produce hepatotoxicity and nephrotoxicity.
    3. Lead to functional damage of the cardiopulmonary system.
    4. Cause profound dissociative personality problems.

51. An older female has a diagnosis of dementia and is taking haloperidol (Haldol) 2 mg HS. The nurse practitioner observes her engaging in a restless, repetitive movement with her legs. She states that, not only does she have ongoing movement, but she also feels jittery. The nurse practitioner would interpret this activity to be:

    1. Ataxia.
    2. Akathisia.
    3. Agitation.
    4. Dyskinesia.

52. What is the best initial treatment plan for a sleep disorder in the elderly client?

    1. Medicate with amitriptyline (Elavil).
    2. Medicate with trazodone (Desyrel).
    3. Discuss the importance of naps daily.
    4. Decrease noise and light in the environment.

53. An elderly client presents with a new symptom of acute confusion over the last 24 hours. Which assessment would be a priority for the nurse practitioner to evaluate during the examination?

    1. Drug history.
    2. Electrocardiogram.
    3. Minimental status exam.
    4. Thyroid profile.

54. The nurse practitioner is aware that the following class of drugs is most likely to precipitate a hypertensive crisis in the elderly.

    1. Narcotic analgesics.
    2. Monoamine oxidase (MAO) inhibitors.
    3. Barbiturates.
    4. Phenothiazines.

55. The nurse practitioner knows that the following class of drugs would have the greatest effect on memory in the elderly client:

    1. Phenothiazines.

    2. Tricyclic antidepressants.

    3. Benzodiazepines.

    4. MAO inhibitors.

56. The nurse practitioner understands that adolescents who use lysergic acid diethylamide (LSD):

    1. Experience withdrawal symptoms within 24 hours.

    2. Develop tolerance quickly and need increased amounts.

    3. Experience flashbacks and depression.

    4. Experience disorientation and delusional feelings.

57. Of the following antidepressants, which one has the most sedating side effects making it a good sleeping agent?

    1. Fluoxetine (Prozac).

    2. Doxepin (Sinequan).

    3. Trazadone (Desyrel).

    4. Paroxetine (Paxil).

58. In the management of acute alcohol withdrawal delirium, a nurse practitioner may want to use all of the following drugs **except**:

    1. Chlordiazepoxide (Librium).

    2. Lorazepam (Ativan).

    3. Thiamine.

    4. Chlorpromazine (Thorazine).

59. The nurse practitioner's physical exam on an adolescent is as follows: disheveled appearance, 5-lb weight loss since last visit 2 months ago, pulse strong and regular at 128, +4 deep tendon reflexes (DTRs), nasal mucosa erythematous and ulcerated. His mother relates that he has been getting in trouble at school, avoids the family, has no appetite, and is not sleeping much at night. The nurse practitioner suspects drug use of:

    1. Heroin.

    2. Marijuana.

    3. LSD.

    4. Crack cocaine.

60. Which laboratory results would be **least** important to assess before placing a client on Lithium?

    1. Thyroid-stimulating hormone, triidothyronine, thyroxine.

    2. Blood urea nitrogen, creatinine.

    3. Urinalysis, electrolytes.

    4. Alanine aminotransferase, aspartate aminotransferase, lactate dehydrogenase.

61. A client comes to the rural clinic having taken an undetermined amount of heroin. Prior to transferring the client to a psychiatric treatment facility, the nurse practitioner anticipates the drug of choice for an opioid overdose is:

    1. Clonidine (Catapres).

    2. Methadone (Dolophine).

    3. Naloxone (Narcan).

    4. Naltrexone HCl (Revia).

62. Benzodiazepines are useful in the treatment of all the disorders below, **except**:

    1. Alcohol withdrawal.

    2. Anxiety.

    3. Obsessive-compulsive disorder.

    4. Seizures.

63. When starting a psychotropic medication in the elderly, a good rule of thumb is:

    1. Start low, go slow.

    2. Higher doses are almost always needed.

    3. Side effects of psychotropic medications will usually not impact other medications.

    4. The same adult dosages can be used initially without any problems.

64. A client is a 20-year, 2-pack-a-day smoker with a history of chronic bronchitis. What is the prescription to give to this client who wishes to stop smoking?

    1. Nicotine polacrilex (Nicorette) gum 2-mg piece, chew for 30 minutes, q1–2h × 6 weeks, then q2–4h × 3 weeks, then q4–8h × 3 weeks, then discontinue.

    2. Nicotine patch (Nicoderm) 21 mg/24 hr qd × 6 weeks, then 14 mg/24 hr qd × 2 weeks, then 7 mg/24 hr qd × 2 weeks, then discontinue.

    3. Bupropion HCl (Zyban) 150 mg qd × 3 days, then 150 mg bid for 7–12 weeks and to stop smoking when medication is started.

    4. Nicotine patch (Nicoderm) 14 mg/24 hr qd × 6 weeks, then 7 mg/24 hr qd × 6 weeks, then discontinue.

65. The nurse practitioner understands the following about the use of benzodiazepines in the older adult:

    1. Withdrawal symptoms may occur within 24 hours of abruptly stopping the medication.

    2. Adverse side effects are minimal and tend to minimize the incidence of falls and other injuries.

    3. Long-acting medications (i.e., chlordiazepoxide [Librium]) are preferred over the shorter acting medications (i.e., lorazepam [Ativan]).

    4. Larger doses are needed to maintain therapeutic levels for the anxious or agitated client.

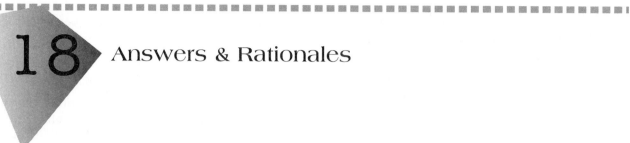

Answers & Rationales

Psychosocial Examination & Diagnostic Tests

1. **(2)** The mental status examination provides a basic assessment of the client's intellectual functioning (reasoning, abstract thinking, memory). The intelligence quotient (IQ) is determined by psychological testing. Psychomotor skill assessment is part of a neurologic examination.

2. **(1)** Delusions are false, fixed beliefs that can be of a persecutory or grandiose nature. In this instance, the client is experiencing a delusion of grandeur. Often elders with a diagnosis of dementia will have delusions, which worsen with acute illnesses. A hallucination is a false sensory experience. An illusion is a misinterpretation of reality. Magical thinking is when the client feels that his/her thoughts or wishes can control other people.

3. **(1)** The client experiencing the auditory hallucination will often look out into space and act as if he/she is listening to someone talking. This is associated with behaviors such as tilting the head, mumbling, and eye movement.

4. **(3)** The Michigan Alcoholism Screening Test (MAST) and the CAGE (Cut down, Annoyed, Guilty, Eye opener) are used to alert providers to possibility of alcoholism.

5. **(3)** Dual diagnosis involves both a psychiatric diagnosis and a substance abuse diagnosis.

6. **(1)** Children with learning disabilities and ADHD are often impulsive, inattentive, and overactive. Usually, children with ADHD do not have lower IQ achievement scores; however, children with a learning disability usually demonstrate a level of educational achievement substantially below that of the IQ.

7. **(2)** Clients who experience confabulation are fabricating events or situations to fill in gaps in their memory, usually in a plausible way, exhibiting signs and symptoms of dementia from chronic alcohol abuse. Confabulation is a common symptom of alcohol amnesic disorder, or Korsakoff's syndrome. Echolalia is the parroting or automatic, meaningless repeating of another's words. Perseveration is the involuntary persistent repetition of an idea or response (e.g., client keeps repeating the same phrase over and over).

8. **(4)** Although it is important to know if the client has ever experienced hallucinations, delusions, or illusions and if they have ever been hospitalized in a psychiatric facility, the single most important factor to ascertain is whether or not the client has contemplated suicide. In addition, determination of a specific plan and the means to do it are also involved in the questioning about suicidal ideation. It is also important for the nurse practitioner to determine if the client regularly takes antidepressants or other medications. Clients may have stopped taking their antidepressant causing an acute exacerbation of their depression, or another medication that they may be taking may be causing an increase in their depression.

9. **(1)** Nicotine is known as the "gateway drug" and is commonly the first drug used by adolescents.

10. **(2)** The other abnormalities are not usually associated with bulimia. The hypochloremia is associated with the purging (self-induced vomiting).

11. **(1)** Habituation exists when the same dose of the drug produces reduced effects and is usually seen with the development of physical dependence on any medication. Addiction occurs when there is a deep-seated psychological need for the drug/medication.

12. **(1)** According to research, self-esteem, along with attitude and morals, are maintained as a client ages. Older adults tend to have a more positive self-image and are more confident when compared to younger adults. Learning ability is maintained although more time is often needed for the early phases of the learning process. Retrieval of information in long-term memory is slower, and short-term memory is diminished.

13. **(3)** Requires the client to compare and tell how two things are alike or different, involving the thought process that is oriented toward the development of an idea without application to a particular object; it is independent of space and time. Today's date assists to determine orientation, the names of past presidents assists to demonstrate long-term memory, and repetition of numbers assists to demonstrate short-term memory.

Psychiatric Disorders

14. **(1)** Confusion can occur in both dementia and depression. However, with dementia, symptoms worsen at night and are commonly referred to as sundowning. Additionally, the nurse practitioner must also ensure that the increased confusion is not a result of an acute illness. Often the only sign or symptom the demented elder may present with is confusion. Usually the culprit is a urinary tract infection. The nurse practitioner should order a urine analysis (UA) to ensure that the confusion is not the result of an acute illness and is reversible.

15. **(4)** The nurse practitioner must first establish trust and rapport with the caller before an assessment can be made. If rapport is not established, the client will hang up the phone.

The nurse practitioner understands that, by keeping the client talking, he/she is prevented from acting out the suicidal threat.

16. **(3)** Impaired concentration and irritability are major characteristics of generalized anxiety disorder. Clients often pace the exam room due to their irritability; they are more focused on the here and now and have low self-esteem.

17. **(2)** Confusion and cognitive function problems (i.e., short-term memory loss) are initial signs of dementia. The severity of the symptoms depends on what stage of cognitive degeneration the client is manifesting. The other options are characteristic of hallucinatory experiences and usually occur later. This client may also be exhibiting signs and symptoms of an acute illness. The culprit is usually a urinary tract infection (UTI) and the nurse practitioner should order a UA to ensure that that cause of the confusion is not related to a reversible cause.

18. **(2)** Cimetidine (Tagamet) is not tolerated well in the elder client, and one of the major side effects is confusion. Anytime a new medication is added to an elder client's medication regimem, an abrupt onset of confusion must be reviewed closely as it may be attributed to the new medication or a drug-drug interaction with an existing medication. Another possibility is the onset of an acute illness, which often manifests as acute confusion in the elder client. Most often the culprit is a UTI; therefore, in addition to a careful medication review, obtaining a UA could also rule out a UTI. When a patient has true dementia, the onset of confusion develops slowly, over a longer period of time, not acutely, which would indicate that there is another underlying problem causing the acute confusion. Attention span and memory may be affected in each diagnosis.

19. **(3)** The nurse's statement acknowledges the client's feelings and is open ended, which promotes open discussion and helps the client clarify his feelings and thoughts. Option #1 is condescending and punitive. Option #2 offers false reassurance. Option #4 tends to discount the client's feelings.

20. **(3)** The characteristics of schizophrenia are delusions, tangential thought, suspiciousness, disorganized behavior, and hallucinations.

21. **(4)** Although clients with a diagnosis of dementia do not usually have altered perceptions that include hallucinations and illusions, it is occasionally seen in those with underlying psychiatric disorders. Dementia normally lasts for months to years and the client never recovers. Delirium is an acute process and is often associated with medications or a systemic illness and is reversible, once the acute problem is addressed and resolved.

22. **(4)** One of the most common reasons for an acute change in mental status in the demented elder client is an acute infection. This is usually an UTI. Usually the demented elder client is incontinent, and, because of the changes of aging, does not recognize the normal signs or symptoms of a UTI (burning, urgency, frequency, suprapubic tenderness). Elders also do not typically run elevated temperatures. The nurse practitioner should order a UA to ensure that an acute infectious process is not the cause of the acute confusion. While waiting for the results of the UA, the nurse practitioner should conduct a medication review to ensure that no new medications have been added or that no new over-the-counter or herbal medications have been added as this is the second largest reason for acute confusion in the elder client.

23. **(2)** The indicators to domestic violence in this case are the multiple vague physical complaints without supporting objective data, the suspected depression, and the reluctance to wait around in the clinic for extended periods of time. This client is on the verge of disclosing if a provider would only ask her about domestic violence.

24. **(1)** Based on the acute confusion state and the incontinence, she is experiencing delirium. This is most likely secondary to sepsis, with the source of infection being a UTI. The fact that she has mental status changes (disoriented to person, place, or time, in addition to the acute confusion, delirium, and incontinence give you the clues to sepsis). Dementia is more insidious versus acute. Depression and psychosis are not consistent with the assessments. The major symptoms in depression would include loss of interest, sleep disorder, decreased appetite, loss of concentration, inactivity, guilt, lack of energy, and potential suicidal thoughts. Psychotic disorders include thoughts and behavior indicating the client is not in touch with reality.

25. **(4)** The laws in most states require the reporting of suspected or actual abuse and neglect of any person considered to be dependent or with a reduced ability to make life choices. Children, disabled individuals, and dependent elderly fall into these categories. Very few states require reporting for adult women unless a weapon is involved; this is a different situation requiring a report.

26. **(3)** The nurse practitioner must determine whether the bruised areas match the type of trauma the parent describes. Bruises in various stages of healing turn different colors and are indicative that the injuries did not occur at the same time, which could be indicative of child abuse.

27. **(4)** Adolescents with anorexia nervosa will severely reduce their nutritional intake by dieting constantly on high fiber and low calories. They usually have an inappropriate body image and may admit to occasional episodes of vomiting.

28. **(1)** Nightmares peak in incidence around ages 3–4 years and are often associated with abandonment issues and posttraumatic stress disorder (following gun shootings, fires, abuse). Night terrors are typically accompanied by gross motor movements (sleepwalking, enuresis), tachypnea, labored breathing, and tachycardia.

29. **(2)** Role playing and planning a rehearsed reply to teasing comments about short stature are helpful tools to deal with this issue. Although humor can be effective, constantly clowning around for attention is not positive coping behavior. Withdrawal (i.e., watching television or reading) is not effective coping and may indicate depression. Spending time and associating only with younger adolescents who are his height is not a positive coping behavior and may hinder normal maturation.

30. **(4)** More than 50% of intravenous cocaine users develop hepatitis, phlebitis, endocarditis, and acquired immunodeficiency syndrome (AIDS). Epistaxis, rhinorrhea, and nasal congestion are seen most often in intranasal users of cocaine. Chest congestion, wheezing, and eventual emphysema occur with chronic free-base (crack) smokers. Although cardiac

arrhythmias, hypertension, and respiratory arrest can occur, they are not the common complications.

31. **(3)** Adults who are depressed typically display findings noted in Options #1, #2, and #4. Adolescents often act out to protect themselves from feelings of vulnerability and dependency. It is important to evaluate signs of anger and frustration in the adolescent because the significance of the behavior may indicate symptoms of depression.

32. **(1)** The newborn exposed to cocaine is often premature, small-for-gestational-age, has low birth weight, and has a low Apgar score. Intrauterine growth retardation occurs along with symptoms of hypertonia, irritability, tremulousness, irregular sleeping patterns, and frequent gaze aversion.

33. **(3)** People with anorexia nervosa will exercise up to 4 hours a day. They are above average intelligence in most cases, suffer from bradycardia, and have decreased libido.

34. **(4)** In a preschool child, it may be difficult to distinguish ADHD, as problems of overactivity, inattention, and negativism are common. Problems with language skill development along with fine motor skills are more likely found with learning disabilities. Active curiosity and negativism are normal behaviors for preschoolers.

35. **(1)** Autism is a developmental disorder that starts early in a child's life and is characterized by avoidance of eye contact, indifference to caregivers, language and communication delays, failure to develop a social smile, repetitive movements, and an excessive need for routine.

36. **(4)** Repetition of whole words and phrases is normal for preschoolers; therefore, it would be inappropriate to refer to a speech pathologist at this time. Parents should not correct or criticize the child as it could contribute to low self-esteem. Verbal exercises are unnecessary and could be very stressful to the child and contribute to low self-esteem.

37. **(3)** The grandmother's concern is warranted. In teenage girls, the most common form of suicide attempt is by drug overdose. The combination of vomiting and confusion suggests a drug overdose, and the nurse practitioner should run a tox screen.

38. **(1)** The nurse practitioner should suspect this client of having a diagnosis of substance-induced mood disorder. It would be appropriate to determine exactly how much, how long, and how often he consumes alcohol or any other drugs. The key points in the situation are the occupational burn out, depressive symptoms, and ineffective coping measures (taking and doing everything to relax, but with no relief).

39. **(2)** This client should be examined by emergency department personnel, many of whom are specially trained to collect the evidence needed to testify in court about rape. The exam should not be done in the office unless the nurse practitioner has been trained in evidence collection and has a rape evidence collection kit. The exam must be done quickly, before evidence is destroyed. The client decides who should be called for support. While she is encouraged to call her parents, she is also offered the support of rape crisis and other resources.

40. **(2)** Bradycardia and excessive salivation are not found with cocaine abuse. There are no drug antagonists that can be used for cocaine overdose, although naloxone is given to reduce the concurrent toxic effects of other narcotic drugs that may be in the client's body system.

41. **(4)** While all of the answers may contribute to a clinician's suspicion of family violence, the admission of genuine fear of a household member is considered an excellent indicator of actual or potential violence and the level of danger in a home. The nurse practitioner should involve Social Services to assist the adolescent female in this situation.

42. **(2)** Woraich's 1994 study failed to demonstrate a link between sugar and behavior or cognitive performance. Further assessment is indicated before labeling as ADHD.

43. **(3)** Dopamine and norepinephine (drugs that stimulate the noradrenergic and dopaminergic receptors) can precipitate mania or hypomania in clients. GABA and acetylcholine may also be neurotransmitters involved in the process. In addition, stimulants such as amphetamines and cocaine can also cause manic-like symptoms.

44. **(3)** Chronic anxiety attacks are not part of the DSM-IV criteria for substance abuse.

45. **(4)** While all of the items listed are appropriate to assess in this patient, it is most important to determine judgment. If he cannot make safe judgments he is at high risk for unsafe behaviors, such as driving, walking along the sidewalk, running bath water, etc.

46. **(1)** The patient needs to be able to easily interpret his surroundings. Shadows or areas of poor lighting will increase the illusions. When in the room, it is important to speak in clear tones and make sure to include the client in the conversations to decrease the paranoia and feelings that people are talking about him. Radio and television may provide too much stimuli and may not be of any assistance in maintaining orientation. Suction equipment is for physical safety, not therapeutic milieu.

47. **(3)** Based on developmental levels, a 6-month-old is not walking or pulling up. A 4-year-old is beginning to run and jump, a 6-year-old is playing outside and riding a bicycle, and a 1-year-old is beginning to pull up and cruise around cabinets and tables.

Pharmacology

48. **(3)** The client is experiencing a rare problem called neuroleptic malignant syndrome. This client would require immediate referral and hospitalization. This can also occur with the medication prochlorperazine (Compazine). Acute dystonia, parkinsonism, and akathisia are associated with extrapyramidal disorder or acute movement disorder. Tardive dyskinesia occurs late in therapy and is often irreversible. Slow worm-like movements of the tongue are the earliest symptom, followed by grimacing, lip smacking, and involuntary limb movements.

49. **(2)** Citalopram (Celexa's) favorable side-effect profile makes it a useful alternative to the traditional tricyclic antidepressants. It has the shortest half-life of the currently marketed serotonin reuptake inhibitors. Amitriptyline (Elavil) has the most anticholinergic and sedating side effects of the antidepressants. There may be pronounced effects on the cardiovascular system (hypotension).

Geropsychiatrists agree it is best to avoid in the elderly; however, low dose (10 mg, PC, qhs) is low cost and can be effective at controlling neuropathic pain. Trazodone (Desyrel) is very sedating for the elderly client. Haloperidol (Haldol) is an antipsychotic medication and is not to be used at all in long-term care facilities.

50. **(1)** Physical dependence can occur, even with low doses of the medication. This is a particular problem in the elderly, who are sensitive to low-dose ranges. If possible, it is better to slowly taper the patient from the anti-anxiety medication; often they can be tapered to a much lower dose.

51. **(2)** Akathisia is a feeling of restlessness. The nurse practitioner should slowly taper the client from the haloperidol (Haldol) 2 mg HS; it is possible that she may not need the medication or that one of the newer atypical anti-psychotics would be more effective with a lesser side effect profile. Clients may complain of a feeling of muscular quivering. Ataxia is a disorder wherein muscular incoordination occurs with voluntary muscular movements. Agitation is a general assessment that may be part of the psychotic behavior. Dyskinesia is a defect in voluntary movement.

52. **(4)** Correction of environmental factors and treatment of underlying iatrogenic and medical problems should be addressed initially. Amitriptyline (Elavil) can cause excessive somnolence. Trazadone (Desyrel) may be of particular use when sleep disturbance is prominent; however, it does not address the best initial plan. The goal is to begin with good sleep hygiene prior to pharmacologic therapy. Eliminating naps during the day may be useful in facilitating sleep.

53. **(1)** Drug-drug interactions are a common cause of acute confusion in the elderly client. This assessment can minimize the need to do further costly interventions if the client only needs medication adjustment. The other options should be included in the plan after the drug history is completed and has been ruled out as a potential problem. The nurse practitioner must always consider that an acute illness, such as a UTI, may be the cause of acute confusion. A UA should also be obtained because the client can quickly progress to sepsis.

54. **(2)** In combination with tyramine-rich foods that have undergone an aging process such as cheese, wine, beer, salami, and yogurt, catecholamines are released from the nerve endings causing a hypertensive crisis. The other drugs listed cause hypotension.

55. **(3)** The benzodiazepines cause sedation and decreased attention, which in turn affects the memory. Although phenothiazines and antidepressants may also cause sedation, they don't affect memory.

56. **(3)** Flashbacks, depression, and psychotic behavior can occur with LSD use. There are no withdrawal symptoms or physical dependence associated with use. Commonly, the adolescent remains oriented but experiences hallucinations and altered bodily sensations.

57. **(3)** Trazadone (Desyrel) has sedation as a side effect, which has made it less popular as an antidepressant; however, it is commonly prescribed for insomnia.

58. **(4)** All of the drugs listed may be used in acute alcohol withdrawal delirium except chlorpromazine (Librium), which is an antipsychotic that has no use in the management plan.

59. **(4)** Often, the first indication of drug use in adolescents is a sudden change in behavior or school performance. Heroin use symptoms are constricted pupils, respiratory depression, needle tracks, and poor nutrition. Marijuana use symptoms are slow reflexes, tachycardia, conjunctival injection, nasal congestion, and increased appetite. LSD use symptoms are dilated pupils, reddened eyes, hypertension, increased appetite, and hallucinations. The use of central nervous system stimulants, like crack cocaine, leads to hypertension, weight loss, anorexia, insomnia, hyperreflexia, and a perforated or ulcerated nasal septum.

60. **(4)** It is **not** important to evaluate liver function before initiating treatment with lithium. However, lithium has adverse side effects on renal, cardiac, and thyroid function. Baseline electrolytes are also important to obtain.

61. **(3)** Naloxone (Narcan) is a narcotic antagonist and is used for the reversal of narcotic depression, including respiratory depression. Clonidine (Catapres) is a central α-agonist and is indicated for treatment of hypertension.

Methadone is used in the treatment of opioid addiction. The Food and Drug Administration (FDA) has placed methadone in a special drug category that allows medically supervised administration of the drug to addicts with chronic, intractable addiction to heroin. The therapeutic classification of naltrexone (Revia) is as a narcotic detoxification adjunct.

62. **(3)** Seizures, alcohol withdrawal, and anxiety are commonly treated with benzodiazepines. They are **not** the first drug of choice for obsessive-compulsive disorder; selective serotonin reuptake inhibitors are usually used.

63. **(1)** The rule of thumb for starting medications in the elder client is to start low and go slow; therefore, dosages should be reduced by 30%–50% to start therapy and gradually increased as necessary. Adverse effects are likely to occur because of slowed drug metabolism, which occurs with aging. These include hypotension, arrhythmias, and sedative and anticholinergic effects.

64. **(2)** A highly nicotine-dependent client benefits from intense counseling and prescription of alternative nicotine delivery during the smoking cessation process. The nicotine patch is usually the preferred form of replacement because the gum is noncontinuous and withdrawal symptoms may occur during nonchewing times. The nicotine patch delivers a fixed dose of nicotine on a continual basis, is applied once daily, and eliminates the gastrointestinal upset that often occurs with the gum. If this client insisted on using the gum, the dose should be 4 mg, not 2 mg. Option #4 is too low a dose to start on this client and is not the correct dosing schedule. Zyban (bupropion HCl) would be used in conjunction with the nicotine patch, and clients are to quit smoking 1–2 weeks after starting the Zyban (bupropion HCl), not immediately.

65. **(1)** Benzodiazepines should be tapered slowly in the older adult. Withdrawal symptoms occur within 24 hours in clients taking the shorter acting medications and may not occur for several days in clients taking long-acting medications. The adverse effects of oversedation—dizziness, confusion, and sometimes hypotension—contribute to falls and other injuries in the elderly. In Option #3, short-acting medications are preferred. Typically, larger doses are not needed but rather small initial doses with gradual increases.

Research & Theory

19

Research

1. When designing a research project that will involve clients, what is the most important point to be included in the written consent to participate?

   1. Directions regarding the use of a black pen.

   2. Anticipated date for publication of the completed research report.

   3. Assurance of privacy and confidentiality.

   4. Number of previously published research studies about this topic.

2. When determining whether to incorporate a new procedure into a clinical practice based on the findings of a recent study, which of the following should be considered?

   1. Statistical significance of the findings.

   2. Statistical relevance of the findings.

   3. Statistical software program used.

   4. Statistical background of the researcher.

3. The research process is similar to the processes that nurse practitioners use to provide client care in that both are decision-making processes that include the steps (in the order presented here) of:

   1. Assessing, teaching, evaluating, and discussing.

   2. Defining, planning, implementing, and charting.

   3. Questioning, evaluating, diagnosing, and teaching.

   4. Assessing, planning, implementing, and evaluating.

4. Both descriptive and inferential statistics are used in research. However, their purposes are different in that:

   1. Inferential statistics are used for assigning participant code numbers.

   2. Descriptive statistics are used for assigning participant code numbers.

   3. Inferential statistics are used for hypothesis testing.

   4. Descriptive statistics are used for hypothesis testing.

5. In an ambulatory care setting, the nurse practitioner might find it difficult to utilize nursing research because:

   1. The demands of providing primary care leave little time for research utilization.

   2. Procedures for research utilization have not been well defined in the literature.

   3. Research published in professional journals is too difficult to access by clinicians.

   4. Ambulatory care settings have little in common with the settings used for most research.

6. The scientific method for conducting research uses the null hypothesis, which is statistically based. What is the correct format for the null hypothesis?

   1. There is no significant difference between two groups.

   2. Group "A" is greater than group "B."

   3. Group "A" is less than group "B."

   4. There is a 95% probability that group "A" is different from group "B."

7. When evaluating claims made on advertisements, such as "Drug X has been used for 5 years with over 1 million doses administered in the United States, Canada, and Great Britain. Drug X stops heartburn, aids in digestion, and prevents esophageal reflux, and is the 'treatment of choice' to relieve GERD," the nurse practitioner realizes that the claim is:

   1. Invalid; there is no control or comparison group, and no statistics are stated.

   2. Valid; there are sufficient numbers of users who have had success.

   3. Invalid; the level of significance is not mentioned to be at the 0.05 level.

   4. Valid; the cohort and Hawthorne effects are operating.

8. Reviewing labor and delivery in the practice, the nurse practitioner notes that pregnant clients who are still in their teens generally seem to go into labor before their due date (as determined by ultrasound), whereas the women in their mid-20s usually go into labor at or after their due date. Which statistical analysis would answer the research question,

"Among pregnant women in a nurse practitioner practice, is there a statistically significant difference between the length of gestation for women age 16–19 compared with women age 23–26?"

   1. Multiple regression.

   2. Chronbach's alpha.

   3. Two-tailed t-test.

   4. Pearson's correlation.

9. The utilization of research in nursing practice can be equated with:

   1. The nursing process.

   2. The change process.

   3. Discharge planning.

   4. Family planning.

10. The nurse practitioner is compiling monthly statistics for the practice, and one of the elements of the analysis is the cultural background of clients. What level of data is cultural background?

    1. Nominal level.

    2. Ordinal level.

    3. Interval level.

    4. Ratio level.

11. A nurse practitioner working with a physician in general practice is compiling end-of-month statistics. The clients who received care range from infants to elderly persons. Which of the following data from the monthly report is most likely to be normally distributed?

    1. Laboratory tests scheduled for the clients.

    2. Gender of the clients.

    3. Primary diagnosis of the clients.

    4. Age of the clients.

12. A nurse practitioner is compiling statistics at the end of the month for a client population ranging from infant to elderly. The practitioner and physician in the general practice want to know the average monthly income of their clients. Which would be the most appropriate statistical measure of the "average income,"

assuming income was exact in dollars and cents?

1. The mean.

2. The median.

3. The mode.

4. The range.

13. A nurse practitioner is evaluating research articles for a utilization project. The majority of the articles report that either random selection or random assignment was used to select the sample for that study. Because certain procedures in research are used across disciplines, what can be assumed for studies where randomization has been used?

1. The ages of the research subjects in these studies will be negatively skewed.

2. The research subjects in these studies will automatically be half male and half female.

3. The ages of the research subjects in these studies will be positively skewed.

4. The researchers were attempting to obtain the most representative sample.

14. The ability to predict outcomes of care is desirable both in research and in practice. If a nurse practitioner wanted to create a theoretic model for a specific aspect of the practice to predict client outcomes, which statistical analysis method would be used to analyze the clinical data?

1. Descriptive statistics.

2. Repeated-measures t-test.

3. Multiple regression.

4. Chi-squared (χ^2) for independent samples.

15. Research articles are being evaluated for a utilization project. What can be done if the nurse practitioner does not understand the statistical procedures used for analysis of data in an article?

1. Assume that the correct procedure was used, and read about the method or consult a statistician for an explanation of the statistics.

2. Assume that the article is beyond the nurse's ability to understand, so set that one aside and go on to the next article.

3. Assume that the correct procedure was used, and instead of reading the results section, read the discussion of the findings section.

4. Assume that the article is beyond the practitioner's ability to understand, and use another person's critique of the reported study.

16. The nurse practitioner has determined that the office procedures for diagnosing and stabilizing new diabetic clients need to be evaluated and possibly changed. Which would be the best choice for the first phase of the evaluation?

1. Design and conduct a double-blind clinical trial.

2. Design and conduct a research utilization project.

3. Design and conduct a research project comparing men and women.

4. Design and conduct a study to test Callista Roy's theoretic model.

17. A nurse practitioner has read a nursing research article in which there were no statistically significant findings. What would be the practitioner's most appropriate response?

1. "Reading this article was a waste of my time."

2. "Because of this article, there is no reason to conduct similar studies."

3. "Reading this article raises new questions for my practice."

4. "Because of this article, I will immediately change my practice."

18. In a recent study the researcher reports that "the statistical analysis used to identify the differences between the two variables was Pearson's correlation." Which of the following most specifically indicates what is **wrong** with this statement?

1. Pearson's correlation can be used only with three or more variables.

2. Pearson's correlation actually identifies the common factors between variables.

3. Pearson's correlation can be used only when there is a single variable.

4. Pearson's correlation actually identifies the relationship between variables.

19. Nurse researchers conduct qualitative research studies because:

    1. Qualitative studies help to identify and define nursing concepts.

    2. With qualitative methods, there are no concerns about the rights of research subjects.

    3. Qualitative approaches provide precise measures for statistical analysis.

    4. Nurse researchers find qualitative research designs easier to use.

20. The normal ranges of blood chemistry values are most similar to which statistical concept?

    1. The standard error.

    2. The mean.

    3. The standard deviation.

    4. The median.

21. The five major sequential steps of research utilization are:

    1. Establish a client relationship, perform a health assessment, make a diagnosis, devise a plan of care, and evaluate the treatment.

    2. Identify the problem, assess published research, design the innovation, evaluate, and decide whether to adopt the innovation.

    3. Review the popular literature, review the practice's clients, summarize of the findings, evaluate, and do client teaching.

    4. Review the client's lab reports, complete a thorough health assessment, diagnose, implement the treatment, and evaluate.

22. Why are both qualitative and quantitative research methods used in nursing research?

    1. Master's-prepared nurses conduct quantitative studies, whereas doctorally prepared nurses conduct qualitative studies.

    2. Master's-prepared nurses conduct qualitative studies, whereas doctorally prepared nurses conduct quantitative studies.

    3. The methods complement each other because they produce different types of findings about the same concepts.

    4. The methods complement each other because they produce the same types of findings about different concepts.

23. Nursing research subscribes to the scientific method for the design of research studies. What is the advantage of this approach?

    1. Nursing research is based on logically constructed arguments.

    2. Nursing research is designed to answer any research question.

    3. Nursing research findings are precise and need not be duplicated.

    4. Nursing research findings are generalizable to all client populations.

24. With the restructuring of health care delivery and a shift in the provision of nonacute care from the hospital to ambulatory care settings and the home, nursing research previously conducted in hospitals:

    1. Now becomes applicable to all in-hospital providers of care.

    2. Remains relevant in the new settings; client care is unchanged.

    3. Should be applied directly to client care provided in the new settings.

    4. May no longer be applicable to the delivery of client care.

25. Nurse researchers strive to substantiate causality so that client outcomes can be consistently predicted. For the nurse practitioner, the ability to predict the outcomes for every client could mean that:

    1. The appropriate treatment would be prescribed for clients.

    2. No further studies would need to be conducted about treatments.

    3. The client's individual qualities would not need to be considered.

    4. Treatments would not need to be individualized for each client.

26. Quantitative research articles always have a section containing descriptive findings because descriptive data analysis:

    1. Provides the basis for making inferences about the findings.

    2. May yield statistically significant findings that were unexpected.

3. Is conducted for predicting client outcomes in nursing settings.

4. Organizes the data for clearer understanding of subjects and variables.

27. What is the difference between univariate and multivariate studies?

1. Number of subjects in the sample.

2. Number of variables being studied.

3. Number of sites for collecting data.

4. Number of statistical hypotheses.

28. The independent variable and the dependent variable of a research study might be thought of as:

1. The cause (the independent variable) and the effect (the dependent variable).

2. The median (the independent variable) and the mode (the dependent variable).

3. The outcome (the independent variable) and the treatment (the dependent variable).

4. The sample (the independent variable) and the population (the dependent variable).

29. Variance is a key statistical concept. How would current research methods change if there were no variance?

1. Nurse researchers would need to increase the sample size in all research studies to 100 research subjects or greater.

2. Since current research methods do not depend on the presence of variance, researchers would not need to change our current methods.

3. Nurse researchers would need to decrease the sample size of all research studies to 15 research subjects.

4. Since current research methods are based on the presence of variance, researchers would not be able to use current methods.

Theory

30. Although nursing theories vary greatly in their perspectives of nursing care, all nursing theorists explicitly incorporate three key concepts that are basic to nursing care, as follows:

1. Individuals, families, and communities.

2. Primary, secondary, and tertiary prevention.

3. Past, present, and future well-being.

4. Person, health, and environment.

31. The theoretic basis for nursing practice is:

1. A relatively new approach to nursing care.

2. Borrowed from other professions such as medicine.

3. As old as formal nursing and began with Florence Nightingale.

4. Unrelated to the conduct of nursing research studies.

32. The verification of the more abstract nursing theories (e.g., of Martha Rogers) is often hampered by:

1. Lack of adequate measures for the theoretic concepts.

2. Prior studies that did not support the theory.

3. Lack of adequate laboratory settings for conducting experiments.

4. Prior studies that were conducted in other countries.

33. Basing nursing practice on nursing theory contributes to the professionalization of nursing practice by:

1. Adapting the medical model to nursing care.

2. Limiting the choice of treatments for clients.

3. Determining what type of clients will be seen by the nurse.

4. Providing a consistent perspective for providing care to clients.

34. A nurse practitioner has decided to incorporate a theoretic nursing model into the ambulatory care practice, which emphasizes clients doing as much as possible to maintain their own health. Which nursing model is most applicable to this setting?

1. Orem's Self-Care Model (Self-Care Deficit Theory of Nursing).

2. Roy's Adaptation Model.

3. Roger's Science of Unitary Human Beings.

4. King's Interacting Systems Model.

35. Which of the following nursing theorist is considered to have general systems theory as the philosophic orientation to her model?

    1. Sister Callista Roy.

    2. Martha Rogers.

    3. Rosemarie Parse.

    4. Betty Neuman.

36. Which nursing theory addresses nursing outcomes in terms of primary, secondary, and tertiary prevention?

    1. Roy's Adapatation Model.

    2. Neuman's Health Care Systems Model.

    3. King's Interacting Systems Framework.

    4. Watson's Human Caring Theory.

37. Which nursing model primarily addresses health promotion?

    1. Watson's Human Science and Human Model of caring.

    2. Neuman's Health Care Systems Model.

    3. Pender's Health Promotion Model.

    4. Roy's Adaptation Model.

19 Answers & Rationales

Research

1. **(3)** By federal law, clients must be assured of their privacy and confidentiality. The other information is interesting and may be included but is not required by federal law.

2. **(1)** In published research reports, of the options listed, only Option #1 is consistently reported by researchers. The clinical relevance is considered, not the statistical relevance. The specific program used does not make a difference because all are based on the same statistical formulas. Researchers frequently work with statistical consultants, so a researcher's background is not a limitation to a published study.

3. **(4)** Only Option #4 contains those elements common to both processes: assessing, planning, implementing, and evaluating.

4. **(3)** Neither type of statistics is used to assign participant code numbers. Descriptive statistics are used to describe the sample.

5. **(1)** Inadequate time can be a barrier to research utilization in any setting. The process of research utilization is well delineated by researchers. With the ever-increasing availability of professional journals via the Internet, access is rarely a problem. A considerable body of research has been conducted in ambulatory care settings.

6. **(1)** The correct format for the null hypothesis is, "There is no significant difference between two groups." The alternate or research hypothesis may take the other forms.

7. **(1)** Even though the claims detail extensive use of "Drug X," there must be statistical evidence, as demonstrated through the use of control or comparison groups that will render a level of significance.

8. **(3)** Only the t-test compares two independent groups on a variable.

9. **(2)** Incorporating research findings into practice often results in a change in practice. The nursing process most resembles conducting research.

10. **(1)** The variable of cultural background is categorical data or nominal-level data.

11. **(4)** The gender and primary diagnosis are nominal-level data. The lab tests would be skewed, whereas the age would approximate the normal curve.

12. **(2)** The median income would be most representative of the average because the income of 50% of the clients is above and 50% is below the median. The mean could be influenced by one client with a very high or very low income. The mode identifies only the income that is reported most often. The range identifies only the lowest and the highest income and does not present an average.

13. **(4)** Randomization is a research technique used to increase the amount of control in any research design. The other three options are false; they do not occur because of randomization.

14. **(3)** Of the options, only multiple regression examines the relationship between two or more variables in a way that permits prediction.

15. **(1)** In reviewing research, it is necessary to understand the statistical methods that the researcher used in order to determine the value of the study findings for the practice setting. The researcher's discussion may not provide the full extent of the findings, and another person's critique may reflect a specific point of view that does not apply in every situation.

16. **(2)** As a first step, a research utilization project would provide a thorough review of the published literature on which to base a change. A full study may not be needed, and testing a theoretic model is not appropriate for this situation.

17. **(3)** The lack of significant findings is an important piece of information about the topic of the research and definitely is not a waste of time. Particularly when findings are nonsignificant, more studies need to be conducted about this topic. Ideally, changes in practice are based on the findings of more than one study.

18. **(4)** Correlations identify the relationships between variables. Two or more variables may be used. Factor analysis is used to identify common factors.

19. **(1)** The purpose of qualitative designs is to identify and define nursing concepts. Qualitative designs do not yield precise measures, are usually not analyzed statistically, are more difficult to use, and carry the same concerns about the rights of subjects as all other research designs.

20. **(3)** The normal ranges of blood chemistry values are based on studies that identified the standard deviation for each blood chemical. The mean and the median are averages, and the standard error is not applicable to this situation.

21. **(2)** This option contains the published steps. All other options are nursing actions taken on behalf of the client (in no particular order).

22. **(3)** The two methods complement each other because they produce different types of findings about the same concepts. The educational preparation of the researcher does not dictate the research method used.

23. **(1)** The scientific method is highly organized and is based on logical reasoning. Findings are rarely precise, and studies do need to be duplicated. Some questions are unanswerable by current research methods. Because of small samples and other limitations, many findings from nursing research are *not* generalizable.

24. **(4)** Such a drastic change in health care delivery may make previous studies no longer applicable to nursing care. Health care restructuring has changed the way client care is provided.

25. **(1)** The ability to always predict client outcomes would mean that every client would receive the exact treatment for that individual. Treatments would still have to be individualized, and individual qualities would need to be considered. Because new treatments are always being devised, there would be a need for ongoing research.

26. **(4)** Descriptive data analysis organizes the data, and it facilitates understanding. Descriptive statistics cannot be used for significance testing or for making inferences; inferential statistics are used. Predictions are made from studies that use inferential statistics.

27. **(2)** Variate refers to the number of variables in the study.

28. **(1)** The independent variable may be considered the cause or the treatment, and the dependent variable may be considered the effect or the outcome. The median, mode, sample, and population are not designations for the independent or the dependent variables.

29. **(4)** All current research and statistical analysis methods rely on the presence of variance or variation; if variance is no longer present, current methods could no longer be used. If there is no variance, a sample of one would be adequate.

Theory

30. **(4)** All current theories incorporate person, health, and environment. Other concepts may or may not be explicitly included in nursing theories.

31. **(3)** The theoretic basis for nursing practice began with Florence Nightingale and has been used in practice and research for more than a century. Nursing theories are specifically developed for nursing.

32. **(1)** The lack of adequate measures for theoretic concepts is a major roadblock in many areas of research, and particularly so with the more abstract theories. Prior studies always provide information about the theory, even when conducted in other countries. More abstract concepts tend not to be studied in laboratory settings.

33. **(4)** Theory-based practice contributes the consistent perspective that permits the comparison of care across settings. This practice does not necessarily limit treatments or determine client types. Theory-based practice specifically eliminates reliance on the medical model.

34. **(1)** Orem's theory focuses on the client participating and being in control of own health care. Roy's model is most appropriate for acute care settings, Roger's for holistic health settings, and King's for a mental health setting.

35. **(4)** Betty Neuman's Health Care Systems Model, Imogene King's Systems Interaction Model, and Dorothy Johnson's Behavioral Systems are based on general systems theory. Roy's Adaptation Model is based on stress and adaptation as the framework. Martha Roger's Science of Unitary Human Beings and Rosemarie Parse's Human Becoming Model are based on a humanistic developmental framework.

36. **(2)** Betty Neuman identified the need to implement nursing interventions through the use of one or more of three preventive modalities: primary, secondary, and tertiary prevention.

37. **(3)** Pender's Health Promotion Model is an excellent nursing model that readily fits into a nurse practitioner's scope of practice.

Issues & Trends

1. The nurse practitioner understands which of the following about the Health Insurance Portability and Accountability Act of 1996 (HIPAA)?

   1. The HIPAA allows health insurance providers to deny insurance to patients because of pre-existing medical conditions.

   2. The HIPAA provides easier access to all providers to obtain secure and private health information.

   3. A National Provider Identifier and Employer Identifier facilitates enrollment, eligibility, and claims processing and provides a mechanism to identify a specific provider, insurer, or patient.

   4. Healthcare organizations, insurers, and payers using electronic storage of patient data and performing claims submission must comply with the Final Rule for National Standards for Electronic Transactions .

2. Considering the four advanced practice roles of clinical nurse specialist, nurse practitioner, certified nurse midwife, and nurse anesthetist, which role became accepted by and included into the practice arena without significant controversy?

   1. Clinical nurse specialist.

   2. Nurse practitioner.

   3. Certified nurse midwife.

   4. Nurse anesthetist.

3. Historically, who was one of the most outspoken opponents of the nurse practitioner role?

   1. Loretta Ford.

   2. Hildegard Peplau.

   3. Martha Rogers.

   4. Dorothea Orem.

4. Who started the first nurse practitioner program?

   1. Hildegard Peplau.

   2. Mary Breckenridge.

   3. Agnes McGee.

   4. Loretta Ford.

5. Which is the most important action in developing health policy skills in the nurse practitioner?

    1. Develop political allies in the U.S. Congress.

    2. Work on a campaign.

    3. Support causes (e.g., teen pregnancy, AIDS).

    4. Write letters and editorials.

6. Which is the **least** important barrier to collaborative advanced nursing practice?

    1. Prescriptive authority.

    2. Reimbursement privileges.

    3. Legal scope of practice.

    4. Political activism.

7. To obtain reimbursement, the nurse practitioner must understand which of the following?

    1. Minimum Nursing Data Set (MNDS).

    2. ICD-9-CM, CPT, and HCPC codes.

    3. HCPC codes and NANDA diagnoses.

    4. Medicare and Medicaid numbers.

8. According to Kurt Lewin, steps in the change process are as follows:

    1. Unsolving, mobilizing, recruiting, and finalizing.

    2. Building relationships, acquiring resources, choosing solution, and stabilizing.

    3. Unfreezing, moving, and refreezing.

    4. Forming, storming, and norming.

9. What was the major impetus for nurse practitioner development?

    1. Need for an expert nurse clinician.

    2. Shortage of primary care physicians.

    3. Trend for specialized nurses to diagnose and manage unstable acute and chronic clients.

    4. Movement of graduate nursing education to diagnosis and treatment of major illness.

10. The nurse practitioner understands that Medicare B provides:

    1. Hospitalization costs for insured patients.

    2. Health insurance benefits for low-income families.

    3. Benefits that cover physicians, nurse practitioners, medical equipment, and outpatient services.

    4. Outpatient laboratory services, radiography services, and skilled nursing care in appropriate facilities.

11. What was the impact of the Balanced Budget Act of 1997 on nurse practitioner practice?

    1. Authorized all states to provide nurse practitioners prescriptive authority.

    2. Provided for only well visits and primary care services.

    3. Prevented a physician from billing 100% for a nurse practitioner's services.

    4. Allowed direct Medicare payments to nurse practitioners in both rural and urban settings.

12. In the clinic the nurse practitioner must resolve a conflict between two medical assistants. The nurse has observed that one assistant is usually pleasant and helpful and the other is often abrasive and angry. What is the most important guideline that the nurse practitioner must observe in resolving such a conflict?

    1. Require the medical assistants to reach a compromise.

    2. Weigh the consequences of each possible solution.

    3. Encourage ventilation of anger and use humor to minimize the conflict.

    4. Deal with issues, not personalities.

13. A nurse practitioner approaches his friend, another nurse practitioner, and tells him that a female physician at the clinic often follows him into the supplies room and tells him how "good looking" he is. Yesterday she patted his hand

and said, "I wish we would get to know each other better. I would make it worth your while—better benefits at the clinic, more money." The staff nurse asks his friend, "What do I do? I don't want to date her, but I don't want to lose my job. I just want her to leave me alone." What would be the friend's best reply?

1. "Tell her that her behavior makes you feel uncomfortable and that you want her to stop."

2. "Go for it; date her and see if you get what she promises."

3. "Go to the human relations office at the agency right away and relate to them the entire situation."

4. "Contact your lawyer and get advice as soon as possible, in case she decides to turn the tables and accuse you of advances."

14. The nurse practitioner understands that "incident to" services are reimbursed at which percentage?

1. 75%

2. 80%

3. 85%

4. 100%

Answers & Rationales

1. **(4)** The four major goals of HIPAA are to ensure health insurance portability by eliminating "job-lock" due to preexisting medical conditions, reduce health care fraud and abuse, enforce standards for health information, and guarantee security and privacy of health information. Because of protests from civil libertarians and others concerned about privacy issues, the National Individual Identifier has been put on hold until some compromise can ensure that no abuses of such an identifier system will occur. The first compliance HIPPA rule relates to national standards for electronic transactions.

2. **(1)** According to the National Commission on Nursing (1983) and the Task Force on Nursing Practice in Hospitals (1983), the clinical nurse specialist (CNS) role was accepted quite rapidly. The psychiatric CNS role is considered the oldest and most highly developed of the CNS specialities and helped initiate the growth of other CNS specialties.

3. **(3)** Martha Rogers argued that the development of the nurse practitioner role was a ploy to lure nurses out of nursing and into medicine, thus weakening and undermining nursing's unique role in health care. This led to a major division within nursing, hindering the establishment of nurse practitioner educational programs within the mainstream of graduate nursing education.

4. **(4)** Loretta Ford, RN, PhD, and Henry Silver, MD, established the first pediatric nurse practitioner program at the University of Colorado. Hildegard Peplau started the first psychiatric CNS program at Rutger's University. Mary Breckenridge established the Frontier Nursing Service in the depressed rural mountain area of Kentucky, which led to training nurse midwives. Agnes McGee is credited with offering the first postgraduate program for the nurse anesthetist role at St. Vincent's Hospital in Portland, Oregon.

5. **(1)** Although all these answers are important for the nurse practitioner in developing policy skills, the most important is developing political allies. Having political allies in decision-making places (legislature) will enable the nurse practitioner to be active and informed regarding issues of regulation, limitations on admitting privileges and prescriptive authority, and managed care.

6. **(4)** Three major issues are central to the expansion of the nurse practitioner role: prescriptive authority, reimbursement privileges, and legal scope of practice. Although political activism is important, it is not specific to collaborative practice.

7. **(2)** The *International Classification of Diseases* (ICD-9-CM) diagnostic codes identify the condition, illness, or injury to be treated and are used for billing insurance carriers. Physicians' Current Procedural Terminology (CPT) codes specify the procedure or medical service given (>7000 terms). Medicare and state Medicaid carriers are required by law to use CPT codes. The Health Care Financing Administration Common Procedure Coding System (HCPC) is used for reporting supplies and medical equipment.

8. **(3)** Lewin described three processes of change. Unfreezing involves "breaking the habit" or "disturbing the equilibrium." Moving involves development of new responses based on new information, with a change in attitudes, feelings, behaviors, or values. Refreezing involves reaching a new status quo by

stabilizing and integrating new behaviors, with appropriate support to maintain the change. Forming, storming, and norming refer to the stages of group process development. Option #2 lists steps in Havelock's change theory.

9. **(2)** According to most sources, the nurse practitioner role developed due to a shortage of primary care physicians in the 1960s and 1970s, when medical specialization was the trend.

10. **(3)** Medicare is regulated by the federal government and includes the services described, plus outpatient laboratory and radiography. Hospitalization costs are covered under Medicare A.

11. **(4)** The Balanced Budget Act is a crucial piece of legislation that allows direct payments to nurse practitioners at "80% of the lesser of either the actual charge or 85% of the fee schedule amount of the same service if provided by a physician." This does not change the "incident to" rule, which allows a physician to bill for 100% of a nurse practitioner's services, provided the physician is in the suite at the time of the service and readily available to provide assistance.

12. **(4)** Conflict must be addressed directly by the nurse practitioner. The personal characteristics of the medical assistants must not enter into the conflict resolution process. The nurse practitioner should determine the issue of conflict and then work on possible solutions to resolve the issue. Compromise, in which both parties must be willing to give up something, is only one method of conflict resolution.

13. **(1)** There are two ways to deal with sexual harassment at work: informally and formally through a grievance procedure. The harassed person should always start with the direct approach and ask the person to **stop**. The male staff nurse should tell the female physician in clear terms that her behavior makes him uncomfortable and that he wants it to stop immediately.

14. **(4)** The nurse practitioner is reimbursed at 100% of "incident to" services. Medicare services provided entirely by the nurse practitioner are reimbursed at 80% of the lesser of the actual charge or 85% of the fee schedule amount of physicians. Medicaid services are reimbursed at 75%.

Legal & Ethical Issues 21

1. An occurrence-form professional liability insurance policy is preferred because:

   1. The amount of insurance money available to pay a claim increases with each renewal of the policy.

   2. The policy proceeds are available to pay claims regardless of when the claim is reported to the carrier.

   3. The carrier will be notified of a potential claim during the policy period.

   4. The coverage is broader than that provided by a claims-made policy form.

2. Early reporting of a potential professional liability claim is advantageous because:

   1. Insurance carriers have a 10-day reporting window, after which the coverage is canceled.

   2. Documents and witnesses needed to defend the claim are more likely to be available at the time of the event.

   3. Insurance premiums will be reduced with a good-faith showing of cooperation with the carrier.

   4. Risk management personnel require such reporting in order to comply with Joint Commission on the Accreditation of Healthcare Organizations (JCAHO) mandates.

3. A nursing practitioner's nursing license may be in jeopardy if:

   1. The practitioner appropriately delegates medication administration to a trusted registered nurse (RN) employee, who administers a fatal dose.

   2. The practitioner delegates client assessment tasks to a licensed practical nurse (LPN) who has been "floated" to the outpatient clinic for the day.

   3. The practitioner provides nursing care services consistent with established standards of practice in the jurisdiction.

   4. The medical assistant in the supervising physician's office exceeds the scope of her authority, but the nurse practitioner takes prompt action to correct the problem.

4. A 46-year-old mentally challenged man who has been diagnosed with colon cancer. Consent for his corrective surgery should be obtained from:

   1. The client himself.

   2. The client's 84-year-old mother, who is his closest relative.

   3. The client's court-appointed guardian.

   4. The administrator of the group home where the client lives.

5. A nurse practitioner has a 75-year-old female client with metastatic cancer. Her affairs are in order; she has arranged all her finances and her own funeral rites. She has systematically secured enough barbiturates to successfully end her life. The client asks the practitioner to mix the drugs for her in some pudding to make them palatable for ingestion. What would be the nurse practitioner's best course of action?

   1. Mix the medications as requested and stay with her while she consumes the preparation.

   2. Consult with family and attending physician to warn them about the client's proposed course of action.

   3. Seek an immediate order for an antidepressant.

   4. Sit down with the client and conduct a physical and psychological needs assessment.

6. The Patient Self-Determination Act (PSDA), passed by the U.S. Congress in 1990, resulted in which of the following policy changes?

   1. Hospitals are mandated to assist every client to create a "living will."

   2. Federally funded managed care organizations (MCOs) are required to inform subscribers about their rights under state law to create "advance directives."

   3. Home health agencies are required to have "do-not-resuscitate" (DNR) orders on file for all terminally ill clients.

   4. Hospitalized clients are obligated to select a surrogate decision maker to make health care decisions for them if they become incapacitated.

7. Both the U.S. Food and Drug Administration (FDA) and Department of Health and Human Services (DHHS) have regulations governing research activities on human subjects. The principal investigator is responsible for:

   1. Securing a signed special research consent form.

   2. Reporting back to the Institutional Review Board if a subject is injured during the course of the study.

   3. Appearing before the Institutional Review Board to present the study and secure approval to proceed with subject recruitment at the facility.

   4. All the above.

8. If served with a summons and complaint (lawsuit documents), the nurse practitioner should take which of the following actions as the first step?

   1. Call the client to determine the basis for the action and nature of the alleged wrongdoing.

   2. Call the client's lawyer (listed on first page of lawsuit) to obtain more information.

   3. Call the insurance company for instructions on how to proceed.

   4. Confer with colleagues and review the chart to determine if notes need to be clarified.

9. A nurse practitioner in an impoverished rural area frequently encounters a female client in a situation of domestic violence with few community options for referral. To address the situation, the practitioner participates in community education forums and fund-raising for a safe house. The nurse's participation is an example of applying what ethical principle?

   1. Autonomy.

   2. Nonmaleficence.

   3. Justice.

   4. Veracity.

10. Nurses practicing in expanded roles should carry professional liability insurance for which of the following reasons?

   1. Premiums are often modest and are a tax-deductible business expense.

   2. Even if the employer insures the nurse practitioner, situations of conflict between employer and nurse may necessitate separate legal counsel.

3. As roles expand, so does the liability potential.

4. All the above.

11. The confidentiality of medical records is always a valid concern, especially with widespread computerization, "smart cards," and fax machines. Release of medical information to third parties is:

1. A "creature of state law," meaning that state statutes control the processing of such requests.

2. Prohibited without the informed consent of the client.

3. Automatic when the requesting party is a third-party payer or insurer.

4. Disallowed if the records contain proof of a diagnosis of acquired immunodeficiency syndrome (AIDS).

12. Which population is **not** included in the definition of disability under the Americans with Disabilities Act (ADA)?

1. Profoundly deaf employees.

2. Persons who are wheelchair bound.

3. Current users of illegal drugs.

4. Persons with mental retardation.

13. If a client is having a problem with a managed care plan, the nurse practitioner can offer to assist in which of the following ways?

1. Suggest that the client contact the customer service department (or "member services") for the care plan to resolve the issue; a formal grievance filing may be necessary.

2. Remind the client, who is a member of the "senior" plan for Medicare recipients, that the client may complain to the federal Office of Personnel Management (OPM).

3. Remind the client that the state's insurance department also investigates complaints against health plans.

4. All the above.

14. Health policy theorist Daniel Callahan believes that the U.S. health care system could be improved by:

1. Making the care of chronically ill clients the first priority so that these individuals are not abandoned by the health care system.

2. Making preventive care the first priority.

3. Maintaining the current allocation of dollars to high-technology care.

4. Leaving the system "as is" and letting market forces determine the allocation of health care dollars.

15. If a piece of equipment malfunctions while being used on a hospitalized client, the risk manager would probably recommend which of the following courses of action?

1. Return the item to the manufacturer with a description of the problem and a request for analysis.

2. Tag and sequester the item at the facility and defer analysis pending risk management review of the litigation potential.

3. Send the item to the biomedical engineering department with a request for immediate equipment breakdown and troubleshooting.

4. Repair the item, either in house or by an outside contracted firm, and return it to service as soon as possible.

16. Nurse expert witnesses are essential in the adjudication of most professional negligence claims against nurses. Which of the following criteria do attorneys use in selecting nurse experts?

1. Appropriate professional education, preferably at the technical level.

2. Relevant and recent professional work experience.

3. Ability to understand and articulate the legal issues involved in the claim.

4. Published authors of medical texts in the clinical subject areas.

17. Which federal law mandates the tracking of implantable medical devices?

1. Administrative Procedures Act (APA).

2. Patient Self-Determination Act (PSDA).

3. Safe Medical Devices Act (SMDA).

4. Omnibus Budget Reconciliation Act (OBRA) of 1987.

18. Which of the following are elements of a broad-based risk management program?

    1. Hazardous materials compliance program as part of a comprehensive safety and security system.

    2. Early-warning/incident reporting program to identify elements of risk.

    3. System of contract review to avoid assuming liabilities that should be borne by others.

    4. All the above.

19. What the type of insurance coverage is purchased (or self-insured) by an organization to address employee job-related injuries?

    1. Professional liability insurance.

    2. Business interruption insurance.

    3. Directors and officers insurance.

    4. Workers' compensation insurance.

20. While driving your personal vehicle on a job-related errand, you are struck by a semitrailer on the interstate. The car is totaled and you are severely injured. Which insurance policies will respond to these losses?

    1. Your personal auto policy and your employer's workers' compensation policy.

    2. The employer's business auto policy and workers' compensation policy.

    3. Your homeowner's policy.

    4. The semitrailer driver's personal auto policy.

21. Nurse practitioners with hospital privileges may be impacted by the part of the Health Care Quality Improvement Act known as the National Practitioner Data Bank (NPDB). Which of the following statements about the Data Bank is **not** true?

    1. Professional liability insurance claims payments made on behalf of nurse practitioners are reported to the NPDB.

    2. The facility granting medical staff privileges must query the NPDB before approving a practitioner's privileges.

    3. The purpose of the NPDB is a nationwide flagging system that provides information about malpractice claims, licensure actions, and restrictions on privileges so that practitioners may not easily move from one jurisdiction to another to escape quality review.

    4. Insurance companies report all malpractice payments made on behalf of affected nurse practitioners within 30 days of the date the payment was made, if the amount of the claim is in excess of $11,000 and no matter how it was settled.

22. In 1985 the U.S. Congress took action against a phenomenon known as "patient dumping" by enacting what was known at the time as the COBRA law, now referred to the Emergency Medical Treatment and Active Labor Act (EMTALA). Which statement about EMTALA is **not true**?

    1. The original purpose of the statute was to prohibit the transfer of uninsured and untreated clients from the emergency department of one hospital to another (usually the county hospital).

    2. Subsequent rules and case law have expanded the statute so that almost any unauthorized transfer of a client from one facility to another is potentially problematic.

    3. To effect a proper transfer, the forwarding facility need not notify or secure the acquiescence of the receiving facility.

    4. The transferring facility must utilize appropriate transport methods and send copies of clients' medical records.

23. A nurse practitioner who wants to effect change in the state's laws regarding the dispensing of prescription medications by nurse practitioners would take this case to the:

    1. State legislature.

    2. State board of nursing.

    3. State board of pharmacy.

    4. Nursing specialty organization.

24. What is the common meaning of "gag clauses" or "gag orders" in managed care?

    1. The managed care organization (MCO) declines to publish, in its subscriber contracts, the treatments that are excluded from coverage under the plan.

    2. The MCO refuses to allow its member services personnel to answer certain subscriber questions about covered benefits.

3. The MCO contracts with providers to disallow providers from offering treatment alternatives that the providers know are not covered by client plans.

4. Providers are prohibited from offering experimental treatment to clients.

25. Under the Safe Medical Devices Act of 1990, which of the following health care providers or organizations are required to report the death of a client to the FDA if the death is related to the use of a medical device?

1. Physician office staff.

2. Hospitals, home health agencies, and ambulance companies.

3. Nurse family members treating clients without compensation.

4. Physicians making home visits.

26. A client receives a medication that was intended for another person. Which is an appropriate way for the nurse practitioner to document this event in the medical record?

1. "Client was given x mg of y drug in error."

2. "X mg of Y drug administered to client. No adverse effects noted. Physician notified."

3. "Client received wrong medication. Incident report filed. Practitioner disciplined."

4. "Practitioner inadvertently administered Y drug to wrong client. Supervisor notified. Family threatening litigation."

27. What is the primary reason that clients give for suing practitioners for medical negligence?

1. The care they received was substandard.

2. The provider made an honest mistake.

3. The client wasn't "heard" when attempting to communicate with the provider.

4. The client participated fully in all aspects of medical decision making, but the results were disappointing.

28. Informed consent is based on the ethical principle of:

1. Beneficence.

2. Respect for persons.

3. Nonmaleficence.

4. Autonomy.

29. The four elements of a professional negligence claim are:

1. Duty, fulfillment of duty, professional relationship, and wrongful act.

2. Professional responsibility, fault, harm to client, and wrongful act.

3. Duty, breach of duty, causal connection between act and harm, and harm to client.

4. Professional relationship, intentional wrongful act, proximate cause, and damage to client.

30. A nurse practitioner is making an initial home health care visit to an elderly woman. Her spouse states that she is often confused; he answers all the questions and dominates the discussion. On the initial assessment the client does seem to be oriented to time, place, and person. Who is the proper party to sign the written form to request/consent for services?

1. Spouse.

2. Client.

3. Attending physician.

4. Home health aide who will be providing continuing care.

31. Why is an expert witness usually required in a nursing negligence case?

1. Knowledge of medical or nursing facts is not considered intuitive to a lay jury.

2. Jurors are allowed to use their "sixth sense" regarding the facts presented to them.

3. Fact witnesses are not able to present an unbiased account of the circumstances in dispute.

4. Appropriately credentialed experts have more credibility in the eyes of lay jurors.

32. The standard of care for a nurse practitioner will be established by an expert witness(es) in a trial. The expert opinion will be based on:

1. National norms for the specialty.

2. Facility policies and procedures.

3. Professional literature.

4. All the above.

33. Alternative dispute resolution (ADR) is a process in which the parties to a dispute resolve their differences outside of a court trial. Advantages to this system of problem solving include all the following **except**:

    1. The parties usually prefer the process because they have their opportunity to be heard in a less formal and less intimidating environment.

    2. The process is often less time-consuming and less costly than traditional litigation.

    3. Damage awards are less likely to include nonfinancial compensation.

    4. Insurers are amenable to working with mediators with a track record of fairness and successful case resolution.

34. The statute of limitations is:

    1. The state law that prescribes the time frames within which a nursing negligence action may be filed.

    2. The law that states that minors have no legal authority to sue nurses for malpractice.

    3. The law that limits the right of clients to sue nurse practitioners for negligent acts.

    4. The federal law that limits a nurse practitioner's right to countersue a client for malicious prosecution.

35. A family nurse practitioner is driving to a nursing seminar on an interstate highway. The practitioner observes a head-on collision and decides to stop to render aid. Which statement is **false** with respect to the practitioner's potential liability for malpractice?

    1. There is no legal obligation to stop to render assistance; if the nurse practitioner had driven by the accident, there would be no liability on the nurse's part.

    2. If appropriate nursing care is provided, gratuitously, the family practitioner will be protected from liability under that state's Good Samaritan Law.

    3. Even if the practitioner acts in a grossly negligent manner, the Good Samaritan Law will shield the nurse from liability.

    4. The protections afforded by the Good Samaritan Law may differ from state to state; the practitioner should research the state's law on the subject.

36. If a nurse practitioner is subpoenaed to appear for a deposition in a nursing negligence case, appropriate preparation is prudent. Which advice from the attorney is **not** appropriate?

    1. "Discreetly chew gum to calm your nerves, and dress for dinner because depositions usually take all day and you won't have time to change."

    2. "Review the client's medical record and other pertinent material before appearing for questioning."

    3. "Take as much time as needed to think about your responses before answering; don't let the other lawyer put words in your mouth."

    4. "Be straightforward and truthful; remember that `I don't know' and `I don't remember' are acceptable responses."

37. Which of the following suggestions for documentation is **not** recommended?

    1. "Carefully document your criticism of a fellow provider's clinical decision in the client's medical record. This will protect you if your treatment decisions need to be defended later."

    2. "Use standard abbreviations in the medical record so that subsequent readers will have no doubt as to your meaning and intent."

    3. "Document telephone conversations with the client and family in the medical record. Be particularly vigilant about recording changes in the client's medications."

    4. "Document noncompliant client behaviors in the medical record; be thorough, yet factual."

38. If a client is under the "age of majority" for the state, what factors would be considered to determine if the client is "emancipated" and able to consent to medical treatment?

    1. Whether the client is married.

    2. Whether the client is in the military.

3. Whether the client is living outside the "care, custody, and control" of a parent or guardian.

4. All the above.

39. In 1987 and 1994 the U.S. Congress updated many of the regulations that govern the provision of long-term care services. What is important for an employer or nurse manager working in the long-term care environment to know?

   1. Nursing assistants working in long-term care facilities must be formally trained and certified.

   2. Clients or residents have specific rights, such as information about their physical condition, medical benefits, and associated costs.

   3. New and swifter sanctions are available to reviewers to impose on facilities with deficiencies.

   4. All the above.

40. A nurse practitioner is employed in a private medical office. There is constant activity at the front desk, with clients checking in for appointments, staff scheduling tests, and telephone advice triage in progress. To preserve client confidentiality, what changes should be implemented?

   1. Orient the fax machine and computer monitor so that persons other than staff cannot read incoming reports and other data.

   2. Do all telephone scheduling from a more secure location, such as a conference room in the back office.

   3. Create a more private space to confer with clients who need follow-up information or explanations of tests or treatments.

   4. All the above.

41. A nurse employer would be well advised to have procedures in place to terminate an employee appropriately. To avoid a charge of discrimination or a claim of wrongful termination, the employer should be particularly sensitive to the protections afforded to select groups. Which of the following groups is **not** a pro-

tected class under the antidiscrimination statutes?

   1. Pregnant women.

   2. Gay men.

   3. Persons age 40 and older.

   4. Handicapped persons.

42. Which activity could be considered grounds for a sexual harassment claim?

   1. A male employee tells an off-color joke to another man. The joke is overheard by a female co-worker who seems to appreciate the humor in it. The joke telling is an isolated incident.

   2. A nurse supervisor conducts an employee performance review. The supervisor does not mention a prior social relationship with the employee. The ratings are appropriate for the level of performance, and the employee receives a salary increase.

   3. A co-ed locker room is decorated with multiple centerfold photos from a popular men's magazine. The female employees find this offensive and have filed several complaints.

   4. A nurse is complimented on her appearance and asked on a date by her boss. She informs the boss that she is married and not seeking another relationship. The incident is forgotten.

43. A comatose female client requires a feeding tube inserted for long-term nutritional needs. Her husband presents the nurse practitioner with a document that he says is his wife's living will. It is signed by him, and he says that it sets out the wishes of his wife with respect to the feeding tube. Why is this living will not a legally binding document?

   1. The wife did not sign the document.

   2. The husband is not authorized to execute a living will on behalf of his wife.

   3. This type of advance directive must be signed by the individual (wife/client) while this person is legally competent to execute documents.

   4. All the above.

44. A nurse practitioner is helping out at a clinic for homeless women. A diabetic client in her third trimester of pregnancy has been reasonably compliant with respect to insulin therapy. Now, however, she has announced her intent to abandon her insulin regimen because she has heard "on the streets" that some drugs are harmful to fetuses. Which option is **not** legally appropriate for the nurse practitioner, as this client's health care provider, to consider?

    1. Seek the support of the clinic's attorney to file a petition for court-ordered treatment for the client.

    2. Attempt to engage the client in dialogue to provide her with accurate medical information.

    3. Detain the client in the homeless shelter and administer the insulin, with or without her consent.

    4. Confer with social services to find an appropriate interim placement for the client until her medical and legal issues can be addressed.

45. What is the purpose of the Americans with Disabilities Act (ADA)?

    1. "Level the playing field" with respect to employment and other opportunities for disabled persons.

    2. Create a federal entitlement program for AIDS patients.

    3. Guarantee wheelchair access to every residential and commercial building.

    4. Authorize interpreters for deaf employees at all private businesses.

46. As a result of the U.S. Supreme Court's ruling on assisted suicide, which of the following is the current state of the law on this topic?

    1. Assisted suicide is still a criminal offense in most jurisdictions.

    2. A physician may prescribe a fatal dose of medication with the concurrence of the ethics committee.

    3. A nurse practitioner may prescribe a fatal dose of medication with the concurrence of the supervising physician.

    4. A pharmacist may instruct a client on how to mix and ingest a fatal dose of prescription medication.

47. A professional negligence or medical malpractice case is a civil action. What is the difference between a civil lawsuit and a criminal lawsuit?

    1. The damages sought in a civil suit are monetary; one private party sues another for money.

    2. If convicted in a criminal case, you are still covered by your professional liability insurer.

    3. In a criminal case, your state sues you for money; other penalties do not apply.

    4. In a civil suit, if you do not prevail, you could be incarcerated.

48. Which of the following is **not** a form of alternative dispute resolution (ADR)?

    1. Mediation.

    2. Binding and nonbinding arbitration.

    3. Settlement conference.

    4. Jury trial.

49. Why is it especially important for nurse practitioners caring for children to have adequate professional liability insurance coverage?

    1. Damages are always higher when a child is the injured party.

    2. Juries tend to award fewer dollars to injured children because the children are eligible for a variety of social programs that cover their medical expenses.

    3. The statute of limitations is often tolled (put on hold) until the minor reaches majority, so the time frame within which the child can file a lawsuit is extended.

    4. Insurers are sensitive to the increased risk posed by minor claimants, so the coverage is difficult to obtain.

50. A health care provider has a duty to disclose certain information to the client as part of the informed consent process. Exceptions to this duty would include all the following **except**:

    1. The client has waived the right to receive the data.

    2. It is a bona fide emergency situation.

    3. The provider believes that the information would be harmful to the client and invokes the therapeutic privilege.

4. The client is 80 years old, and elderly persons are unable to comprehend complex medical facts.

51. Before deciding to provide a detailed reference on a former employee, it would be important for the nurse supervisor to consider which of the following?

    1. The requirements of the human resources department should be determined.

    2. If the comments are perceived as negative and the former employee becomes aware of them, the nurse could be subjected to suit for defamation.

    3. If the employee exhibits unsafe client care practices, it may be wiser to risk legal action from the employee than to subject future clients to this unsafe practitioner.

    4. All the above.

52. What is the primary purpose of a preemployment physical examination?

    1. Identify existing health problems that might adversely affect the company's insurance rates.

    2. Determine the mental status of the applicant.

    3. Determine if the applicant is physically capable of doing the job.

    4. Document any existing disabilities and recommend accommodations.

53. A nurse practitioner involved in work-related surveillance knows that the records related to this activity must be held for how many years after employment?

    1. 5 years.

    2. 25 years.

    3. 30 years.

    4. Can be destroyed only after the employee's death.

54. When treating a work-related injury, what is the nurse practitioner required to do?

    1. Document thoroughly because of the high probability of legal action.

    2. Communicate directly with the client's employer.

3. File a report with the industrial commission documenting the injury and treatment.

4. Notify the Occupational Safety and Health Administration (OSHA).

55. Which of the following situations would be considered reportable under the Occupational and Safety Health Act?

    1. 3-cm abrasion of forearm.

    2. Warehouse worker with back strain reassigned to office work for a week.

    3. Twisted ankle that responded to ice and Ace wrap.

    4. Minor closed head injury with no loss of consciousness.

56. The purpose of an OSHA 200 log is to record:

    1. Occupational injuries and illnesses.

    2. Only work-related deaths.

    3. Dangerous workplace situations.

    4. Lost work days.

57. The American Disabilities Act (ADA) regulates how employers treat disabled persons. Under the ADA, disability is defined as a physical or mental impairment that substantially limits one or more major life activities of an individual, or a record of a situation in which an individual is regarded as having such an impairment. What would be included under this definition?

    1. History of addiction.

    2. Paralysis.

    3. Bipolar disorder.

    4. All the above.

58. Bioethical practice dilemmas are best described as situations in which proposed treatment alternatives are:

    1. Ranked from most acceptable to least acceptable.

    2. Not appealing to involved parties.

    3. Lacking acceptance by anyone.

    4. Less-than-perfect approaches to the situation.

Answers & Rationales

1. **(2)** The most important advantage of an occurrence policy is that the coverage is available regardless of how long it takes to become aware of a claim (the long "tail" of a medical malpractice claim). The limits do not automatically increase. The carrier need not be notified during the policy period, as is required with claims-made coverage. The coverage under each policy may be as broad as the carrier allows.

2. **(2)** Fact witnesses and necessary paperwork are always easier to discover the sooner they are sought after a medical misadventure. Memories are fresh, and documents are less likely to be misplaced or destroyed. No rigid reporting window is required by insurance carriers, although they do want to be notified in a timely manner. Insurance premiums may be reduced if the insured's track record is clean (i.e., no claims), but not by mere compliance with policy requirements. Risk management employees prefer early notification so that damage control efforts may be implemented promptly, not for regulatory reasons.

3. **(2)** Assessment skills are presumed to be within the purview of the professional nurse, not those with fewer years of nursing education. Also, in this scenario, the LPN is an unknown entity to the delegator. Delegating to the LPN should be done cautiously after determining that person's skill level. The practitioner's license is not in jeopardy if the nurse delegated appropriately, as in Option #1, but an error was made and is attributed to the delegatee. Activities in Options #3 and #4 are appropriate for the role.

4. **(3)** The client's capacity to consent is questionable, so alternatives must be sought. If the client has a court-appointed guardian, that

person is the decision maker. The court has already made a determination of the client's legal incapacity and appointed the person to whom the nurse will look for consent. If there were no guardian, the practitioner would analyze whether the client himself may be able to consent or whether to look to his mother as the most appropriate surrogate decision maker. The group home employee has no automatic legal authority to consent to treatment for any resident.

5. **(4)** Assisted suicide is still a criminal activity in most states (and in legal limbo in others). Circumventing the client may seem to be an appealing option, but it substitutes paternalism for the autonomy we all claim as our due. A diagnosis of depression cannot be made with inadequate data; the necessary information can be determined only by conferring with the client herself.

6. **(2)** MCOs are one group of health care organizations impacted by this law. All subscribers must be provided with the stated information at the time of enrollment. Advance directive documents, although extremely helpful in the health care setting, are never mandatory.

7. **(4)** These are the basic requirements for conducting research at health care facilities.

8. **(3)** Insurance carriers are thoroughly familiar with the processes of handling a claim. They will assist with every step, first by meeting their obligation to put the nurse practitioner in contact with a lawyer. Conferring with the client or the client's lawyer is never a wise move. Colleagues can only offer moral support at this stage; the lawyer is the professional of choice at this time. The nurse practitioner

must never consider altering a record; it can turn a defensible case into a nondefensible one.

9. **(3)** Lobbying for underserved clients is an example of justice, which is the duty to treat all clients fairly, without regard to age, socioeconomic status, or other variables. Autonomy is the client's right to self-determination without outside control. Nonmaleficence is the duty to prevent or avoid doing harm, whether intentional or unintentional. Veracity is the duty to tell the truth.

10. **(4)** These are all valid reasons to protect assets in the event of litigation. In an opposing view regarding the need for professional liability insurance, some professionals think that, if there are few assets to protect, insurance is an unnecessary expense. Nurses with professional liability coverage ("deep pockets") could be retained as defendants in a case for a longer time.

11. **(1)** State law must be examined to define the circumstances under which confidential medical information may be disclosed. There may be additional requirements imposed by federal regulations (e.g., the handling of certain psychiatric records), but the bulk of the rule making on this issue is accomplished at the state level. Exceptions to the requirement of client consent include communicable disease reporting to public health authorities and court-ordered record production. Third-party payers, although powerful with their fiscal controls, must produce some proof of client consent to acquire records. An AIDS diagnosis does not shield a record from production, although many states have enacted extra levels of protection for this information. Again, knowledge of state laws is crucial.

12. **(3)** ADA does not protect this population. In fact, employers may test for illegal drug use; this is not considered a medical examination, which ordinarily is subject to specific requirements under the law.

13. **(4)** These are all ways to achieve satisfaction from a health plan. The nurse practitioner could also offer to help explain clinical issues to personnel who may not be clinically oriented.

14. **(1)** Callahan believes that health care priorities need to be reevaluated. He advocates spending first on chronic care (those who cannot be cured), then preventive care, and lastly on the high-cost, high-tech modalities that benefit few but consume enormous resources.

15. **(2)** The best immediate solution is to identify the item and remove it from service to avoid further client injury. Then the risk manager, in consultation with the facility's attorneys and insurers, will determine how to proceed with equipment analysis. Returning the item to the manufacturer removes it from the nurse's control and diminishes the opportunity to defend against a charge of user error. Immediate repair may fail to uncover the real cause of the client injury and impair a successful defense of a claim. If the litigation potential is high, the parties may want to pool their efforts (and costs) to conduct a third-party review of the equipment. If litigation is likely, it is also likely that the manufacturer and others in the distribution chain will be co-defendants with the facility and staff.

16. **(2)** The level of education preferred is that of the master's degree, not the associate degree conferred on the technical nurse. The legal issues are the province of the attorneys and the judge; the nurse is expected to be the expert in the clinical issues. Published authorship on nursing issues do add an aura of credibility; specific work experience coupled with the educational credentials are more desirable.

17. **(3)** APA describes the workings of federal agencies. PSDA deals with advance directives, and OBRA (1987) changed the rule dealing with long-term care.

18. **(4)** These and other elements combine to produce a program of systematic risk identification, analysis, treatment, and evaluation, with the overall goal of loss prevention.

19. **(4)** Liability insurance is acquired to protect the organization from suits by clients arising from negligent acts of employees. Business interruption coverage is usually purchased in tandem with fire insurance. It reimburses an organization for losses sustained while the business is partially or completely shut down after a catastrophic event. The organization's management team (CEO and senior staff) is insured against losses based on business

judgment errors through directors and officers (D&O) coverage. Workers' compensation is the line of coverage that protects employees after on-the-job injuries. It is a no-fault system (negligence is not a factor) that covers employee medical bills and pays a percentage of wages while an employee is unable to work.

20. **(1)** You were driving your personal vehicle, so your own auto insurer is "primary" (i.e., responds first to a loss). Since you were on company business, your injuries were sustained "within the course and scope of your employment," so there is coverage under the employer's workers' compensation policy for your medical bills and wage replacement. Depending on the circumstances and policy definitions, there could be some "excess" or additional coverage available under the employer's auto policy, but in no event would that carrier be primarily responsible for your losses. This is not the type of incident that homeowner's insurance is intended to cover. The semitrailer, presumably in use as a business vehicle, would not be insured under a driver's personal auto policy.

21. **(4)** The intent of the National Practitioner Data Bank (NPDB) is to improve the quality of health care by encouraging state licensing boards, hospitals and other health care entities and professional societies to identify and discipline those who engage in unprofessional behavior and to restrict the ability of incompetent physicians, dentists, and other health care practitioners to move from state to state without disclosure or discovery of previous medical malpractice payment and adverse action history. Adverse actions can involve licensure, clinical privileges, professional society membership, and exclusions from Medicare and Medicaid.

22. **(3)** The forwarding facility needs to know whether the receiving facility has space for the new arrival and, more importantly, the ability to treat the particular illness for which the client needs therapy. A familiar example of a client transfer is that of the burn victim, for whom specialty care is mandatory, and the locations of that specialty care are usually limited.

23. **(1)** Health care policy within the states is codified or enacted into law by the respective state legislature. The boards should have significant input in the process, providing the

research data and expert "testimony" that the legislature needs to make informed decisions. Nursing organizations should also be willing to provide background information and nurse experts to educate the lawmakers.

24. **(3)** MCOs' cost-containment strategy is enhanced if providers practice within the treatment guidelines suggested by the plans. Providers who inform clients that a certain treatment regimen is the preferred alternative create difficulties if that alternative is excluded from coverage. MCOs usually clearly set out the exclusions in the plan documents, and member services personnel are expected to be able to explain the coverage to subscribers. Experimental treatment, if excluded, would be listed as such in the plan documents.

25. **(2)** These are three of the agencies required to report. Events occurring in the other settings are exempt from reporting requirements under this federal law.

26. **(2)** This is the most factual note; the writer does not apportionate blame or assume liability. The other notes would be "red flags" for a chart reviewer. The mention of an incident report makes it virtually impossible to protect these documents from disclosure, especially in those jurisdictions still affording protection to these internal early warning documents that seek to alert risk management personnel to a potential claim.

27. **(3)** Clients are often unable to evaluate the quality of the care they receive, but they do react to the way in which the care is delivered. Client perceptions of rudeness or "uncaring" actions by the provider often spur clients to pursue legal action. Clients tend to be more forgiving of less-than-optimal outcomes if they have been involved in the process and are treated with respect.

28. **(4)** Making one's own decisions is the basis for informed consent and the ethical underpinning of the Patient Self-Determination Act. "Doing good" (Option #1) and its corollary, "avoiding harm" (Option #3), are ethics principles usually cited as the basis for other health care activities, such as maintaining professional competency. Respect for persons is a more global ethical principle supporting much of a nurse's personal philosophy of caring.

29. **(3)** Usually phrased as duty, breach, proximate cause, and damages, these are the four elements of proof required to prevail in a medical negligence action. Intentional acts are not synonymous with negligent acts. Duty presumes a professional relationship and obligation to provide services. The breach is the error or mistake ascribed to the provider that results in the harm to the client.

30. **(2)** A competent adult client is the person to whom the nurse practitioner looks for consent to treat. A surrogate decision maker is sought only when the client is unable to consent. Individual state laws must be checked for selection and priority of surrogate decision makers.

31. **(1)** Lay jurors are not expected to know the clinical facts and circumstances involved in a professional negligence claim. The expert witness is necessary to educate the jurors about the medical facts and to testify to the standard of care to be applied. Witnesses with direct involvement in the case are no less credible because of their involvement; their testimony and personal bias, if any, will be evaluated by the jurors in the context of their roles.

32. **(4)** With respect to nursing specialties, the standard of care is usually a national one. Facility policies, books, and journals are important to review, and physician input may be sought. In some cases, physicians may even be allowed to testify about the standard of care.

33. **(3)** One particular advantage of ADR is the flexibility of the system. In mediation, for example, the mediator can assist with crafting a solution package that meets all the needs of a party, including such an apology from the health care provider. Money is not always the only answer. Insurers' goals, however, usually do focus on cash: avoiding huge damage awards to plaintiffs. If a mediator is successful in facilitating case settlements, the costs are usually significantly lower than the costs of a court trial. Insurers focusing on the bottom line are not averse to these advantages.

34. **(1)** Statutes of limitations set out each state's rules for the timing of the filing of lawsuits, including malpractice actions. These statutes are procedural laws in that they describe the "how-to" parameters within which legal rights may be exercised. Minority is considered a legal disability; other state laws usually define it and describe its effects. Rights to sue are not governed by statutes of limitations.

35. **(3)** Statutes may indeed differ from state to state with respect to the breadth of the protection, but most will protect a nurse who renders aid, without expectation of compensation, in a competent manner. Gross negligence will usually void the statutory protections.

36. **(1)** A professional appearance boosts credibility as a witness. Inappropriate attire and gum chewing detract from the nurse's professional demeanor. Preparation is critical before the practitioner's words are recorded and transcribed as part of the official litigation transcript. The nurse should review documents but should refrain from bringing any materials to the deposition without the attorney's approval. The nurse should always ask for clarification of ambiguous questions. Speculation is not appropriate. Questions about professional work history are always asked, so a copy of the practitioner's curriculum vitae (CV) is a useful tool to bring to a deposition.

37. **(1)** Jousting in the client's medical record is never a good approach; it provides fodder for plaintiffs' lawyers and does not contribute to quality nursing care. The nurse practitioner who has a conflict with another provider should deal with the provider directly, preferably in person. Another arena for resolving such disputes is the quality review process.

38. **(4)** All these factors enter into an analysis of whether it is appropriate to accept a minor's consent to treatment. Another factor to consider is the type of treatment sought. Some states have statutes allowing minors to consent to specific therapies, such as treatment for venereal disease.

39. **(4)** Long-term care is a specialized area with layers of regulatory requirements, most stemming from the federal government. Nurses who work in this environment need to be vigilant about learning the rules and maintaining compliance. Ongoing, effective communication with regulators is essential.

40. **(4)** Nurse practitioners tend to become careless with information management and the way they interact with clients and their personal data. The often wide-open and frantic front desk atmosphere of an office does little to calm client fears that their information will be too easily accessible to those without a need to know.

41. **(2)** Sexual preference is not a protected classification. The other options refer to groups for whom different federal laws provide varying degrees of protection. It is prudent to check with a business attorney to determine if the policies drafted for the office are in compliance with federal guidelines. The Equal Employment Opportunity Commission (EEOC), which enforces the laws, publishes guidelines about the various statutes. These publications are available, either free or at minimal cost, from the agency. Some may be available on the Internet.

42. **(3)** This seems to fit the criteria for a hostile environment, a form of sexual harassment. The harassment seems to be pervasive and longstanding; the women have complained, and apparently no action has been taken. The isolated incident and single date request do not rise to the level of harassment. The participants did not find the actions objectionable, and job performance was not affected. In Option #2, although the potential was there for the nurse to use the prior relationship either to downgrade the employee or to deny a benefit, this result did not occur.

43. **(4)** Advance directives are documents crafted by individuals who personally decide how they wish their future health care decisions to be handled. The documents must be prepared while the signer is fully capable of understanding their content and importance. Since the wife in this scenario is already comatose, she has missed her opportunity to prepare advance directives. This does not mean that the spouse is unable to decide on her medical treatment, only that a different consent process needs to be employed.

44. **(3)** This option would create liability potential for the nurse practitioner under at least two legal theories, battery and false imprisonment. Option #2 would be the first prong of a planned approach to convince this client that she needs the prescribed medical therapy. Option #4 would be the next choice. Court-ordered treatment is a consideration with a viable fetus.

45. **(1)** This is the overall goal of ADA. It is not another entitlement program, and it cannot impose wheelchair ramp requirements on every building owner in America. Access ramps and interpreters may be required as a "reasonable accommodation" to qualified people in certain defined circumstances. No across-the-board mandate exists for these types of aid to the handicapped population.

46. **(1)** The Supreme Court essentially deferred to the states to legislate on this topic. In most states the activity is not permitted. In one of the states involved in the high court's case, a statute permitting assisted suicide is being challenged. Nurse practitioners need to look at their state laws on this topic for guidance. The providers referenced in Options #2, #3, and #4 would act at their peril if their state laws followed the current majority view.

47. **(1)** The purpose of a medical malpractice action is to make the claimant whole by the awarding of money damages. The award compensates the claimant or plaintiff for the wrong (or tort) he or she has suffered at the hands of the defendant. On the criminal side, the state sues on behalf of society for violations of society's criminal laws. The punishment is fines, imprisonment, or both. Professional liability insurance usually excludes criminal and intentional acts, so coverage for these types of activities is unlikely.

48. **(4)** The full-blown jury trial is what ADR seeks to avoid. Mediation and arbitration are the most well-known forms of ADR. Some jurisdictions use the settlement conference as a technique to attempt settlement after a lawsuit has been filed but before a trial begins. A summary jury trial is a private, shortened version in which the parties share evidence and derive a sense of the strengths and weaknesses of each side's position. ADR hybrids include "med-arb," in which a proceeding starts out as a mediation, but if the case does not settle, it is referred to an arbitrator for resolution.

49. **(3)** This is the so-called "long tail" of professional liability; there is always a time lag from the date of injury to the date a claimant files a malpractice action. In the case of an infant, the time lag may be many years because of the statute of limitations. This extends the period of potential risk to the

nurse who cares for children. Although a sympathy factor may be involved when jurors decide damages awards, the judgment is usually proportional to the injury and not the age of the claimant. Insurance coverage for pediatric providers is no less available than for other specialties; insurers adjust premiums to account for the level of risk.

50. **(4)** All clients are entitled to medical information to make an informed decision about treatment. Age, in and of itself, is not an exclusionary criterion. Providers may treat in the other circumstances.

51. **(4)** If the human resources department has established guidelines for the handling of references, it would be wise to follow them. It is also an effective mechanism to deflect potentially problematic queries by passing requests to the department most equipped to handle them. Most employers will be very circumspect about the information released, often limiting the data to dates of employment only. Without protective state legislation, employers should be prudent about sharing comments on former employees' work histories.

52. **(3)** The purpose is to determine the appropriateness of the applicant for the job. Identifying health problems to prevent hiring

an individual is discriminatory. The mental status and disabilities may also be a part of the preemployment physical but are not the primary purpose.

53. **(3)** OSHA requires that these records must be held for 30 years after termination of employment.

54. **(3)** It is required by law that a report of any work-related injury be filed with the industrial commission of the state in which the injury occurred.

55. **(2)** OSHA requires the report of any injury or illness that requires more than first-aid treatment and/or involves loss of work time, limited work status, loss of consciousness, or death.

56. **(1)** The purpose is to record occupational injuries and illnesses, including mortality reports and lost workdays, which could also reveal dangerous working conditions.

57. **(4)** All the conditions listed would qualify under ADA and may require accommodation in the workplace.

58. **(4)** The crux of a bioethical dilemma is that the proposed solutions are not perfect and therefore create some aspect of moral conflict.

Fred
Tom 2917 Carlisle & Candelaria
Suit 210
NJ Rie